Statistics for Social and Behavioral Sciences

Advisors:
S.E. Fienberg W.J. van der Linden

Statistics for Social and Behavioral Sciences

Matthias von Davier
Claus H. Carstensen

Multivariate and Mixture Distribution Rasch Models

Extensions and Applications

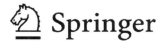 Springer

Matthias von Davier
Rosedale Road
Educational Testing Service
Princeton, NJ 08541
USA
mvondavier@ets.org

Claus H. Carstensen (Editors)
Leibniz-Institut für die Pädagogik
der Naturwissenschaften (IPN)
University of Kiel, Institute for Science
   Education
Kiel 24098
Germany
carstensen@ipn.uni-kiel.de

Advisors:
Stephen E. Fienberg
Department of Statistics
Carnegie Mellon University
Pittsburgh, PA 15213-3890
USA

Wim J. van der Linden
Department of Measurement and Data
   Analysis
Faculty of Behavioral Sciences
University of Twente
7500 AE Enschede
The Netherlands

Library of Congress Control Number: 2006926461

ISBN-10: 0-387-32916-1
ISBN-13: 978-0387-32916-1

Printed on acid-free paper.

9 8 7 6 5 4 3 2 1

springer.com

Preface

This volume gathers together a set of extensions of the Rasch model, one of the most prominent models for measurement in educational research and social science developed by Danish mathematician Georg Rasch. The idea for this volume emerged during a meeting of the Psychometric Society in Monterey, CA. At that meeting, friends and colleagues discussed news about the impending retirement of Dr. Jürgen Rost, an important innovator and mentor in this field. To recognize Jürgen's contributions, we decided to produce a collection of research on extending the Rasch model as well as embedding the Rasch model in more complex statistical models, an area that is receiving broad interest in many fields of social sciences at the current time.

This collection contains 22 chapters by recognized international experts in the field. The contributions cover topics ranging from general model extensions to application in fields as diverse as cognition, personality, organizational and sports psychology, and health sciences and education.

The Rasch model is designed for categorical data, often collected as examinees' responses to multiple tasks such as cognitive items from psychological tests or from educational assessments. The Rasch model's elegant mathematical form is suitable for extensions that allow for greater flexibility in handling complex samples of examinees and collections of tasks from different domains. In these extensions, the Rasch model is enhanced by additional structural elements that account either for differences between diverse populations or for differences among observed variables.

Research on extending well-known statistical tools such as regression, mixture distribution, and hierarchical linear models has led to the adoption of Rasch model features to handle categorical observed variables. We maintain both perspectives in the volume and show how these merged models—Rasch models with a more complex item or population structure—are derived either from the Rasch model or from a structural model, how they are estimated, and where they are applied.

This volume is centered on extensions of the Rasch model to multiple dimensions and complex samples of examinees and/or item responses. Therefore, applications of the unidimensional Rasch model for simple random samples are not specifically mentioned. Such cases can be found in volumes geared toward applying the Rasch model. More importantly, simple data collection designs can be treated as special cases of the extensions presented here, so that data suitable for the ordinary Rasch model can be analyzed with virtually all the extensions presented in this volume.

Thanks goes to our respective families, who helped us a lot with their encouragement and support: thank you Alina, Barbara, Thomas, and Luis! We are also deeply grateful to our academic teacher, Jürgen Rost, who introduced us to the fascinating field of extended Rasch models. We would also like to thank our professional affiliations and colleagues for making this project possible by providing resources and support. We thank Daniel Eignor for the excellent help on clarifying and better organizing a lot of our writing, and thanks go to Kim Fryer for the superb editorial support and to Henning Voigtländer for helping to convert and typeset many contributed chapters. Most of all, the diversity and coverage of topics presented in this volume would not have been possible without the excellent contributors in their roles as authors and reviewers for this volume.

Matthias von Davier
Princeton, NJ, USA

Claus H. Carstensen
Kiel, Germany

March 2006

List of Contributors

Raymond J. Adams
Assessment Research Centre (ARC)
Faculty of Education
University of Melbourne
Victoria 3010 Australia
r.adams@unimelb.edu.au

Keith A. Boughton
CTB/McGraw-Hill
20 Ryan Ranch Road
Monterey, CA 93940, USA
keith_boughton@ctb.com

Dirk Büsch
Universität Bremen
Fachbereich 9 - Kulturwissenschaften
Studiengang Sport
dbuesch@uni-bremen.de

Claus H. Carstensen
Leibniz Institute for
Science Education
Olshausenstrasse 62
24098 Kiel, Germany
carstensen@ipn.uni-kiel.de

Yuk Fai Cheong
Division of Educational Studies
Emory University
1784 North Decatur Road, Suite 240
Atlanta, GA 30322
ycheong@emory.edu

Karl Bang Christensen
Arbejdsmiljøinstituttet
Lersø Parkallé 105
2100 Copenhagen, Denmark
kbc@ami.dk

Matthias von Davier
Educational Testing Service
Rosedale Road
Princeton, NJ 08541, USA
mvondavier@ets.org

Karen Draney
Graduate School of Education
University of California at Berkeley
4415 Tolman Hall
Berkeley, CA 94720
kdraney@berkeley.edu

Clemens Draxler
Leibniz Institute for
Science Education
Olshausenstrasse 62
24098 Kiel, Germany
draxler@ipn.uni-kiel.de

Michael Eid
Institut für Psychologie
Freie Universität Berlin
Habelschwerdter Allee 45
D-14195 Berlin
Germany
michael.eid@pse.unige.ch

Susan E. Embretson
School of Psychology
Georgia Institute of Psychology
654 Cherry Street
Atlanta, Georgia USA 30332
susan.embretson@psych.gatech.edu

Anton K. Formann
Fakultät für Psychologie
Universität Wien
Liebiggasse 5
A-1010 Wien, AUSTRIA
anton.formann@univie.ac.at

Cees A. W. Glas
Faculty of Educational Science and
Technology
University of Twente
PO Box 217
7500 AE Enschede, The Netherlands
glas@edte.utwente.nl

Judith Glück
Fakultät für Psychologie
Universität Wien
Liebiggasse 5
A-1010 Wien, AUSTRIA
judith.glueck@univie.ac.at

Shelby J. Haberman
Educational Testing Service
Rosedale Road
Princeton, NJ 08541, USA
shaberman@ets.org

Chun-Wei Huang
WestEd
730 Harrison Street
San Francisco, CA 94107
chuang@wested.org

Akihito Kamata
Department of Educational
Psychology & Learning Systems
Florida State University
Tallahassee, FL 32306, U.S.A.
kamata@coe.fsu.edu

Henk Kelderman
Vrije Universiteit
Department of Psychology and
Pedagogics
Van der Boechorststraat 1
1081 BT Amsterdam
The Netherlands
h.kelderman@psy.vu.nl

Svend Kreiner
Biostatistisk afdeling Institut for
Folkesundhedsvidenskab
Øster Farimagsgade 5 opg. B
Postboks 2099
1014 Copenhagen, Denmark
S.Kreiner@biostat.ku.dk

Klaus D. Kubinger
Fakultät für Psychologie
Universität Wien
Liebiggasse 5
A-1010 Wien, AUSTRIA
klaus.kubinger@univie.ac.at

Thorsten Meiser
Institut für Psychologie
Universität Jena
Humboldtstr. 11
D-07743 Jena, Germany
thorsten.meiser@uni-jena.de

Robert J. Mislevy
University of Maryland at
College Park
Department of Measurement,
Statistics and Evaluation
Benjamin 1230-C
College Park, MD 20742
rmislevy@umd.edu

Carl P.M. Rijkes
Bogortuin 145
1019PE Amsterdam
The Netherlands
h.kelderman@psy.vu.nl

Jürgen Rost
Leibniz Institute for
Science Education
Olshausenstrasse 62
24098 Kiel, Germany
an@j-rost.de

Bernd Strauss
Westfälische Wilhelms-Universität
Münster
Institut für Sportwissenschaft
Horstmarer Landweg 62b
D-48149 Münster
bstrauss@uni-muenster.de

Christiane Spiel
Fakultät für Psychologie
Universität Wien
Liebiggasse 5
A-1010 Wien, AUSTRIA
christiane.spiel@univie.ac.at

Gershon Tenenbaum
Department of Educational
Psychology & Learning Systems
Florida State University
Tallahassee, FL 32306, U.S.A.
tenenbau@mail.coe.fsu.edu

Mark Wilson
Graduate School of Education
University of California at Berkeley
4415 Tolman Hall
Berkeley, CA 94720
MarkW@berkeley.edu

Margaret L. Wu
Assessment Research Centre (ARC)
Faculty of Education
University of Melbourne
Victoria 3010 Australia
mlwu@unimelb.edu.au

Kentaro Yamamoto
Educational Testing Service
Rosedale Road
Princeton, NJ 08541, USA
kyamamoto@ets.org

Michael Zickar
Bowling Green State University
Department of Psychology
Bowling Green, OH 43403, USA
mzickar@bgnet.bgsu.edu

Contents

Introduction: Extending the Rasch Model

Matthias von Davier[1], Jürgen Rost[2], and Claus H. Carstensen[2]

[1] Educational Testing Service
[2] Leibniz Institute for Science Education, Kiel

1.1 Introduction

The present volume is a collection of chapters on research and development work on extensions of the Rasch model (RM; Rasch, 1960) that have focused on relaxing some fundamental constraints of the original RM, while preserving many of the unique features of the model. More specifically, the volume presents extensions of the RM in which certain homogeneity assumptions on the item level and the population level have been relaxed. With these two types of assumption intact, the original RM decomposes the probability of item responses in two independent components: an item-specific difficulty parameter that is constant across all examinees in the population, and one ability parameter for each examinee that is the same across all items in a given assessment.

These homogeneity assumptions, however, are the ones not met in many practical applications of the RM, since either some or all of the items may function differently in different subpopulations, or the responses of subjects to these items may depend on more than one latent trait. This turns out to be an issue, for example, if item types are mixed, if the content of items varies somewhat, and/or if items are assessed in complex populations of examinees that come from different backgrounds such as different educational systems.

The volume addresses these issues in two ways, first by presenting chapters on recent extensions to the RM and second by providing chapters on applications of these extensions in educational or psychological contexts. The model extensions presented here have been actively developed and studied by various researchers, who have contributed to pioneering theoretical developments on extending the RM to multiple populations and multidimensional abilities. These researchers are often long-term advocates of applying these models to substantial research questions in the social sciences. Many researchers with backgrounds in other well-established statistical fields likewise took the RM as a basis for extending "their" models, frequently with a specific substantive question in mind. Several chapters in this volume are contributed by the original developers of such model extensions, who took a mathematical model and made it more flexible to suit applied research questions.

This direction of development—from a theory-driven substantive research question or a hypothesis to a model extension that reflects this theory—is guiding the structure of most contributions in this volume. The different chapters describe this process by referring to exemplary theories or research questions under investigation, then outline the required features of the model extension used to investigate these questions, and finally describe the path taken to extend or choose a model and to plan and carry out the analysis. To reflect this interplay between substantive theory and model development, the first part of this volume includes papers presenting work on extending MRMs and multiple group RMs—relaxing the person homogeneity assumptions—as well as multivariate RMs that relax the item homogeneity assumption to fit typical questions arising in applied research. The second part of this volume consists of chapters that present the models developed in the first part in a variety of applications in empirical educational research and a number of areas of psychological research.

1.1.1 The Rasch Model

This section introduces a basic set of assumptions and a general framework for latent variable models for item response data. The conventions introduced here can be found in most subsequent chapters, except where the extensions developed in subsequent chapters are more easily derived using a different notation.

Assume there are n examinees, $E_1, \ldots, E_n$, drawn randomly from a population, who respond to a set of I test items. Let $x_{vi} \in \{0, 1, \ldots, m_i\}$ denote the integer-coded response of examinee v to item i, that is, the actual behavioral response is mapped to an element of a set of successive integers starting from 0.

If the responses to item i take on only the two values 0 and 1, we speak of dichotomous data and refer to the dichotomous RM; if the responses can take on more than two integer values, say $x_{\cdot i} \in \{0, 1, 2, 3, 4\}$, the RM has to be specified for polytomous ordinal data to model responses of this type appropriately. In this volume, both the dichotomous RM and the RM for polytomous data will be used frequently, and it will often not be explicitly specified whether item responses are assumed to be dichotomous or polytomous. We ensure that this will not lead to ambiguities by using a specific method of introducing the RM in a mathematical form that can be used for both dichotomous and polytomous data while meeting certain common foundational assumptions of the RM.

Given the above definitions, denote the observed item responses of an examinee v by $\boldsymbol{x}_v = (x_{v1}, \ldots, x_{vI})$, that is, a vector with integer components in the finite space $\Omega_{\boldsymbol{x}} = \prod_{i=1}^{I} \{0, \ldots, m_i\}$ of possible response patterns for these I test items. The RM is derived by assuming certain unobserved quantities in addition to the observed quantities $x_{v1}, \ldots, x_{vI}$ for each examinee v and each item i, and by specifying certain assumptions about the relation of these, yet to be specified, unobserved quantities to the probability of observing a response pattern $\boldsymbol{x} \in \Omega_{\boldsymbol{x}}$.

The dichotomous RM assumes that there is a real-valued parameter θ_v for each examinee, referred to as person parameter, and real-valued β_i for each item, subsequently referred to as item difficulty. For the probability of a response x_{vi}, the RM assumes

$$P_{vi}(X = x_{vi}) = P(x_{vi}|\theta_v, \beta_i) = \frac{\exp(x_{vi}(\theta_v - \beta_i))}{1 + \exp(\theta_v - \beta_i)} \tag{1.1}$$

for all examinees $v = 1, \ldots, N$ and all items $i = 1, \ldots, I$.

This equation can easily be extended to polytomous responses by writing the model as

$$P(x_{vi}|\theta_v, \beta_{i\cdot}) = \frac{\exp\left(x_{vi}\theta_v - \beta_{ix_{vi}}\right)}{1 + \sum_{x=1}^{m_i} \exp\left(x\theta_v - \beta_{ix}\right)} \tag{1.2}$$

with real-valued β_{ix} for $i = 1, \ldots, I$ and $x = 1, \ldots, m_i$ and θ_v real-valued as above. The model as defined in Equation 1.2 is suitable for observed variables $x_{vi} \in \{0, \ldots, m_i\}$ with an integer $m_i > 0$.

The definition of the RM ensures that the probability of responding with category x rather than with $x - 1$ is strictly increasing with increasing person parameter θ. For the item parameters, strictly decreasing monotonicity holds, with increasing difficulty threshold γ_{ix}, a response in the upper (x) of two adjacent categories $(x, x - 1)$ decreases in probability. These *monotonicity properties (MO)* are among the defining characteristics of the RM.

For the second defining characteristic, it is convenient to write

$$\alpha(\theta_v, \beta_{i\cdot}) = -\ln\left(1 + \sum_{x=1}^{m_i} \exp(x\theta_v - \beta_{ix})\right)$$

and to write the RM as

$$P(X = x_{vi}|\theta_v, \beta_{i\cdot}) = \exp\left(x_{vi}\theta_v - \beta_{ix_{iv}} + \alpha(\theta_v, \beta_{i\cdot})\right). \tag{1.3}$$

In addition to the monotonicity in item and person parameters, the RM assumes *local independence (LI)*, i.e., it is assumed that, for an examinee with person parameter θ, the responses $\boldsymbol{x} = (x_1, \ldots, x_I)$ are independently distributed given θ. That is,

$$P(\boldsymbol{x}|\theta) = \prod_{i=1}^{I} P(X = x_i|\theta, \beta_i)$$

for all θ. This, with the above definitions, yields after some elementary transformations

$$P(\boldsymbol{x}|\theta) = \exp(t_v\theta)\exp(\boldsymbol{\alpha}(\theta,\boldsymbol{\beta}))\exp\left(\sum_{i=1}^{I}\beta_{ix_{iv}}\right) \qquad (1.4)$$

with $t_v = \sum_{i=1}^{I} x_{vi}$ and $\boldsymbol{\alpha}(\theta_v,\boldsymbol{\beta}) = \sum_{i=1}^{I} \alpha(\theta_v,\beta_i.)$.

Note that in Equation 1.4, the probability of a response pattern $\boldsymbol{x}$ in the RM has been written as a product of three terms. Note that one of the terms, $\exp(\alpha(\theta,\beta))$, does not depend on the observed data, and another one is the same for all response patterns that share the same total score t. This property will be used in the next section, which talks about conditional inferences in the RM.

To estimate parameters, maximum likelihood methods can be applied. Initial approaches to the estimation problem have been based on maximizing a likelihood function for the observed data matrix $(x_{vi})_{i=1...I,v=1...N}$ jointly for the θ_v and the β_{ix} parameters. To avoid undesirable properties of the joint estimation (Neyman & Scott, 1948), later approaches applied modified likelihood equations that eliminated the person parameter θ and thus allow one to maximize for the item parameters only. By eliminating the "nuisance" parameters θ_v, which are increasing in number with sample size N, the consistency of item parameter estimates can be ensured. This is done either by assuming a distribution for the person parameter θ and integrating over this distribution (marginal maximum likelihood—MML) or by conditioning on some available observed quantity, a sufficient statistic (Bickel & Doksum, 1977) that allows one to eliminate the nuisance parameters.

MML estimation is prevalent in more general IRT models since these often do not have simple sufficient statistics. However, the specific form of the RM as given in Equations 1.1 and 1.2 ensures that the total score t_v is a sufficient statistic for the person parameter θ_v, and similarly for the item-category totals. This property of the RM, the *sufficiency of total (ST) scores* for the item and person parameters, is the third defining characteristic of RMs. The impact of this sufficiency is elaborated on in the following subsection on the conditional (on total score) form used in the conditional maximum likelihood estimation (CML) of the RM.

1.1.2 Conditional Inferences in the Rasch Model

The sufficiency of the total score *(ST)* ensures that the RM can be written in a conditional form, based on the observed distribution of the sufficient statistic. The conditional form of the RM no longer contains the person parameter and can be used to draw conditional inferences about model data fit and to estimate item parameters without assumptions about the distribution of person parameters in the population by plugging in the observed counts of the total score.

The derivation of the RM in conditional form is based on Equation 1.4. For a given θ, the probability of observing a total score t is

$$P(t|\theta) = \sum_{x|t} P(x|\theta),$$

which is the sum over all conditional probabilities of response patterns x with the same total score t. As it is easily seen in Equation 1.4, all probabilities in the above sum share the terms $\exp(t\theta)$ and $\exp(\alpha(\theta, \beta))$, since these do not depend on the specific response pattern x, but only on θ and t (and β, which is of lesser concern at this point).

Conditional inference in the RM uses the specific form of $P(x|\theta)$ from Equation 1.4, which separates terms that depend on the observed data x from terms that depend only on the total score t or do not at all depend on the observed data. Then, after some algebra, we may write

$$P(x|t, \theta) = \frac{P(x|\theta)}{P(t|\theta)} = \frac{\exp(-\sum_{i=1}^{I} \beta_{ix_i})}{\sum_{x'|t} \exp(-\sum_{i=1}^{I} \beta_{ix_i'})}.$$

The right-hand side of the above expression is independent of θ and contains only the response vector x and the item parameters β. Integrating over the person parameter distribution using $P(x|t) = \int_\theta P(x|t, \theta) p(\theta) d\theta$ yields

$$P(x|t) = \frac{\exp(-\sum_{i=1}^{I} \beta_{ix_i})}{\sum_{x'|t} \exp(-\sum_{i=1}^{I} \beta_{ix_i'})}, \tag{1.5}$$

which is the probability of a response vector x in the conditional form of the RM. This is not to be confused with the integration over the ability distribution commonly used for more general IRT models in conjunction with MML estimation methods (Bock & Aitkin, 1981). In contrast to MML estimation, the integration mentioned above to arrive at the expression in Equation 1.5 does not actually take place during estimation; it is utilized as an algebraic equivalence to get rid of the θ on the left side of the expression.

In this conditional form of the RM, we have an expression for the probability of a response pattern x, given total score t that is independent of θ. This eliminates the need either to estimate the ability θ for each examinee or to assume a specific form of ability distribution when estimating item parameters.

The conditional form of the RM is quite useful when item parameters have to be estimated from observed data. The independence of specific assumptions about the ability distribution is ensured in the conditional estimation of parameters. This sets the RM apart from other models for item response data, since most other models such as the two- and three-parameter item response theory (IRT) models need additional assumptions about the distribution of person parameters for estimating item parameters.

Conditional inferences play an important role in the RM (Fischer & Molenaar, 1995) and in many of the extensions of the RM presented in this volume. These extensions preserve the defining characteristics of the RM in a way that enables one to use the RM (or its extensions) in conditional form.

1.1.3 Some Notation for Extended Rasch Models

This section introduces notation that allows one to specify the RM in the presence of multiple populations and for multiple scales simultaneously. Using this approach, many extensions presented in this volume can be viewed as models that assume that the RM holds, with the qualifying condition that it holds with a different set of parameters in different populations or with a different ability (person) parameter for each of a set of distinguishable subsets (scales) of test items.

Assume that there is a many-to-one classification g that maps the person index v to $v \to g(v) = c \in \{1, \dots, C\}$, so that each examinee v is member of exactly one of C populations (classes, groups). In the ordinary RM, $C = 1$, and therefore, the population index c is not needed. Also, assume that there is a real-valued θ_{vk} for all v and multiple scales $k = 1, \dots, K$, and let $\boldsymbol{\theta}_v = (\theta_{v1}, \dots, \theta_{vK})$ be the k-dimensional person parameter.

Let $\boldsymbol{x}_v = (x_{v1}, \dots, x_{vI})$ be the vector of observed responses for examinee $v \in \{1, \dots, N\}$. As above, the categorical responses x_{vi} may be dichotomous or polytomous ordinal responses, i.e., assume $x_{vi} \in \{0, \dots, m_i\}$. Note that we keep most of the notation intact; v denotes the examinee index, and N is the total number of observations. Since there is more than one set of items, the index k denotes the scale, and the items $i = 1, \dots, I$ are mapped onto the k scales.

One additional constructive element has to be included. Each item may belong to exactly one component of ability, say the kth component of $\boldsymbol{\theta}$, or it may be considered an item that taps into one or more of the K-person parameter components. In the case that the items belong to more than one ability component k, we speak about *within-item multidimensionality*. Otherwise, if each item belongs to exactly one ability component, we talk about *between-item multidimensionality* (compare also Chapter 4 in this volume).

Within-item multidimensionality refers to the assumption that responses to each item may require multiple ability components (more than one skill or ability component is required for each item) while between-item multidimensionality refers to the assumption that each item can be solved using only one skill, but different subsets of items may require different skills.

For the case of within-item multidimensionality, each item i is characterized by a vector $\boldsymbol{q}_i = (q_{i1}, \dots, q_{iK})$ that represents the load of each scale on the ith item. The collection of these vectors into a matrix Q represents the design of the assessment instrument. The matrix Q determines which items load on which scales. In the RMs presented here, this design matrix consists of zeros and ones, predetermined by the researcher. More specifically, the Q-matrix entries are a hypothesized structure of relationships between required skills and items, and the matrix entries (loadings) are fixed, not estimated.

Therefore, we may write for the case of within-item multidimensionality

$$P_i(x|\boldsymbol{\theta}_v, c = g(v)) = \frac{\exp\left(x(\boldsymbol{q}_i^T \boldsymbol{\theta}_v) - \beta_{ixc}\right)}{1 + \sum_{y=1}^{m_i} \exp\left(y(\boldsymbol{q}_i^T \boldsymbol{\theta}_v) - \beta_{iyc}\right)}$$

with $\boldsymbol{q}_i^T \boldsymbol{\theta} = \sum_k q_{ik}\theta_k$.

For the case of between-item multidimensionality (each item "loads" on one scale only), we can define the probability of a response x to item i in scale k by an examinee v with $c = g(v)$ as

$$P_i(x|\boldsymbol{\theta}_v, c = g(v)) = \frac{\exp(x\theta_{vk} - \beta_{ixc})}{1 + \sum_{y=1}^{m_i} \exp(y\theta_{vk} - \beta_{iyc})}$$

with real-valued β_{ixc} for $x = 1, \ldots, m_i$, and $\beta_{i0c} = 0$. The two definitions above are compatible, since the between-item multidimensionality is a special case of the within-item multidimensionality. If each item loads on only one scale, the cross product $\boldsymbol{q}_i^T \boldsymbol{\theta}$ reduces to the one term $\theta_{\cdot k}$ for which $q_{ik} = 1$, since all other $q_{ik'}$ are equal to 0.

Obviously, if c and k were not present, the above equation would resemble the ordinary RM from the previous section. Many of the extensions treated in this volume can be expressed in ways that add a population index (like c), or a scale index (like k) to the ordinary RM.

In the equations, the probability of the outcome depends on v only through $\boldsymbol{\theta}_v$ and through $c = g(v)$, so that we may write

$$P_i(x|\boldsymbol{\theta}, c) = \frac{\exp\left(x(\boldsymbol{q}_i^T \boldsymbol{\theta}) - \beta_{ixc}\right)}{1 + \sum_{y=1}^{m_i} \exp\left(y(\boldsymbol{q}_i^T \boldsymbol{\theta}) - \beta_{iyc}\right)} \tag{1.6}$$

by omitting the v in the equation. This holds, since all examinees v, v' with identical $\boldsymbol{\theta}_v = \boldsymbol{\theta}_{v'}$ and $c = g(v) = g(v')$ have the same response probabilities in the model above.

For a response vector $\boldsymbol{x} = (x_1, \ldots, x_I)$, the probability of this variable is defined by Equation 1.6 above and the usual assumption of local independence, that is,

$$P(\boldsymbol{x}|\boldsymbol{\theta}, c) = \prod_{i=1}^{I} P_i(x_i|\boldsymbol{\theta}, c)$$

with the same definitions as before, i.e, $\boldsymbol{\theta} = (\theta_1, \ldots, \theta_K)$ and $c \in \{1, \ldots, C\}$, and $P_i(x_i|\boldsymbol{\theta}, c)$ as defined above.

For between-item multidimensionality, the conditional form of the RM is easily derived in this framework as well, but it will be obviously dependent on the scale k and the population c. In that case, the conditional RM becomes

$$P(\boldsymbol{x}_k|t_k, c) = \frac{\exp(-\sum_{i|k(i)=k} \beta_{ix_ic})}{\sum_{\boldsymbol{x}_k'|t_k} \exp(-\sum_{i|k(i)=k} \beta_{kix_{ki}'c})} \tag{1.7}$$

with $\boldsymbol{x}_k$ denoting the projection of the response vector that contains only items of scale k. The total scale score t_k is the corresponding sum over only those items belonging to the kth scale. The conditional RM for scale k in population c allows one to estimate item parameters for this scale in this population, using conditional maximum likelihood estimation methods (Fischer & Molenaar, 1995; von Davier & Rost, 1995).

1.1.4 Are These Extensions Still Rasch Models?

Critics of extensions such as the ones presented in this volume may argue that these models are no longer RMs, since some basic assumptions of the original model are modified. Even within the group of researchers who use the original RM, there are arguments as to what is the right way to do so. In this volume, the majority of extensions of the RM are based on the assumption that the original RM holds in exhaustive and mutually exclusive subsets of the item universe and the examinee population. This means that each examinee belongs to one subpopulation where the RM holds, possibly with a unique set of item parameters. The same is true for most extensions presented here for each item; that is, it is assumed that each of the items belongs to one subset (subscale) for which the original RM holds, but there may be more than one subscale. A Rasch purist could still analyze these subscales separately, or analyze subpopulations separately in this case. Such an approach would retain all the assumptions of the RM by using a more constrained definition of the target population and/or the item universe. However, if a joint analysis is desired, an extended model that accommodates differences between items and subpopulations is required.

The first rule of statistical modeling is that no model ever "really"' fits the data. This is true and can be shown empirically by rigorously testing models in sufficiently large samples. Still, there is hope in the sense that some models provide useful summaries of data, so that these summaries are predictive for some outside variable that was assessed concurrently or even some future outcome. Model extensions are aimed at improving these capabilities; they are aimed at improving predictions by including a more complex description of the observed variables (that is, the item responses), the examinees involved, or both. This more complex description relates to an increased number of model parameters that often make either items' response functions or population distributions more flexible.

Which of these extensions are legitimate? And for whom? This may often depend on which *group (or subpopulation)* the researcher who judges these extensions belongs in (von Davier, 2006). There are, of course, common statistical issues that pose problems for any model extension, such as a lack of identifiability, which all professional groups would agree disqualifies a model from further consideration. Apart from these, the selection of which extensions are permissible, and which catapult the specific model outside of the group of "extended" RMs stays somewhat subjective.

As mentioned above, most extensions in this volume maintain basic features of the RM such as the conditional sufficiency of raw scores (either in subpopulations, or as subscores based on subsets of items), the conditional independence assumption, and the monotonicity assumption. Conditional independence is given up in only one of the chapters, mainly to account for differences in point-biserial correlations among items, which would otherwise be modeled by allowing a discrimination parameter. Monotone increasing characteristic functions, in both item easiness (negative difficulty) and in the person parameter, are the basis for all the models presented in this volume.

Maybe more interesting than the question whether the extensions presented here may still be called (extended) RMs is whether these models add value to the statistical analysis of item response data. In many cases, adding parameters to a model and increasing model-data fit is easy to do, but the added value of doing so has to be well established in order to justify the added complexity for the given purpose of the analysis. Molenaar (1997) has expressed this in very understandable terms that may be paraphrased as "IRT models are great, even if they never fit the data. But does it matter?" The RM (and its extensions) set the stage for answering Molenaar's question. However, the question whether it matters has to be qualified as, "Does it matter for the specific purpose one has in mind?"

Applications aimed at variance decomposition using background variables ask a different question, and therefore may require consideration of a different type of model extension, than applications aimed at deriving a rank order of students applying to a higher-education facility. The former purpose is explanatory and tests hypotheses about relationships between variables, whereas the latter classifies students as admitted versus not admitted. One application is concerned with the best possible representation of variance components, whereas the other is concerned with the best possible point estimate for each student in order to provide the most accurate classification, given data and model. The chapters in this volume derive extensions of the RM with specific purposes in mind. The reader is kindly asked to view the chapters with that in mind, in order to see the scope of applicability of the specific extensions and to explore the different fields in which the simple and elegant form of the RM has proven useful as the foundational basis for a more complex statistical model.

1.2 Overview and Structure of This Volume

Most if not all extensions presented in this volume were created after encountering the need to model data that are more complex than the RM in its "pure" form can handle. Some extensions address specific questions and were driven by some specific research context, whereas other extensions address more general considerations as to which model assumptions may limit the applicability of the RM to more complex assessment data.

The chapters within this volume introduce specific extensions or applications and cross reference to other appropriate chapters. References to work published outside this volume are also provided to encourage further reading and to provide a broader view of this area of research as consisting of interconnected fields. In this view, it is less important whether a statistical tool such as hierarchical linear models uses the RM for categorical dependent variables or whether the RM adopts a more complex population structure that reminds one of a hierarchical linear model. We hope that it becomes evident that no matter what prompted a particular development, the merger of the RM with other statistical methods creates interesting, useful, and rigorously testable models with applications in a variety of fields. This approach should provide some guidance for readers and help them to build a cognitive map of the different extensions of the RM.

This format is applied to the more general chapters as well as to the more applied chapters, which either contain an overview of relevant applications or illustrate certain extensions using exemplary studies from various areas of research.

1.2.1 General Rasch Model Extensions

The first part of this volume covers the ideas guiding these model extensions and tries to create a framework that helps the reader understand the specific tools these model extensions provide for researchers. These more conceptual chapters are an attempt to showcase more generally some ways to think about deriving model extensions from demands that cannot be fulfilled by a model that assumes a very strict structure. This part also contains a chapter that provides some insight into how the expected payoff of extending the RM can be tested.

The first chapter in this part (Chapter 2) is the most conceptual in the sense that it lays out what kind of inferences require models that include strong homogeneity assumptions. Chapter 3 outlines how evidence for the need for more complex models can be collected and evaluated statistically. This chapter introduces procedures for testing whether the added complexity of extended RMs actually helps to describe and understand the data better. This, in our understanding, is a fundamental requirement of analysis with complex statistical models, since the added complexity requires more resources for reporting as well as additional effort for researchers who want to make sense of the results or who want to use the outcomes in subsequent analysis. Chapter 4 presents an overview of flexible families of multivariate RMs. These multivariate RMs are based on the assumption that there is a hypothesis about the dimensional structure of each observed variable, i.e., each item is related to one or more of the multiple abilities through a design matrix defined a priori. This design matrix is often referred to as a Q-matrix in models for student profiles (Tatsuoka, 1983) and resembles the structural basis for a confirmatory analysis of a multivariate model. Chapter 5 introduces a very useful way to specify, estimate, and study extensions of RMs. This chapter shows how RMs and their extensions can be framed in terms of loglinear models and how these models can be estimated using software for loglinear models. The final chapter (Chapter 6) in the first part of this volume describes the family of discrete mixture distribution RMs (mixed Rasch models, [MRMs]; Rost, 1990; von Davier & Rost, 1995) and HYBRID RMs. This chapter provides an outline of the basis for these models as derived from IRT and the RM and as integrated with latent class analysis (LCA). This unique way of modeling offers tools to, among other things, handle differential item functioning (DIF) as well as to test for multidimensionality in the context of discrete mixture distribution models.

1.2.2 Model Extensions for Specific Purposes

The second part of the volume covers models that were created in response to a specific problem or research question. Overlap with the first part is intentional, since some of the extensions treated here, even if originally developed for a specific research question, grew into a broader class of models with applications in a variety of fields.

The first chapter in this part (Chapter 7) describes a model that allows one to study developmental processes using repeated measures. This chapter introduces the saltus model, an extension of the RM that allows one to study changes in difficulty of tasks over different developmental stages. Chapter 8 in this part introduces stochastically ordered MRMs for identifying diagnostic cutscores. Chapter 9 is dedicated to an extension of the HYBRID model that allows one to study speededness phenomena in detail. This chapter modifies mixture distribution RMs introduced in the first part of the volume by imposing complex equality constraints on them to model the switch between systematic and random response at a certain point in the response process. Chapter 10 is a specialization of the multidimensional approach also already introduced in the first part of the volume. This chapter covers different types of potential applications of these multidimensional RMs. The fifth chapter in Part II, Chapter 11, relates the RM and the MRM to discrete latent trait models, namely to located latent-class models, and compares parameter estimates from these different latent-variable models.

The following chapter (Chapter 12) introduces MRMs for longitudinal data. Interestingly, several contributions in this volume use loglinear models, initially described in Chapter 5, as the common language to describe developments based on multivariate or mixture-distribution Rasch models. These loglinear models with unobserved grouping variables are a useful tool that lends itself nicely to treating this kind of missing-data problem. Chapter 13 extends the RM to allow for differences in discriminations across the range of items by introducing an interaction rather than a slope parameter. In contrast to the two-parameter logistic model, the interaction model used in Chapter 13 retains some of the conditional inference features of the RM. The final chapter in Part II (Chapter 14) is an extension of the RM to complex samples from hierarchically organized populations that do not lend themselves easily to drawing simple random samples. This situation is often encountered in large-scale educational assessments and other survey assessments. Here we might also assume the development from the other side of the statistical toolbox, namely that the model basis was a hierarchical linear model that was extended by a Rasch-type measurement model.

1.2.3 Applications of Extended Rasch Models

The third part of this volume is dedicated to chapters that provide insight into exemplary applications of extended RMs in various fields of research. There is a strong link between these chapters and the previous parts, since the applied work shows how statistical tools that are based on the RM can help to pose and answer specific questions on data from complex assessments and or populations.

The first chapter in this part (Chapter 15) presents a variety of applications of extended RMs such as mixture distribution RMs in the area of cognitive psychology. Chapter 16 applies mixture RMs to the task of detecting faking and response distortions with the aim of identifying candidates who try to present themselves in a specific way. Chapter 17 talks about applications of multidimensional RMs in an international educational survey assessment.

Chapter 18 talks about applications of RMs and extensions of RMs to studying developmental issues. This chapter presents an overview of areas of application and the limitations of these approaches. Chapter 19 compares an item response model that uses a parsimonious way to account for guessing by estimating a constrained three-parameter logistic model with the application of mixture-distribution RMs to identify and correct for guessing behavior.

Chapter 20 covers extended RMs developed for modeling strategy shifts. This chapter extends previous work on strategy differences and helps one to understand how such complex models can be conveniently specified in the framework of loglinear models. Chapter 21 integrates principles of graphical models and mixture distribution RMs and presents an application to health science data. The last chapter in this volume (Chapter 22) presents some applications of RMs and extensions of RMs to data from sports science and applied psychology in the motor domains.

Part I

Multivariate and Mixture Rasch Models

Measurement Models as Narrative Structures

Robert Mislevy[1] and Chun-Wei Huang[2]

[1] University of Maryland
[2] WestEd

2.1 Introduction

An active area in psychometric research has been developing models that address strategies by which examinees respond to tasks. One purpose of this chapter is to describe some of these models and the relationships among them. The other is to lay out a framework for discussing topics of this sort, foregrounding the interplay between the technical affordances of the probability-based psychometric models and the substantive arguments they are meant to support.

The framework consists of a narrative structure overlaid by a model that supports probability-based reasoning. The narrative component is a specialization of Toulmin's (1958) general argument structure to assessment arguments (Mislevy, 2003). The component that supports probability-based reasoning is the measurement model (Mislevy, 1994; Mislevy & Gitomer, 1996). It is through the narrative structure connecting them to real-world phenomena that the formal variables and conditional distributions in measurement models acquire situated meanings. The key feature of the measurement models we discuss is that the narrative space has been extended beyond the measurement theme that characterizes trait/differential psychology, to include relationships among the ways people process information and features of tasks that interact with their problem-solving—themes that have emerged from the information-processing research in cognitive psychology in the tradition of Newell and Simon's (1972) classic *Human Problem Solving*.

Section 2.2 reviews Toulmin's structure for arguments and its application to educational and psychological testing. Section 2.3 describes the extension to probability-based models and illustrates with the basic Rasch model (RM) for dichotomous items (Rasch, 1960). Section 2.4 describes themes that are the basis of extensions from basic measurement models such as the RM, including mixtures, differential item functioning (DIF), multiple groups of examinees, and covariates for tasks based on theories of problem-solving. Section 2.5 describes a number of these models and relates the structures of the probability models to the structures of the narratives they embody. Section 2.6 concludes with a comment about contrasting aims of psychometric modeling.

2.2 Assessment Arguments and Measurement Models

Toulmin (1958) proposed a schema for how we use substantive theories and accumulated experience to reason from particular data to particular claims. Figure 2.1 outlines the structure of a simple argument. The *claim* (C) is a proposition we wish to support with *data* (D). The arrow represents inference, which is justified by a *warrant* (W), a generalization that justifies the inference from the particular data to the particular claim. Theory and experience—both personal and formal, such as empirical studies and prior research findings—provide *backing* (B) for the warrant. In any particular case we reason back through the warrant, so we may need to qualify our conclusions because there may be *alternative explanations* (A) for the data, which may in turn be supported or uncut by *rebuttal data* (R).

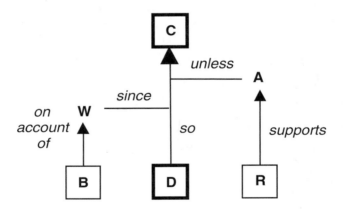

Fig. 2.1. Toulmin's structure for arguments. Reasoning flows from data (D) to claim (C) by justification of a warrant (W), which in turn is supported by backing (B). The inference may need to be qualified by alternative explanations (A), which may have rebuttal evidence (R) to support them.

The foundation of an educational or psychological assessment argument is a concept of the nature of proficiency (e.g., knowledge, ability, propensity to act in certain ways in certain situations). It determines the nature of every element in the argument structure and the rationale that orchestrates them as a coherent argument. As Messick (1994) asks, what kinds of things might one wish say about persons? What kinds of things does one need to see an examinee say or do in what kinds of situations? How are they related? The answers to these questions become claims, data, and warrants respectively in assessment arguments.

In particular, there are myriad aspects of persons, situations, and persons' actions within situations to which we might attend, and ways in which we might characterize them. The conception of proficiency shapes which of these will constitute data. An assessment argument generally includes three classes of data: aspects of the circumstances in which the person is acting, over which an assessment designer generally has principal influence; aspects of the person's behavior in the situations, over which the person has principal influence; and additional knowledge about the person's history or relationship to the observational situation that may be further required. These latter factors are essential to assessment in practice, even though they are often tacit, embedded in forms and practices.

To illustrate, consider a kind of task often used to assess spatial rotation (Cooper & Shepard, 1973). A subject is first shown a target figure, in this case a nonisosceles right triangle with a certain angle, then a second version of the target, rotated by a specified number of degrees from the target (Figure 2.2). The subject must indicate whether the stimulus is identical to the target or a mirror image of it. Lower response latencies are usually taken as evidence of higher proficiency for tasks like these, but we will use correctness: More-proficient subjects are posited to be more likely to make correct responses than less-proficient subjects. The Toulmin diagram for an assessment argument based on Sue's correct response to an item of this type is shown in Figure 2.3. Data about the item are each triangle's acute angle, the rotation from the target, and whether the stimulus is the same or different. Data about the subject, such as gender and ethnicity, may not be available to the analyst but are not relevant in the basic measurement models illustrated here. Reasoning back through the warrant, the claim is that Sue has a high level of proficiency in spatial rotation, based on the observation of this item response. We will address alternative explanations in the next section.

Of course a single item provides meager information, so spatial rotation tests generally consists of many items of the same kind. As such, the same warrant applies in each case, as shown in Figure 2.4. Reasoning back through the same substantive warrant is called for, of course, and it is clear that more information is available. How is the evidence contained in the data across tasks to be synthesized, and how might we use this richer body of evidence to phrase more refined claims? This is where probability-based models come in.

2.3 The Role of Probability Models

2.3.1 From Arguments to Probability Models

Recognizing assessment as an evidentiary argument, one would like a mechanism to reason back up through the warrant, from data about what ex-

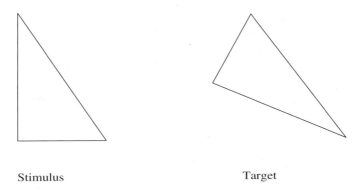

Stimulus   Target

Fig. 2.2. A spatial rotation item

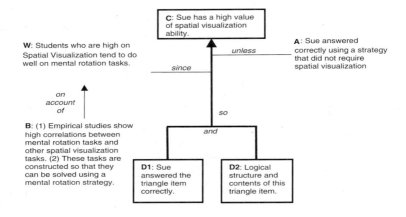

Fig. 2.3. Toulmin diagram for one assessment task. Note that the warrant requires a conjunction of data about the nature of Sue's performance and the nature of the performance situation.

aminees say, do, or make, to claims about their knowledge and proficiencies more broadly conceived. Probability-based reasoning supports coherent reverse reasoning, specifically through Bayes's theorem. We construct a probability model that approximates key features of the situation in terms of variables and their interrelationships. Figure 2.5 shows the structure of an IRT model for the similar-tasks example described earlier. Details appear in the following section; we first address features illustrated here that are common to, and characteristic of, psychometric models more generally.

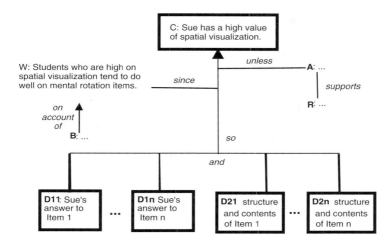

Fig. 2.4. Toulmin diagram for several tasks of the same kind. The same general warrant is employed, as adapted to the particulars of each piece of data as they fit into the same scheme.

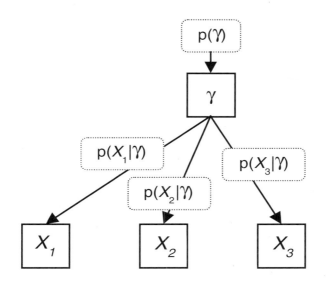

Fig. 2.5. Graph for an item response theory (IRT) model

There is an important difference between the variables in a probability model and the corresponding entities, claims, and data in a Toulmin diagram.

A claim in a Toulmin diagram is a particular proposition that one seeks to support; a datum is a particular proposition about an aspect of an observation. A variable addresses not only the particular claim or observation, but also other claims or observations that could be entertained. As a datum in an argument, one might say that the response to Item j is correct. As a value of the item response variable X_j, we would say that the value of X_j is "correct" or 1 *as opposed to* "incorrect" or 0. If you know what the value of the variable is, you also know what it is not.

Whereas a claim in a Toulmin diagram is a particular proposition, a proficiency variable γ in a psychometric model characterizes ranges or potential values for selected aspects of proficiency. The possible values of the unobservable, possibly vector-valued, γ correspond to different states, levels, or configurations of proficiency. In Figure 2.1, the generic γ takes the particular form of a real-valued scalar θ that characterizes an examinee's propensity to make correct rather than incorrect responses. As formal entities, these variables can correspond to aspects of proficiency cast in trait, behavioral, information-processing, developmental, sociocultural, or any psychological perspective; that same perspective will drive the nature of observations and the relationships between them (Mislevy, 2003)—that is, the view of proficiency in the space of narratives a given probability model is constructed to support. A probability distribution over γ indicates knowledge at a given point in time about what the value of γ might be. The prior probability distribution $p(\gamma)$ expresses what is known about a person's value of γ before responses or values of covariates are known.

A possibly vector-valued observable variable X characterizes selected aspects of a person's response. X's are modeled as depending in probability on the person variables through conditional probabilities $p(x|\gamma)$. In this formulation the direction of reasoning flows, like the substantive warrant, in a deductive direction, that is, expectations for what observables might be if person variables were known.

The support for a substantive claim is expressed in terms of a probability distribution that represents a degree of belief about corresponding values of γ. The situated meaning of such a claim arises from the nature of the observations that it is posited to affect and the substantive grounding of the model. Once such a model is fit and parameters have been estimated from initial data (pretest data, or "calibration" data), Bayes's theorem can be used to update belief about person variables in light of task performances:

$$p(\gamma|x) = \frac{p(x|\gamma)\,p(\gamma)}{p(x)}.$$

The probability model becomes an additional component of a warrant that permits a quantitative expression of support for claims, and affords the calculus of probability to synthesize multiple, possibly conflicting, possibly overlapping, pieces of evidence. These advantages do not come for free. Additional backing is required for the probability-based aspects of the warrant, in the form of the pretest data. Additional alternative explanations for good or poor performance are introduced in connection with model misspecification and data errors.

Shafer (1976) defines a "frame of discernment" as all of the possible subsets of combinations of values that the variables in an inferential problem at a given point in time might take. The term "frame" emphasizes how a frame of discernment circumscribes the universe in which inference will take place. The term "discernment" emphasizes how a frame of discernment reflects purposive choices about what is important to recognize in the inferential situation, how to categorize observations, and from what perspective and at what level of detail variables should be defined.

Powerful methods are available for reasoning in probability models, for example, coherent updating of belief about any subset of variables, given new information about any other subset, clear expression of degree of support for claims expressed in terms of values of γ's or X's, and the capability to express relationships of considerable subtlety and complexity (Schum, 1994), as might arise in simulation-based assessments tapping many aspects of knowledge and producing complex performances with sequential dependencies. These advantages obtain only for inferences that can be expressed in terms of a model's frame of discernment, however. The structure of the relationships embodied in a model may be quite flexible, but they effectively lay out the narrative space of stories that can be told, in terms of all the possible values that the variables might take. Questions concerning features of situations or patterns of interactions outside this universe of discourse cannot be asked, let alone answered. And to the extent that unmodeled patterns do exist in the real-world setting, they can distort inferences made through the model. We return to this issue in Section 2.5 in connection with multiple problem-solving strategies.

Model criticism tools do help deal with these problems. Tests of overall model fit are available. Even more useful are tests for particular suspected departures, such as adequacy across subsets of the data partitioned by features not in the model. Some patterns of observables—for example, a given person's pattern of responses—may be so improbable under the model as to cast doubt on using the model for that individual, even if the model fits well in general.

2.3.2 Example: The Rasch Model for Dichotomous Items

The Rasch IRT model for dichotomous items (RM: Rasch, 1960) posits that a probability of response to Item j given θ takes the following form:

$$\mathrm{P}\left(X_j = 1|\theta, b_j\right) = \Psi\left(\theta - b_j\right), \qquad (2.1)$$

where $\Psi\left(\cdot\right) \equiv \exp\left(\cdot\right)/[1 + \exp\left(\cdot\right)]$ is the cumulative logistic probability distribution, θ is a one-dimensional measure of proficiency, b_j is a difficulty parameter for Item j, and x_j is 1 if right and 0 if wrong. Under the usual IRT assumption of conditional independence, the probability of a vector of responses to n items is

$$P(x_1, \ldots, x_n | \theta, \beta_1, \ldots, \beta_n) = \prod_{i=1}^{n} P(x_j | \theta, \beta_j). \tag{2.2}$$

The RM corresponds to a narrative space in which persons may differ as to their probability of answering items correctly, specified by θ; items may differ as to their probabilities of being answered correctly, specified by β_j; and the probability of the outcome when a person with proficiency θ attempts Item j is given by (2.1). Exactly the same difference in log odds (i.e., $\ln(p/(1 - p))$) obtains when we compute differences between two given persons for any item across the collection for which the model is presumed to hold. The only difference among persons that can be expressed in the model is as to their overall propensity; all persons with the same evidence about the their θ's (in the case of a test, all persons with the same total score) are indistinguishable through the lens of the RM.

These main-effects patterns for comparing persons and similarly for comparing items render the RM a probabilistic version of a fundamental measurement model (Campbell, 1920), specifically, a conjoint measurement model as described by Luce & Tukey (1964) (see Perline et al., 1979, Fischer, 1968, Keats, 1971; Michell, 1997, 1999, and Roskam & Jansen, 1984). Although high-θ persons sometimes answer low-β items incorrectly and vice versa, patterns in which some items are systematically easier for some people than others lie outside the narrative space of the RM. The narrative theme of fundamental measurement accords well with the trait or differential-psychological perspective.

Model criticism tools such as item fit and person fit indices (e.g., Meijer & Sijtsma, 2001) allow the analyst to detect situations in which items do not appear to be equally difficult given overall proficiency for different groups of persons, or a person's response patterns are so unlike those of most people with similar overall proficiencies that the same substantive interpretation is not supported. In this way the item-level probabilistic framework grounds much stronger inference than the still-widespread practice of treating all examinees with the same total score as equivalent, without regard for systematic patterns within the data that would argue otherwise.

The basic RM does not encompass covariates q_j for items or w_i for persons. It is not an explanatory model, in the sense of De Boeck & Wilson (2004): Considerations of correlates of person proficiency and item difficulty, and thus substantive explanations of its character and probabilistic tests of conjectures to this effect, lie outside the model. Tests of whether β's are invariant across distinguishable groups of students and examinations of the relationships between item difficulties and item features are starting points for some of the extensions we discuss in Section 2.5. Such issues are there incorporated into measurement models, and the larger universe of inference that can be addressed in them supports a correspondingly larger narrative space.

2.4 Modeling Solution Processes

The "cognitive revolution" of the 1960s and 1970s, exemplified by *Human Information Processing* (Newell & Simon, 1972), called attention to the nature of knowledge, and how people acquire and use it. How do people represent the information in a situation? What operations and strategies do they use to solve problems? What aspects of problems make them difficult, or call for various knowledge or processes? Strong parallels to computation and artificial intelligence appear in the use of rules, production systems, task decompositions, and means–ends analyses. The key insight is modeling problem-solving in these terms in light of the capabilities and the limitations of human thought and memory that are revealed by psychological experiments.

Among the tools developed to study cognitive processes is cognitive task analysis (CTA). CTA is a disciplined process of investigating the knowledge structures and strategies that individuals at targeted levels of ability use to solve specific types of tasks, through observable evidence of those structures and strategies. A CTA seeks to expose (a) essential features of task situations for eliciting certain behaviors; (b) internal representations of task situations; (c) the relationship between problem-solving behavior and internal representation; (d) processes used to solve problems; and (e) task characteristics that impact problem-solving processes and task difficulty (Newell & Simon, 1972).

In the 1970s, researchers such as Carroll (1976) and Sternberg (1977) studied test items in these terms as psychological tasks. Others, including Whitely (1976) and Tatsuoka (Klein et al., 1981), designed aptitude- and achievement-test items around features motivated by theories of knowledge and performance in a given domain. For example, the cognitive model for processing documents (Mosenthal & Kirsch, 1991) indicates that the difficulty of a task will be driven by (a) features of the document in question, such as the number of organizing categories, (b) features of the directive, such the number of features that must be matched, and (c) the correspondence between the two, as determined by the degree to which the document has been designed to facilitate the inference that must be drawn. In the third edition of the influential volume *Educational Measurement* (Linn, 1989), Snow & Lohman (1989) assert that

> Summary test scores, and factors based on them, have often been thought of as "signs" indicating the presence of underlying, latent traits. ... An alternative interpretation of test scores as samples of cognitive processes and contents, and of correlations as indicating the similarity or overlap of this sampling, is equally justifiable and could be theoretically more useful. The evidence from cognitive psychology suggests that test performances are comprised of complex assemblies of component information-processing actions that are adapted to task requirements during performance (p. 317).

Even when considering performances on familiar tasks, the cognitive perspective entails a new narrative space, in order to cast claims about persons, to characterize relevant features of tasks, and to express conjectures about relationships between task features and person performances. A new narrative space in turn entails a new frame of discernment, to bring into the probabilistic model those features and relationships that are central to the discourse of cognitive explanation but were irrelevant for the strict purpose of measuring traits.

We may distinguish five cases for modeling strategy use (extending a list given by Junker, 1999):

Case 0: No explicit modeling of strategies (basic IRT models)
Case 1: Common strategy presumed across persons.
Case 2: Strategy may differ between persons
Case 3: Strategy may differ between tasks, within persons
Case 4: Strategy may change within task, within persons

The RM discussed in Section 3.2 is an example of Case 0. Models below include Case 1 (the linear logistic test model, or LLTM), Case 2 (mixtures of RMs, mixtures of LLTMs), and Case 3 (the Andersen/RM).

2.5 A Space of Models

This section describes a number of cognitively motivated extensions of IRT. Enough research has been done along these lines that a comprehensive review is beyond the scope of this chapter presentation. We confine attention to tasks with single right/wrong responses, for example, and to extensions of the RM. We will illustrate three notable extensions of the narrative space: Story lines that reflect aspects of how persons solve tasks, how features of tasks influence their difficulty under a given approach, and that an observer may or may not know about the approach a person is taking for a given task. Interest lies in how these themes are incorporated into parameters and structures of conditional probability distributions. The models described below are ordered approximately in terms of increasing complexity. A strict linear order does not exist, but cases in which one model can be viewed as an extension of models discussed previously will be noted.

2.5.1 Differential Item Functioning (DIF)

As noted in Section 2.3.2, it is a common practice in educational and psychological testing to sum over item responses and treat all examinees with the same total score as interchangeable with respect to whatever the test is purported to "measure." It is a matter of some importance that similar scores for students of different demographic groups based on, say, gender and race/ethnicity reflect similar performances on the items that comprise a test. Also as noted in Section 3.2, probability-based IRT models, such as the RM, make it possible to test whether the patterns in a given data set support this interpretation (Thissen et al., 1993). Differential item functioning (DIF) means that typical performance on certain items varies substantially across groups among students with similar overall proficiency. That is, the difficulties of items vary across known groups of students.

A model that incorporates DIF with respect to manifest groups of students thus incorporates an observed student covariate w into the probability model:

$$P\left(X_j = 1 | \theta, w, b._j\right) = \Psi\left(\theta - b_{wj}\right), \tag{2.3}$$

where the item difficulty now depends on group membership, as indicated by the group index w on group-specific item parameters b_{wj}. It may be the case that only certain items exhibit DIF across groups. Nevertheless, substantive interpretations of examinees' performances, and by extension their proficiencies, are incomplete without taking their group membership into account. Equation 2.3 affords no substantive explanation for these differences. It is compelling to examine the items that differentiate the groups. Is it that background knowledge differs among different groups of people? Are different people using different strategies to solve items? Conjectures about patterns suggested by substantive knowledge about items can be incorporated using the approach discussed in Section 2.5.3.

It may be found that the RM fits well within the classes determined by partitioning persons and responses on the basis of w. In these circumstances one again obtains measurement models in the sense of probabilistic versions of conjoint measurement.

2.5.2 Mixtures of Rasch Models

The not-uncommon finding of DIF among manifest groups raises the possibility that this phenomenon may be occurring even when the analyst does not happen to know persons' values on the appropriate grouping variable. Mixture distribution of RMs (e.g., Kelderman & Macready, 1990; Rost, 1990) incorporate an *unobserved* student covariate ϕ into the probability model:

$$P\left(X_j = 1 | \theta, \phi, b_j\right) = \Psi\left(\theta - b_{\phi j}\right), \tag{2.4}$$

where the interpretation is the same as in the DIF model (2.3) except that now which group a given student belongs to is not known with certainty. Equation 2.4 can be described in terms of latent trait models within a latent class model. Given a student's pattern of observed responses and estimates of the group-specific item parameters, one uses Bayes's theorem to compute the posterior probability that the student belongs to each of the possible latent groups. A mixture IRT model obtains when patterns of relative difficulty for certain items appear to differ in a consistent manner in subsets of a data set.

As with DIF models, it is compelling to examine the items that differentiate the groups discovered in an application of a mixture model.

Although the probabilistic version of conjoint measurement would hold within groups, and this narrative theme could be used in discussing results, the mixture model of (2.4) is not itself a measurement model in this strict sense. Whether such models ought to be called measurement models is an open question.

Glück et al. (2002) provide an interesting example of a mixture RM to study the effects of strategy training for spatial rotation tasks. Pretest and posttest subsets of data are distinguished, and within time points propor- tions of students using a true rotational strategy and a less-effective pattern- matching strategy. The efficacy of each strategy as applied to three kinds of tasks could be predicted, so that when unrestricted-mixture Rasch models were fit it was possible to identify resulting classes with strategies. They found that almost all of the students who used the pattern strategy at the pretest had switched to a spatial strategy at the posttest, after receiving training to that effect.

2.5.3 The LLTM

In the linear logistic test model (LLTM; Scheiblechner, 1972; Fischer, 1983), cognitively based features of items and persons' probabilities of response are related through a so-called Q-matrix (Tatsuoka, 1983): q_{jk} indicates the degree to which feature k applies to item j. In simple cases, q_{jk} is 1 if feature k is present in item j and 0 if not. The LLTM extends the Rasch model by positing a linear structure for the β_j's:

$$\beta_j = \sum_k q_{jk}\eta_k = q_j'\eta, \qquad (2.5)$$

where η_k is a contribution to item difficulty entailed by feature k. Features can refer to a requirement for applying a particular skill, using a particular piece of information, carrying out a procedure, or some surface feature of an item—exactly the kinds of elements that Newell & Simon (1972) sought to uncover in cognitive task analysis as correlates of task difficulty.

The LLTM supports probability-based reasoning for a narrative space that addresses conjectures about the reasons that items are difficult and the na- ture of proficiency. In particular, any given value of θ can now be interpreted in terms of expected performance in situations described by their theoreti- cally relevant features. The LLTM is a measurement model in the sense of probabilistic conjoint measurement, so it supports the narrative theme of fun- damental measurement in the comparison of persons.

As an example, Fischer (1983) used the LLTM to model the difficulty of multistep calculus items, as a function of how many times each of seven differentiation formulas had to be applied. He used statistical tests to deter- mine how well the smaller set of features accounted for empirical patterns of difficulty, and whether repeated applications of a rule contribute additional increments to difficulty (they didn't). A relaxed version of (2.4), the random-weights LLTM (RW-LLTM; Rijmen & De Boeck, 2002), allows items with the same features to differ in difficulty, presumably due to nonmodeled item features. Sheehan & Mislevy (1990) fit the RW-LLTM to a data set using features based on the Mosenthal & Kirsch (1991) cognitive analysis of document literacy tasks described in Section 2.4.

One can argue that models such as the LLTM marked a realization of the call for the synthesis of the "two disciplines" of psychology (Cronbach, 1957), the experimental and the correlational, for they bring substantive theory, task design, and measurement modeling into a unified framework (Embretson, 1985a, 1998). When items are generated in accordance with theory and patterns among responses can be predicted and tested against that theory, every item provides a new test of the theory (Bejar, 2002). Note that the reach of the basic LLTM extends only to final responses, not the identities or the sequences of processes that persons may carry out during the course of solution.

Behavior at this more detailed level is central to cognitive task analysis, and inferences at this level are required in many intelligent tutoring systems to provide feedback or select instruction (e.g., Martin & van Lehn, 1995). This so-called model tracing lies below the level that can be addressed in the narrative space supported by the LLTM, but in favorable cases the patterns LLTM can address will appear as emergent phenomena in overall performance. Steps in the direction of model tracing are seen, for example, in the Embretson (1985b) model for multistep problems: Each step produces a result to be modeled in terms of RM or LLTM-like structures, and the final product is a stochastic outcome of step-level outcomes.

2.5.4 Multiple-Group LLTM

By combining elements of the DIF model (2.3) and the LLTM (2.5), one obtains a model that supports narratives about how items with different features are differentially difficult to members of different manifest groups:

$$P\left(X_j = 1|\theta, w, b_j\right) = \Psi\left(\theta - b_{wj}\right),$$

where

$$\beta_{wj} = \sum_k q_{wjk}\eta_{wk} = q'_j \eta_w. \qquad (2.6)$$

Equation 2.6 shows that the both codings of item covariates, q_{wjk}, and contributions to item difficulty, η_{wk}, can differ across groups. That is, both which features of items are relevant and how they are relevant can differ, presumably in accordance with a substantive theory that underlies the intended narrative space. Spada & McGaw (1985), for example, define groups in terms of educational treatments and pre- and posttest occasions, and item features in terms of curricular elements.

2.5.5 Multivariate Structured Models

Providing theoretically derived multidimensional characterizations of persons' knowledge and skills is called cognitive diagnosis (Nichols et al., 1995). Three features of cognitive diagnostic models are of interest here: First, the model space, hence the supported narrative space, supports qualified claims about persons, i.e., claims that have the word "but" in them; for example, "Steven is familiar with the strategy of space-splitting but he is not sufficiently familiar with the canopy system to apply it there." Rather than claims about overall proficiency in a domain, a multidimensional model accounts for persons' performance in terms of profiles of knowledge and skill. Second, the tasks used to provide observations can be complex in that each depends on one or more of these dimensions of proficiency, and different tasks may impose different profiles of demand on them. Third, as with task design under the LLTM, substantive theory guides the construction of both the tasks themselves and the probability model for analyzing the ensuing performances. The narrative depends on a conception of how persons with different levels or configurations of proficiency are likely to act in different ways in settings with different cognitively relevant features.

Most cognitively based multidimensional IRT models posit compensatory or conjunctive combinations of proficiencies to determine response probabilities. The reader interested in conjunctive models is referred to Junker & Sijtsma (2001). In compensatory models, proficiencies combine so that a lack in one proficiency can be made up with an excess in another proficiency, that is, $a'_j\theta = a_{j1}\theta_1 + \cdots + a_{jD}\theta_D$, where θ is a D-dimensional vector. The a_{jd}'s indicate the extent to which proficiency d is required to succeed on item j. The A-matrix indicating examinee proficiency requirements is analogous to a Q-matrix specification of task features. A is estimated in some models (Ackerman, 1994), but in applications more strongly grounded in cognitive theory the a's are treated as known, their values depending on the knowledge and skill requirements that have been designed into each item. As an example, the Adams, Wilson, & Wang (1997) multidimensional random coefficients multinomial logit model (MRCMLM, Chapter 4 in this volume) is a multivariate generalization of the LLTM. Under the MRCMLM, the probability of a correct response is modeled as

$$\Pr\left(X_j = 1 \,|\, \theta, \eta, a_j, q_j\right) = \Psi\left(a'_j\theta + q'_j\eta\right). \tag{2.7}$$

De Boeck and his colleagues (e.g., Hoskins & De Boeck, 1995; Janssen & De Boeck, 1997; Rijmen & De Boeck, 2002) have carried out an active program of research using such models to investigate hypotheses about the psychological processes underlying item performance. In the extension of the MRCMLM to polytomous responses, each response category has its own a and q vectors to indicate which aspects of proficiency are evidenced in that response and which features of the category context contribute to its occurrence. Different aspects of proficiency may be involved in different responses to a given item, and different item features can be associated with different combinations of proficiencies.

Structured multivariate models such as the MRCMLM provide the means to solve a thorny problem in task-based language assessment (Mislevy, Steinberg, & Almond, 2002). Real-world language use draws simultaneously on several aspects of competence: from phonemic and morphological, through lexical and syntactic, to pragmatic, substantive, and cultural (Bachman, 1990). Research has shed light on factors that increase challenge in each aspect, such as the complexity of sentence structures and the familiarity of the content. The challenge a task presents to a given person depends on both of what Robinson (1984) calls "complexity factors" and "difficulty factors." The former is associated with features such as syntactic complexity and time pressure, though information-processing arguments increase the load for most people. The latter he associates with features by which a task is rendered differentially hard or easy for particular persons, such as familiarity with content and prior experience with the genre.

Tasks differ from one to another with regard to the mix of demands they offer and the degree to which these demands interact with persons. How might one make sense of such complex data? The frame of discernment of multivariate structured models can support claims of the desired structure: Within the probability model, one can (a) characterize task demands with respect to complexity factors via a Q-matrix, (b) define a multivariate θ in terms of aspects of proficiency along which persons may differ with respect to planned variations in tasks tapping Robinson's "difficulty factors," and (c) indicate through an A-matrix which dimensions of θ are involved to what degrees for each observable variable. A model so constructed embodies generalizations about how persons with different profiles of language proficiencies are likely to act in situations with specified features—again, the direction of reasoning that accords with a warrant. From patterns of performance across tasks with different profiles of demand, the analyst applies Bayes' theorem to infer a person's profile of proficiency. We have argued elsewhere that the key to applying such models is defining from the beginning a joint narrative space for desired inferences, a design space for tasks to support claims so framed, and a structured probability model for responses that accords with the narrative and design spaces (Mislevy, Steinberg, Breyer, et al., 2002).

2.5.6 Structured Mixture Models

Cognitive task analyses reveal that different subjects apply different strategies to the same problems (Simon, 1975), including familiar item types from educational and psychological testing (Kyllonen, Lohman, & Snow, 1984). Further, comparisons of experts' and novices' problem-solving suggest that the sophistication with which one chooses and monitors strategy use develops as expertise grows. Strategy use is therefore a potential target for inference in assessment. This section considers Case 2 models for solution strategies, or structured mixture models.

The narrative themes embodied in mixed strategy models (e.g., Wilson, 1989; Mislevy & Verhelst, 1990) are these: Different persons may use different strategies but are presumed to use the same strategy for all items. It is not known which strategy a person is using. Features of tasks that render them difficult are posited for each strategy.

Structured mixture models incorporate multiple Q-matrices to differentiate the strategies that may be used to solve the test items. Consider the case of M strategies; each person applies one of them to all items, and item difficulty under strategy m depends on features of the task that are relevant under this strategy in accordance with an LLTM structure. Specifically, the difficulty of item j under strategy m is $b_{jm} = \sum_k q_{jmk}\eta_{mk}$. Define for each person the vector parameter $\phi_i = (\phi_{i1}, \ldots, \phi_{iM})$, where $\phi_{im} = 1$ if person i uses strategy m and 0 if not, and denote the proficiency of person i under strategy m as θ_{im}. The probability of a correct response under such a model takes the form

$$\Pr\left(X_{ij} = 1 \,|\theta_i, \phi_i, q_j, \eta\right) = \prod_m \left[\Psi\left(\theta_{im} - \sum_k q_{jmk}\eta_{mk}\right)\right]^{\phi_i}. \qquad (2.8)$$

As a first example, the Wilson (1989) saltus model (Chapter 7 in this volume) addresses developing proficiency that occurs in Piagetian stages. Balance beam tasks are a familiar example (Siegler, 1981). Movement to a new stage involves the acquisition of a new rule, so that certain classes of tasks becomes relatively easier. The saltus model posits that an RM holds across all items for persons at a given stage, but that these models may differ from one stage to another by shift parameters that depend on stage membership and its effect on items in each item class. Figure 2.6 illustrates a saltus model for three stages, and Table 2.1 shows one way of parameterizing the Q-matrices and η's. (The illustrated model is a special case of the saltus model in which each group of tasks becomes easier by a given amount once a student reaches a particular stage, and the shifts for that task group are zero before that stage and constrained to equality across groups thereafter. In an unrestricted saltus model, the shift parameters for a group of tasks may vary from stage to stage.)

As a second example, consider the finding that subjects may solve putative mental rotation items such as the one shown as Figure 2.2 either by the anticipated rotation strategy or by a feature-based analytic strategy (Hochberg & Gellman, 1977). Mislevy et al. (1991) modeled response times in this situation in terms of a mixture of the two strategies. The analytic strategy checks which direction, clockwise or counterclockwise from the right angle, one finds the sharper angle in the stimulus and target triangles. Difficulty is posited to increase linearly with degree of rotation under the rotational strategy (Shepard & Meltzer, 1971), but to depend mainly on the acuteness of the angle

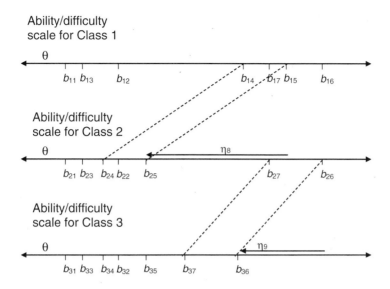

Fig. 2.6. Three saltus RMs

under the analytic strategy. The task in Figure 2.2 would thus be relatively difficult under the rotational strategy but easy under the analytic strategy.

As a third and final example, cognitive analysis by Tatsuoka and her colleagues (Klein et al., 1981) found that the 530 middle-school students she studied characteristically solved mixed-number subtraction problems using one of two strategies:

Method A: Convert mixed numbers to improper fractions, subtract, then reduce if necessary.

Method B: Separate mixed numbers into whole-number and fractional parts, subtract as two subproblems, borrowing one from the minuend whole number if necessary, and then reduce if necessary.

Tatsuoka (1983) further detailed the subprocesses required for solution under each method, and identified the attributes of items that called for the use of subprocesses under each strategy. An item like $7\frac{2}{3} - 5\frac{1}{3}$ is hard under Method A but easy under Method B; an item like $2\frac{1}{3} - 1\frac{2}{3}$ is the opposite. A response vector with most of the first kind of item right and the second kind wrong shifts belief toward Method B. The opposite pattern shifts belief toward the use of Method A. Note that these response patterns constitute noise, in the form of conflicting evidence, in an overall proficiency model, but constitute evidence about strategy usage under the mixture model. The narrative space of how students might be solving problems differently, and

Table 2.1. Saltus Q-matrices and η's for an example with seven items and three stages

Q-matrix for Class 1 Item	η_1	η_2	η_3	η_4	η_5	η_6	η_7	η_8	η_9
1	1	0	0	0	0	0	0	0	0
2	0	1	0	0	0	0	0	0	0
3	0	0	1	0	0	0	0	0	0
4	0	0	0	1	0	0	0	0	0
5	0	0	0	0	1	0	0	0	0
6	0	0	0	0	0	1	0	0	0
7	0	0	0	0	0	0	1	0	0

Q-matrix for Class 2 Item	η_1	η_2	η_3	η_4	η_5	η_6	η_7	η_8	η_9
1	1	0	0	0	0	0	0	0	0
2	0	1	0	0	0	0	0	0	0
3	0	0	1	0	0	0	0	0	0
4	0	0	0	1	0	0	0	1	0
5	0	0	0	0	1	0	0	1	0
6	0	0	0	0	0	1	0	0	0
7	0	0	0	0	0	0	1	0	0

Q-matrix for Class 3 Item	η_1	η_2	η_3	η_4	η_5	η_6	η_7	η_8	η_9
1	1	0	0	0	0	0	0	0	0
2	0	1	0	0	0	0	0	0	0
3	0	0	1	0	0	0	0	0	0
4	0	0	0	1	0	0	0	1	0
5	0	0	0	0	1	0	0	1	0
6	0	0	0	0	0	1	0	0	1
7	0	0	0	0	0	0	1	0	1

η_1: Difficulty parameter for Item 1 in Class 1
η_2: Difficulty parameter for Item 2 in Class 1
η_3: Difficulty parameter for Item 3 in Class 1
η_4: Difficulty parameter for Item 4 in Class 1
η_5: Difficulty parameter for Item 5 in Class 1
η_6: Difficulty parameter for Item 6 in Class 1
η_7: Difficulty parameter for Item 7 in Class 1
η_8: Shift for Items 4 and 5 for examinees in Classes 2 and 3
η_9: Shift for Items 6 and 7 for examinees in Class 3

how an observer might see patterns that suggest which, ground a conjecture that cannot be framed within the overall proficiency model.

2.5.7 A Model for Within-Person Mixtures of Strategy Use

The final model we discuss concerns a Case 3 instance of modeling strategy use. The narrative themes are these: A known fixed set of strategies exists to solve tasks in a given domain. A person may be using any of the strategies to solve a given task, although persons differ in their propensities to use different strategies, and tasks differ, by virtue of their features, to provoke the use of different strategies. It is observed which strategy a person uses to solve each task. The inference of interest is, for each person, their propensities to use each of the strategies.

Examples of domains of tasks in which this narrative space applies can be found in science, where strategies correspond to conceptions and misconceptions in the domain that have been revealed by cognitive research (McCloskey, 1983). Researchers have developed assessments in which tasks present situations, and multiple-choice options for predictions or explanations correspond to particular misconceptions. The Hestenes et al. (1992) force concept inventory (FCI) is an example. Figure 2.5.7 gives two examples of the kind of items found on the FCI, both based on Newton's third law: "For every action, there is an equal and opposite reaction." The first tends to evoke the Newtonian response because it is a paradigmatic third-law situation. The second is equivalent to an expert, but tends to evoke the response based on a common misconception, namely that the truck exerts more force than the fly because it has a greater mass.

C.-W. Huang (2003) used an RM studied by Andersen (1973a) to analyze responses to the FCI, for which responses could all be classified into three approaches to force and motion problems: Newtonian, impetus theory, and nonscientific response. The response of Examinee i to Item j is coded as 1, 2, or 3, for the approach used. Each examinee is characterized by three parameters θ_{ik} indicating propensities to use each approach, and each item is characterized by three parameters indicating propensities to evoke each approach. Strategy choice is modeled as

$$\Pr\left(X_{ij} = k \,|\theta_i, \beta_j\right) = \frac{\exp\left(\theta_{ik} - \beta_{jk}\right)}{\sum\limits_{m=1}^{3} \exp\left(\theta_{im} - \beta_{jm}\right)}. \tag{2.9}$$

We may note that this model assumes that strategy use can be ascertained as an observable for each task, and that the categorization of strategies is exhaustive. Note also that the model addresses strategy approach only, not proficiency in using a given strategy. Were proficiency within strategy also a target of inference, then data concerning strategy application, such as correctness, would additionally be required. It would be modeled jointly with strategy choice, through a model such as the RM where the proficiency for a given strategy applied only to tasks in which the student was observed to have used that strategy. Further, if task features related to difficulty under the various strategies were available, then the within-strategy proficiency models could feature LLTM-like structures for task difficulties, or MRCMLM-like structures if the models were multivariate.

What are the forces at the instant of impact?

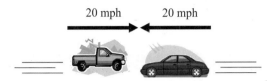

A. The truck exerts the same amount of force on
the car as the car exerts on the truck.
B. The car exerts more force on the truck than the
truck exerts on the car.
C. The truck exerts more force on the car than the
car exerts on the truck.
D. There's no force because they both stop.

What are the forces at the instant of impact?

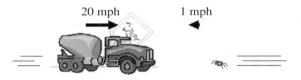

A. The truck exerts the same amount of force on
the fly as the fly exerts on the truck.
B. The fly exerts more force on the truck than the
truck exerts on the fly
C. The truck exerts more force on the fly than the
fly exerts on the truck.
D. There's no force because they both stop.

Fig. 2.7. Two items testing misconceptions about Newton's third law

2.6 Closing Comment

Before the advent of item response theory, total scores on putatively similar
tasks were taken a fortiori to be operationally defined measures—of what,
and in what sense of measurement to be determined partially through the
thinking that led to the construction of the items and partly through correlations with other scores. Both issues lie outside the scope of the classical test
theoretic model generally used to model uncertainty associated with persons'
scores. Michell (2000) argues that this practice constitutes an abrogation of
responsibility on the part of those who wish to contend that test scores are

measures of quantitative psychological traits, where "measurement" is meant in the classical sense of the term (Campbell, 1920).

Developments in psychometric models and in cognitive research have moved the debate forward in ways both anticipated and unanticipated. A case can be made that the family of RMs does embody the axioms of fundamental measure in a falsifiable probabilistic model. Hence the claim of a quantitative measured trait can be put to the test in any given data set. The question is becoming not so much whether scores reflect fundamentally measured attributes as whether the measurement narrative is sufficiently well approximated to ground applied work. As research provides insight into the nature of human capabilities, extensions of psychometric models bring hypothesized data patterns into the probabilistic models where they too can be put to the test. The methodological tools to address the question whether psychological attributes are quantitative, and to explore their nature with experiments and statistical tests. But the same research reveals that much that is important in the acquisition and use of knowledge is better expressed in terms other than common measured attributes. Now that tools have at last been developed to address the fundamental questions of trait psychology, a future may lie in using those tools for inferences that lie beyond its narrative space.

3

Testing Generalized Rasch Models

Cees A.W. Glas

University of Twente

3.1 Introduction

Item response theory (IRT) models provide a useful and well-founded framework for measurement in the social sciences. The family of IRT models is still expanding (see, for instance, De Boeck & Wilson, 2004; Skrondal & Rabe-Hesketh, 2004), so characterization of the family of IRT models is not easy. But to provide some demarcation, IRT models can be defined as stochastic models for multiway data, usually two-way data consisting of responses of persons to items. An essential feature in this definition of IRT models is parameter separation, that is, the influences of the various factors, say items and persons, on the responses are modeled by distinct sets of parameters. (It must be mentioned here that some authors define IRT more broadly to include models that are not necessarily based on parameter separation, such as the distance model by Lazarsfeld (1950b), and the BTL model by Bradley & Terry (1952), but these models are beyond the scope of this chapter.)

The Rasch model (RM, Rasch, 1960) is just one of many IRT models. However, the RM has a special place in the family of IRT models because it represents an approach to measurement in the social sciences that sets it apart from the rest of IRT. The two approaches can be labeled the measurement approach (for the RM) and the model-fitting approach (for the rest of IRT). The idea of the model-fitting approach is that the test is a given entity constructed by experts in some educational, psychological, or sociological domain, and the role of the psychometrician is to find a statistical model that is acceptable for making inferences about the students' proficiencies and to attach some measure of reliability to these inferences. The approach is well documented by Lord (1980). The measurement approach starts with a theoretical construct and a set of measurement desiderata, and a measurement instrument is constructed that fits the measurement model. The measurement desiderata usually lead to the RM (see, for instance, Fischer, 1995a).

The RM is a quite strict model, so evaluation of model fit has a long tradition (Andersen, 1973c; Martin-Löf, 1970; Molenaar, 1983; Kelderman,

1984, 1989; Glas, 1988; Glas & Verhelst, 1989, 1995; Klauer, 1989; Ponocny, 2000, 2001). The aim of the present chapter is to present a general framework for testing the class of models that is the topic of this volume: the class of generalized RMs. Therefore, we will start with a definition of this class. A generalized RM is a model in which the likelihood function given the response patterns $\boldsymbol{x}_v$ $(v = 1, \ldots, N)$ can be written as

$$L(\theta, \beta, \lambda, \phi) = \prod_v p(\boldsymbol{x}_v | \theta_v, \beta) g(\theta_v | \lambda, \mathbf{y}_v) h(\beta | \phi, \mathbf{z})$$

$$= \prod_v \exp(\boldsymbol{x}_v^t \mathbf{A} \theta_v - \boldsymbol{x}_v^t \mathbf{B} \beta) c(\theta_v, \beta) g(\theta_v | \lambda, \mathbf{y}_v) h(\beta | \phi, \mathbf{z}), \quad (3.1)$$

where $\theta_v = (\theta_{v1}, \ldots, \theta_{vQ})$ is a vector of the person's ability parameters, β is a vector of item parameters, and $\mathbf{A}$ and $\mathbf{B}$ are matrices of fixed integer scoring weights. Further, $c(\theta_v, \beta)$ is a function of the parameters θ_v, β and independent of $\boldsymbol{x}_v$, and $g(\theta_v | \lambda, \mathbf{y}_v)$ and $h(\beta | \phi, \mathbf{z})$ are the (possibly degenerate) densities of the person and item parameters, with parameters λ and ϕ. These densities might depend on covariates $\mathbf{y}_v$ and $\mathbf{z}$. In this chapter, the factor $p(\boldsymbol{x}_v | \theta_v, \beta)$ will be called the Rasch measurement model and the factor $g(\theta_v | \lambda, \mathbf{y}_v) h(\beta | \phi, \mathbf{z})$ the structural model. It is assumed that persons are independent, so the complete likelihood is the product over persons. Local independence between the person's responses is not assumed to include some interesting models by Jannarone (1986) that lack this assumption. Further, no assumption about the format of the responses has been made yet, so the RM for speed tests (Rasch, 1960) and other models for continuous responses (Mellenbergh, 1994) are also included in this definition.

A general approach to testing this model will be worked out in three estimation settings: the conditional maximum likelihood (CML) framework, the marginal maximum likelihood (MML) framework, and a Bayesian framework that will be labeled the MCMC framework (the Markov chain Monte Carlo framework) for reasons that will become apparent below. The reason for considering three estimation frameworks is that all three have their specific ranges of application. In the CML framework, the structural model does not play a role in the analyses, so this approach is especially suited to evaluate the appropriateness of the measurement model. In MML, the structural model does play a role, so this approach is suited for testing hypotheses concerning the measurement and structural model simultaneously. Below, it will be explained that the feasibility of the MML approach is limited by the dimensionality of the structural model. If the dimensionality becomes too high, Bayesian methods based on MCMC become important.

Most hypotheses concerning the structural model can be easily tested using likelihood ratio tests and their Bayesian analogues. These tests are omnipresent in this volume, and they will not be treated in this chapter. In this chapter, the focus is on the fit of the measurement model, with and without the presence of a structural model. Fit of the measurement model can be viewed from two perspectives: the items and the respondents. In the first case, for every item, residuals (differences between predictions from the estimated model and observations) and item-fit statistics are computed to assess whether the item violates the model. In the second case, residuals and person-fit statistics are computed for every person to assess whether the responses to the items follow the model.

The most important assumptions evaluated from the perspective of item fit are subpopulation invariance (the violation is often labeled differential item functioning, or DIF), the form of the item response function, and local stochastic independence. The first assumption entails that the item responses can be described by the same parameters in all possible subpopulations. Subpopulations are defined on the basis of background variables that should not be relevant in a specific testing situation. One might think of gender, race, age, or socioeconomic status. The second assumption addressed is the form of the item response function that describes the relation between the latent variable and the observable responses to items. Evaluation of the appropriateness of the item response function is usually done by comparing observed and expected item response frequencies given some measure of the latent trait level. The third assumption targeted is local stochastic independence. The assumption entails that responses to different items are independent given the latent trait value. Then, the proposed latent variables completely describe the responses and no additional variables are necessary to describe the responses. The most important assumption evaluated from the perspective of person fit is the invariance of the ability parameter over subtests, but also local independence can be evaluated using person-fit tests.

A final remark in this introduction pertains to the relation between formal tests of model fit and residual analyses. A well-known problem with formal tests of model fit is that they tend to reject the model too often even for moderate sample sizes. That is, their power (the probability of rejection when the model is violated) grows very fast as a function of the sample size. As a result, small deviations from the IRT model may cause a rejection of the model, while these deviations may hardly have practical consequences in the foreseen application of the model. Inspection of the magnitude of the residuals can shed light on the severity of the model violation. The reason for addressing the problem of evaluation of model fit in the framework of formal model tests is that the alternative hypotheses in these model tests clarify which model assumptions are exactly targeted by the residuals. This will be explained further below.

3.2 A Basic Example in a CML Framework

As an introduction, consider a test of model fit for the standard unidimensional RM for dichotomously scored items. The test focuses on the appropriateness of the item characteristic curve (ICC), that is, on the probability of a correct response as a function of a unidimensional ability parameter θ. The idea of the test is to partition the latent ability continuum into a number of segments, and to evaluate whether an item's ICC conforms to the form predicted by the RM. A problem with this idea is that it requires the partitioning of the sample of respondents based on their ability estimates. The derivation of the asymptotic distribution of a test statistic with a partitioning of respondents based on estimates of θ proves very difficult. Therefore, the partitioning of the sample of respondents will be based on the number-correct scores, which are sufficient statistics for the ability parameters. Several statistics can be used to evaluate whether the responses in the subgroups match the predictions derived from the RM. For instance, Andersen (1973c) proposed a likelihood ratio test, where the CML value obtained in the total sample is compared with CML values obtained in the subgroups. In the present chapter, we will outline an approach that is based on the difference between the expected and observed frequencies in the subgroups $g = 1, \ldots, G$. The test is based on the residuals

$$d_{gi} = n_{gi} - E(N_{gi} \mid \mathbf{r}, \hat{\beta}), \qquad (3.2)$$

where n_{gi} is the count of the number of persons belonging to score level g and giving a correct response to item i, and $E(N_{gi} \mid \mathbf{r}, \hat{\beta})$ is the expected value given the respondents' sum scores $\mathbf{r}$ and the CML estimates of the item parameters. The test statistic is defined as

$$S_i = \mathbf{d}_i^t \, \mathbf{W}_i^{-1} \, \mathbf{d}_i, \qquad (3.3)$$

where $\mathbf{d}_i$ is the vector of elements d_{gi}, for $g = 1, \ldots, G - 1$, and $\mathbf{W}_i^{-1}$ is the inverse of the estimated covariance matrix of $\mathbf{d}_i$. The fact that one of the subgroups is not included in $\mathbf{d}_i$ will be explained below. The S_i test has an asymptotic χ^2 distribution with $df = G - 1$ (Glas & Verhelst, 1995).

The exact covariance matrix of $\mathbf{d}_i$, which is $\mathbf{W}_i$, is needed to derive the asymptotic distribution of the statistic. Often, this matrix is replaced by a diagonal matrix where only the diagonal elements of $\mathbf{W}_i$ are included as nonzero elements. In that case, the statistic simplifies to a Pearson's X^2 statistic. Examples in the CML framework for the RM are the tests proposed by van den Wollenberg (1982). Although replacing $\mathbf{W}_i$ by a covariance matrix slightly simplifies the computations, claims about the distribution of the statistic are completely based on simulation studies and the generalization to statistics for more complicated IRT models is problematic.

The approach sketched in this section has two advantages over using a likelihood ratio test. First, the parameters need not be estimated in every subgroup. And, second, the approach can be generalized to other model violations and estimation frameworks. In the next section, the principle of the approach will be outlined.

3.3 Lagrange Multiplier Tests for Evaluating the Fit of IRT Models

IRT models are based on a number of assumptions. The most important are parameter invariance and local independence. Testing these two assumptions for all items and persons using likelihood ratio statistics is problematic because every alternative model for every model violation for every person and each item would have to be estimated. A simple alternative is to estimate the model only once and to produce a number of tables of residuals that are informative with respect to specific model violations. The LM test provides a rationale for the choice of the residuals.

The LM test is grounded as follows. Consider some general parametrized model, and a special case of the general model, the so-called restricted model. The restricted model was derived from the general model by imposing constraints on the parameter space. In many instances, this was accomplished by setting one or more parameters of the general model to constants. The LM test is based on the evaluation of the first–order partial derivatives of the log-likelihood function of the general model, evaluated using the maximum likelihood estimates of the restricted model. The unrestricted elements of the vector of first-order derivatives are equal to zero, because their values originate from solving the likelihood equations. The magnitudes of the elements of the vector of first-order partial derivatives corresponding to restricted parameters determine the value of the statistic: the closer they are to zero, the better the model fit.

More formally, the principle can be described as follows. Consider a general model with parameters $\boldsymbol{\eta}$. In the applications presented below, the special model was derived from the general model by setting one or more parameters to zero. So if the vector of the parameters of the general model, say $\boldsymbol{\eta}$, is partitioned $\boldsymbol{\eta} = (\boldsymbol{\eta}_1, \boldsymbol{\eta}_2)$, the null hypothesis entails $\boldsymbol{\eta}_2 = 0$. Let $\mathbf{h}(\boldsymbol{\eta})$ be the first-order partial derivatives of the log-likelihood of the general model, that is, $\mathbf{h}(\boldsymbol{\eta}) = \partial \log L(\boldsymbol{\eta})/\partial\boldsymbol{\eta}$. This vector of partial derivatives gauges the change of the log-likelihood as a function of local changes in $\boldsymbol{\eta}$. Let the vector of partial derivatives $\mathbf{h}(\boldsymbol{\eta})$ be partitioned as $(\mathbf{h}(\boldsymbol{\eta}_1), \mathbf{h}(\boldsymbol{\eta}_2))$. Then the test is based on the statistic

$$\mathrm{LM} = \mathbf{h}(\boldsymbol{\eta}_2)'\boldsymbol{\Sigma}^{-1}\mathbf{h}(\eta_2), \qquad (3.4)$$

where

$$\boldsymbol{\Sigma} = \boldsymbol{\Sigma}_{22} - \boldsymbol{\Sigma}_{21}\boldsymbol{\Sigma}_{11}^{-1}\boldsymbol{\Sigma}_{12} \qquad (3.5)$$

and

$$\boldsymbol{\Sigma}_{pq} = -\frac{\partial^2 \log L(\boldsymbol{\eta})}{\partial\eta_p\partial\boldsymbol{\eta}'_q},$$

for $p = 1, 2$ and $q = 1, 2$. The matrix $\boldsymbol{\Sigma}$ in (3.5) can be viewed as the asymptotic covariance matrix of $\mathbf{h}(\boldsymbol{\eta}_2)$ with $\boldsymbol{\eta}_1$ estimated and the matrix $\boldsymbol{\Sigma}_{22}$ is the asymptotic covariance matrix of $\mathbf{h}(\boldsymbol{\eta}_2)$ with $\boldsymbol{\eta}_1$ known. Further, $\boldsymbol{\Sigma}_{11}^{-1}$ is the asymptotic covariance matrix of the estimate of $\boldsymbol{\eta}_1$, so the term $\boldsymbol{\Sigma}_{21}\boldsymbol{\Sigma}_{11}^{-1}\boldsymbol{\Sigma}_{12}$ accounts for the influence of the estimation of $\boldsymbol{\eta}_1$ on the covariance matrix of $\mathbf{h}(\boldsymbol{\eta}_2)$. The LM statistic has an asymptotic χ^2-distribution with degrees of freedom equal to the number of parameters in $\boldsymbol{\eta}_2$ (Aitchison & Silvey, 1958).

In the next section, the LM test will first be applied to the evaluation of person fit. Then, in the following two sections, LM item-fit tests will be presented in the CML and MML frameworks, respectively. Then, in the last section before the discussion section, it will be shown how the basic idea of the LM test can be generalized to a Bayesian framework.

3.4 An LM Test for Person Fit

Smith (1985, 1986) introduced a Pearson-type test statistic for the RM for evaluating the constancy of the ability parameter across subtests. To perform the test, the set of test items is divided into S nonoverlapping subtests denoted by A_s $(s = 1, \ldots, S)$. Then the hypothesis that the same ability parameter θ_v accounts for the responses in all subsets can be tested with a statistic defined by

$$UB = \frac{1}{S-1} \sum_{s=1}^{S} \frac{\left[\sum_{i \in A_s} [x_{vi} - P_i(\theta_v)]\right]^2}{\sum_{i \in A_s} P_i(\theta_v)\left[1 - P_i(\theta_v)\right]}, \tag{3.6}$$

where $P_i(\theta_v)$ is the probability of a correct response in the RM.

Dagohoy (2005) proposes an LM statistic that is closely related to the UB statistic. It can be derived by assuming an alternative model where the ability parameter differs across the test, that is, for $s > 1$, it is assumed that

$$P_i(\theta_v) = P(X_{vi} = 1 \mid \theta_v, i \in A_s) = \frac{\exp[\theta_v + \theta_{vs} - \beta_i]}{1 + \exp[\theta_v + \theta_{vs} - \beta_i]}. \tag{3.7}$$

For $s = 1$, we assume the RM, so the responses on the first subtest are used as a base line for θ. In practice, a response pattern is too short to test whether more than two ability parameters are involved. Therefore, the response pattern is usually partitioned into two parts, that is, $S = 2$. Further, assume that the item parameters are known. Then the log-likelihood is given by

$$\log L = \sum_{i=1}^{k} x_{vi} \log P_i(\theta_v) + (1 - x_{vi}) \log(1 - P_i(\theta_v)). \tag{3.8}$$

Taking the first-order derivative of the likelihood of the response pattern with respect to θ_s results in

$$h = \frac{\partial \log L}{\partial \theta_s} = \sum_{i \in A_s} [x_{vi} - P_i(\theta)].$$

For the second-order derivatives of the log-likelihood we obtain

$$\sigma_{11} = -\frac{\partial^2 \log L}{\partial \theta^2} = \sum_{i=1}^{k} P_i(\theta) \left[1 - P_i(\theta)\right],$$

$$\sigma_{22} = -\frac{\partial^2 \log L}{\partial \theta_s^2} = \sum_{i \in A_s} P_i(\theta) \left[1 - P_i(\theta)\right],$$

$$\sigma_{12} = -\frac{\partial^2 \log L}{\partial \theta \partial \theta_s} = -\sum_{i \in A_s} P_i(\theta) \left[1 - P_i(\theta)\right].$$

Inserting these formulas into (3.4) and (3.5) gives an LM statistic for testing the constancy of the ability parameter over the two partial response patterns as

$$LM = \frac{h^2}{\sigma_{22} - \sigma_{12}^2/\sigma_{11}}. \tag{3.9}$$

This LM statistic has an asymptotic χ^2-distribution with one degree of freedom. Note that (3.9) is equivalent to (3.6), except for the term $-\sigma_{12}^2/\sigma_{11}$ in the denominator. It is exactly this term that represents the loss in the variance of h caused by the estimation of θ.

3.5 The CML Framework

In this section, it will be shown how the test given by Equation 3.3 fits the LM-test framework. But first, it will be sketched how the LM and CML frameworks connect in general.

3.5.1 The General Formulation

In the definition of generalized RMs given in (3.1), no assumptions about local independence and about the format of the responses have been made. However, most models do make the assumption of local independence and assume that the items are scored in discrete categories. In these cases, the measurement model $\exp(\boldsymbol{x}_v^t \mathbf{A} \boldsymbol{\theta}_v - \boldsymbol{x}_v^t \mathbf{B} \beta) c(\boldsymbol{\theta}_v, \beta)$ in (3.1) specializes to a product over items, and $\boldsymbol{x}_v$ is defined as the concatenation of item response vectors $\boldsymbol{x}_{vi}$ with entries x_{vij}, $j = 1, \ldots, m_i$, which are equal to one if the response was in category j and zero otherwise. Note that the measurement model $\exp(\boldsymbol{x}_v^t \mathbf{A} \boldsymbol{\theta}_v - \boldsymbol{x}_v^t \mathbf{B} \beta) c(\boldsymbol{\theta}_v, \beta)$ is an exponential family model with sufficient statistics $\mathbf{r}_v$ and $\mathbf{s}_v$ defined by $\mathbf{r}_v^t = \boldsymbol{x}_v^t \mathbf{A}$ and $\mathbf{s}_v^t = \boldsymbol{x}_v^t \mathbf{B}$, respectively. Let $\mathbb{B}(\mathbf{r})$ stand for the set of all possible response patterns $\boldsymbol{x}_v$ resulting in a value $\mathbf{r}$ for the sufficient statistic for θ. Conditioning on the sufficient statistic for the ability parameters results in a conditional response probability given by

$$p(\boldsymbol{x}_v|\mathbf{r}_v,\beta) = \frac{p(\boldsymbol{x}_v|\theta_v,\beta)g(\theta_v|\lambda,\mathbf{y}_v)h(\beta|\phi,\mathbf{z})}{\sum_{\mathbb{B}(\mathbf{r})}p(\boldsymbol{x}_v|\theta_v,\beta)g(\theta_v|\lambda,\mathbf{y}_v)h(\beta|\phi,\mathbf{z})}$$

$$= \frac{\exp(-\boldsymbol{x}_v^t\mathbf{B}\beta)}{\sum_{\mathbb{B}(\mathbf{r})}\exp(-\boldsymbol{x}_v^t\mathbf{B}\beta)}, \qquad (3.10)$$

which does not depend on the ability parameters θ and the structural models $g(\theta_v|\lambda,\mathbf{y}_v)$ and $h(\beta|\phi,\mathbf{z})$. The denominator is usually called an elementary symmetric function. Also, the conditional likelihood is an exponential family model, and estimation of the item parameters β amounts to equating the observed values of the sufficient statistics with their expected values (see, for instance, Andersen, 1980). So the estimation equations are given by

$$s_{ij} = E(S_{ij}|\mathbf{r},\beta),$$

for $i = 1,\ldots,I$ and $j = 1,\ldots,m_i$, with

$$E(S_{ij}|\mathbf{r},\beta) = \sum_v E(X_{ij}|\mathbf{r}_v,\beta)$$

$$= \sum_v \frac{\sum_{\mathbb{B}(\mathbf{r},ij)}\exp(-\boldsymbol{x}_v^t\mathbf{B}\beta)}{\sum_{\mathbb{B}(\mathbf{r})}\exp(-\boldsymbol{x}_v^t\mathbf{B}\beta)}, \qquad (3.11)$$

where $\mathbb{B}(\mathbf{r},ij)$ is the set of all possible response patterns resulting in a score $\mathbf{r}$ with $x_{ij} = 1$.

An LM test for the appropriateness of the ICCs can be derived by posing an alternative measurement model

$$\exp(\boldsymbol{x}_v^t\mathbf{A}\theta_v - \boldsymbol{x}_v^t\mathbf{B}\beta + \boldsymbol{x}_v^t\mathbf{D}\delta)c(\theta_v,\beta,\delta) \qquad (3.12)$$

such that the additional parameters δ represent some model violation, and introduce the null hypothesis $\delta = \mathbf{0}$.

3.5.2 Some Examples Pertaining to the Rasch Model

In 3.2, an example of an LM test for the appropriateness of the ICCs was given. The alternative model underlying the test is given by

$$P(X_{vi} = 1|g(r_v^{(i)}) = g) = \frac{\exp(\theta_v - \beta_i + \delta_{gi})}{1 + \exp(\theta_v - \beta_i + \delta_{gi})}, \qquad (3.13)$$

where $r_v^{(i)}$ stands for the number-correct score ignoring item i, and $g(r_v^{(i)})$ stands for the score-level group to which person v belongs. Note that δ_{gi} can be seen as a shift either of the item parameter or in the ability parameter. This shift is a function of the score level. So the additional parameters gauge the extent to which the ICC given in (3.13) is appropriate for all subgroups g. The fact that only $G - 1$ parameters δ_{gi} are present in the model entails that group G is used as a base line. In fact, the alternative model would not be identified if it had G parameters δ_{gi}. The connection between the alternative model (3.13) and the residuals (3.2) can be established by evaluating the first order derivatives of the likelihood function with respect to δ_{gi}. However, the derivation is straightforward after we note that the model defined by (3.12) and the model derived from it by conditioning on $\boldsymbol{x}_v^t \mathbf{A} \boldsymbol{\theta}_v$ are also exponential family models. Therefore, here too the first-order derivative has the form of the difference between an observed value and an expectation of a sufficient statistic. Since δ_{gi} can be seen as an additional item parameter, analogous to (3.11), it immediately follows that

$$E(N_{ig}|\mathbf{r}, \beta) = \sum_{v|g(r_v^{(i)})=g} E(X_{vi}|\mathbf{r}_v, \beta),$$

where the summation is over all persons with a partial sum score such that $g(r_v^{(i)}) = g$. For a derivation of the covariance matrix $\mathbf{W}$, one is referred to Glas (1988) (see also Glas & Verhelst, 1995).

Using the same rationale, test statistics can also be derived for DIF and local stochastic independence. DIF can be defined as a difference in item responses between equally proficient members of two or more groups. If the groups are labeled $g = 1, \ldots, G$, and indicator variables y_{vg} are defined as equal to one if the person belongs to subgroup g and zero otherwise, an alternative model can be defined as

$$P(X_{vi} = 1 | y_{vg} = 1) = \frac{\exp(\theta_v - \beta_i + \delta_{gi})}{1 + \exp(\theta_v - \beta_i + \delta_{gi})}. \tag{3.14}$$

Again, one of the groups must be used as a base line.

Local independence can be evaluated by posing an alternative model in which the response on item i depends on the response on some other item k. So we have

$$P(X_{vi} = 1 | X_{vk} = x_{vk}) = \frac{\exp(\theta_v - \beta_i + x_{vk}\delta)}{1 + \exp(\theta_v - \beta_i + x_{vk}\delta)}. \tag{3.15}$$

Also, the tests with these two alternative models can be based on LM-statistics that are differences between observed and expected frequencies. The test for DIF is based on the observed frequencies of correct item responses in the subgroups g, and the test for local independence is based on the number of simultaneous correct responses to the two items. For further details, refer to Glas (1988) (see also Glas & Verhelst, 1995).

Interestingly, the model given by (3.15) is a special case of a family of models proposed by Jannarone (1986) and Kelderman (1984) in which local independence can be violated. Since all the models in that family are exponential family models of the form given by (3.10), special versions such as (3.15) can be tested against more general versions using an LM test in a CML framework. One could, for instance, test the hypothesis that the probability of a correct response depends on the responses on a set of items rather than on the response to one item, say the previous item.

A final remark pertains to the practical application of the test. If the test length is k items, there are potentially $k(k-1)/2$ combinations of items that can be tested for dependence. Huge output can be avoided by defining a limited number of pairs on theoretical grounds. However, usually these theoretical grounds are not available, and in these cases it is a reasonable choice to test for dependence in pairs of consecutive items.

3.6 The MML framework

3.6.1 The General Formulation

Marginal maximum likelihood (MML) is probably the most frequently used method for the estimation of the parameters of IRT models. For the 1PL, 2PL, and 3PL models, the theory was developed by such authors as Bock & Aitkin (1981) and Mislevy (1984, 1986). Under the label "full information factor analysis," a multidimensional version of the 2PL and 3PL normal ogive model was developed by Bock, Gibbons, & Muraki (1988).

MML estimation derives its name from maximizing a log-likelihood that is marginalized with respect to θ, rather than maximizing the joint log-likelihood of all model parameters. Let $\boldsymbol{\eta}$ be a vector of all item parameters β and ϕ and population parameters λ. Then the marginal likelihood of $\boldsymbol{\eta}$ is given by

$$L(\boldsymbol{\eta}) = h(\beta|\phi, \mathbf{z}) \prod_v \int \cdots \int p(\boldsymbol{x}_v|\theta_v, \beta)g(\theta_v|\lambda, \mathbf{y}_v)d\theta_v \ .$$

$$= h(\beta|\phi, \mathbf{z}) \prod_v \int \cdots \int \exp(\boldsymbol{x}_v^t \mathbf{A}\theta_v - \boldsymbol{x}_v^t \mathbf{B}\beta)c(\theta_v, \beta)g(\theta_v|\lambda, \mathbf{y}_v)d\theta_v \ .$$

The reason for maximizing the marginal rather than the joint likelihood is that maximizing the latter does not lead to consistent estimates. This is related to the fact that the number of person parameters grows in proportion to the number of observations, and in general, this leads to inconsistency (Neyman & Scott, 1948). Simulation studies by Fischer & Scheiblechner (1970) show that these inconsistencies can indeed occur in IRT models. One way to deal with the problem is removing the person parameters by conditioning on their sufficient statistics. The result is the CML framework sketched above. The other approach is marginalizing over the person parameters. The marginal likelihood equations for $\boldsymbol{\eta}$ can be easily derived using Fisher's identity (Glas, 1992, 1999). The first-order derivatives with respect to $\boldsymbol{\eta}$ can be written as

$$\mathbf{h}(\boldsymbol{\eta}) = \frac{\partial}{\partial \boldsymbol{\eta}} \log L(\boldsymbol{\eta}) = \sum_v E(\omega_v(\boldsymbol{\eta}) \mid \boldsymbol{x}_v, \boldsymbol{\eta}) \ , \qquad (3.16)$$

with

$$\omega_v(\boldsymbol{\eta}) = \frac{\partial}{\partial\boldsymbol{\eta}} \log p(\boldsymbol{x}_v, \theta_v \mid \boldsymbol{\eta}), \tag{3.17}$$

where the expectation is with respect to the posterior distribution $p(\theta_v \mid \boldsymbol{x}_v, \boldsymbol{\eta})$. The identities in (3.16) and (3.17) are closely related to the EM-algorithm (Dempster et al., 1977), which is an algorithm for finding the maximum of a likelihood marginalized over unobserved data. The present application fits this framework when the response patterns are viewed as observed data and the ability parameters as unobserved data. Together they are referred to as the complete data. The EM algorithm is applicable in situations in which direct inference based on the marginal likelihood is complicated, and the complete data likelihood equations, i.e., equations based on $\omega_v(\boldsymbol{\eta})$, are easily solved. The core of the algorithm is that given some estimate of $\boldsymbol{\eta}$, say $\boldsymbol{\eta}^*$, the estimate can be improved by solving $\sum_v E(\omega_v(\boldsymbol{\eta}) \mid \boldsymbol{x}_v, \boldsymbol{\eta}^*) = 0$ with respect to $\boldsymbol{\eta}$. Then this new estimate becomes $\boldsymbol{\eta}^*$ and the process is iterated until convergence. Also the standard errors are easily derived in this framework: Mislevy (1986) points out that the information matrix can be approximated as

$$\mathbf{H}(\boldsymbol{\eta}, \boldsymbol{\eta}) \approx \sum_v E(\omega_v(\boldsymbol{\eta}) \mid \boldsymbol{x}_v, \boldsymbol{\eta}) E(\omega_v(\boldsymbol{\eta}) \mid \boldsymbol{x}_v, \boldsymbol{\eta})^t, \tag{3.18}$$

and the standard errors are the diagonal elements of the inverse of this matrix.

3.6.2 An Example Pertaining to the Partial Credit Model

Application of this framework to the derivation of estimation equations will be clarified using the partial credit model (PCM; Masters, 1982), extended with the assumption that the person parameters have a normal distribution mean μ and standard deviation σ.

In the PCM, the probability of answering in a certain category is dependent on the latent ability of the respondent θ_v and the item parameters β_{ij}, $j = 1, \ldots, m_i$. The item category response function is given by

$$P_{ij}(\theta_v) = P(X_{vij} = 1 \mid \theta_v, \beta_i) = \frac{\exp(j\theta_v - \beta_{ij})}{1 + \sum_{h=1}^{m_i} \exp(h\theta_v - \beta_{ih})}. \tag{3.19}$$

The item parameters defined by $\eta_{ij} = \beta_{ij} - \beta_{i(j-1)}$ are sometimes called step parameters (Masters, 1982). The η_{ij} are the points on the θ scale at which the curves of $P_{i,j-1}(\theta)$ and $P_{ij}(\theta)$ intersect. These two curves intersect only once, and the intersection can occur anywhere along the θ scale.

The likelihood equations are obtained by equating (3.16) to zero. Since the PCM is an exponential family model, the expressions for (3.17) again are the difference between the observed values of the sufficient statistics and the expected values of the sufficient statistics, so we have

$$\omega_v(\beta_{ij}) = -x_{vij} + P_{ij}(\theta_v),$$

and inserting the expressions into (3.16) and equating the resulting expressions to zero results in

$$s_{ij} = \sum_v E\left(\,P_{ij}(\theta_v)\mid \boldsymbol{x}_v, \boldsymbol{\eta}\,\right).$$

To derive the likelihood equations for the population parameters, the first-order derivatives of the log of the density of the ability parameters $g(\theta; \mu, \sigma)$ are needed. In the present case, $g(\theta; \mu, \sigma)$ is the well-known expression for the normal distribution with mean μ and standard deviation σ, so it is easily verified that these derivatives are given by

$$\omega_v(\mu) = \frac{(\theta_v - \mu)}{\sigma^2}$$

and

$$\omega_v(\sigma) = \frac{(\theta_v - \mu)^2 - \sigma^2}{\sigma^3}.$$

The likelihood equations are again found upon inserting these expressions in (3.16) and equating the resulting expressions to zero. Usually, the location of the latent scale is identified by setting μ to zero, in which case the associated estimation equation is not relevant.

Glas (1999) proposed an LM test for the PCM to evaluate the appropriateness of the item response functions. Also in this case, this could in principle be done by estimating the respondents' latent variables θ, ordering them according to size, and evaluating the difference between manifest item response proportions and the theoretical response probabilities. However, test statistics based on partitioning the sample of respondents using estimates rather than of observable statistics have very poor properties (see, for instance, Orlando & Thissen, 2000, or Glas & Suarez-Falcon, 2003). Therefore, here we consider a test based on a partitioning of the respondents on the basis of their total scores. The test is performed for every item. Let the item of interest be labeled i, while the other items are labeled $k = 1, \ldots, i-1, i+1, \ldots, I$. Let $x^{(i)}$ be the response pattern without item i, and let $r_v^{(i)}$ be the sum score on this partial response pattern, that is,

$$r_v^{(i)} = \sum_{k \neq i} \sum_j j x_{vgj}.$$

The possible scores will be partitioned into G_i disjoint subtests, according to the score level. The index i indicates that the partitioning can be different for each item. As an alternative to the model under the null hypothesis, that is, the PCM, we consider a model in which the probability of scoring in category j of item i, conditional on a partial sums score in subset g $(g = 1, \ldots, G_i)$ is given by

$$P(X_{vij} = 1 \mid g, \theta_v, \beta_i, \delta_{gi}) = \frac{\exp(j\theta_v + j\delta_{gi} - \beta_{ij})}{1 + \sum_{h=1}^{m_i} \exp(h\theta_v + h\delta_{gi} - \beta_{ih})}, \qquad (3.20)$$

for $j = 1, \ldots, m_i$. Under the null model, the additional parameter δ_{gi} is equal to zero. Notice that parameter δ_{gi} is multiplied by j, so the term $j\delta_{gi}$ has a function that is analogous to the function of $j\theta_v$. Therefore, the alternative model entails that the latent parameter θ is insufficient to describe the responses, and some shift related to the response level must be incorporated. The first-order derivatives with respect to δ_{gi} are given by

$$- \sum_{v|g} \sum_j jx_{vij} + \sum_{v|g} \sum_j jE(P_{ij}(\theta) \mid \boldsymbol{x}_v, \beta_i), \qquad (3.21)$$

for $i = 1, \ldots, k$, and $g = 1, \ldots, G_i$. So if both terms in (3.21) are divided by the number of respondents in group g it can be seen that the test is based on the difference between the observed average score on item i in score level group g, and its posterior expectation. The expected value is computed using the PCM without the additional parameters, that is, using the null model. If the difference between the observed and expected values is large, it means that the PCM model did not fit the data. The additional parameter δ_{gi} is necessary to fit the model, so the null hypothesis, $\delta_{gi} = 0$, is rejected. An important detail is that the alternative model has to be identified. This can be accomplished by setting the first additional parameters, say δ_{1g}, equal to zero. So the LM statistic given by (3.4) is based on $G_i - 1$ residuals, and it has an asymptotic χ^2-distribution with $g_i - 1$ degrees of freedom (Glas, 1999).

It should be noted that it is essentially the residuals that give insight into the model fit. The associated formal test of model fit based on a statistic with a known (asymptotic) distribution is relevant only for moderate sample sizes. For large sample sizes, these tests become less interesting, because their power then becomes so large that even the smallest deviations from the model become significant. In these cases, the effect size becomes more important than the significance probability of the test.

The testing procedure is illustrated with a small example from a Belgian school effectiveness study. In this survey, the achievement on mathematics and Dutch language ability were measured along with academic self esteem, well-being at school, and concentration during lessons. The example presented here pertains to the scale for "academic self esteem." The scale consisted of 9 questions, such as "If I may choose, I would rather go to another school," "My fellow pupils can learn better than I can," and "In the classroom I am often thinking about things that are not related to the subject matter" (these items are translated from Dutch). Each item of the three scales had five response categories: "strongly disagree," "disagree," "neutral," "agree," and "strongly agree." The analysis presented pertains to the responses of 1942 pupils on the second time point. For more details, refer to Marvelde et al. (2006).

First, MML estimates were computed. Then, for every item, an LM statistic was computed to evaluate the fit of the ICCs. To compute the statistics,

Table 3.1. Evaluation of fit of item response functions

		Group 1		Group 2		Group 3		Group 4	
i	LM	Pr.	Obs	Exp	Obs	Exp	Obs	Exp	Obs	Exp
1	6.5	.09	1.30	1.28	1.69	1.71	1.90	1.93	2.29	2.24
2	5.3	.15	0.37	0.37	0.67	0.69	1.05	1.00	1.53	1.57
3	2.3	.50	0.71	0.72	1.16	1.18	1.56	1.54	2.07	2.06
4	0.5	.92	0.86	0.87	1.28	1.26	1.58	1.57	2.03	2.05
5	12.8	.01	0.39	0.38	0.76	0.78	1.08	1.05	1.41	1.45
6	5.1	.16	0.35	0.36	0.74	0.72	0.98	0.98	1.36	1.38
7	8.5	.04	0.68	0.71	1.21	1.17	1.47	1.46	1.83	1.86
8	1.1	.77	0.77	0.77	1.15	1.14	1.42	1.42	1.90	1.92
9	10.1	.02	1.62	1.60	1.90	1.87	2.02	2.03	2.18	2.23

the sample of respondents was divided into four subgroups of approximately equal sample size. Subgroup 1 contained respondents with a score $r_v^{(i)} \leq 7$, respondents in subgroup 2 had $8 \leq r_v^{(i)} \leq 10$, group 3 had respondents who obtained scores $11 \leq r_v^{(i)} \leq 13$, and respondents of group 4 had $r_v^{(i)} \geq 14$. The results are given in Table 3.1. Note that 3 of the 9 LM tests were significant at a 5% significance level. The observed and the expected average item scores in the subgroups are shown under the headings "Obs" and "Exp," respectively. Note that the observed average scores increased with the score level of the group. Further, it can be seen that the observed and expected values were quite close: the largest absolute difference was .05 and the mean absolute difference was approximately .02. So, even though the number of significant tests was larger than should be expected given the significance level, the fit between the expected and observed scores is such that the conclusion that the data fit the model is justified.

3.7 The MCMC Framework

In the introduction of this chapter, it was indicated that CML has its main application in the evaluation of the measurement model, while MML has its main application in the evaluation of the measurement model in the presence of a structural model. However, the computation of MML estimates becomes quite difficult when the dimensionality of the latent parameter space becomes high. For instance, consider a multidimensional version of the RM given by

$$P(X_{vi} = 1 \mid \theta_v, \beta_i) = \frac{\exp(\sum_{q=1}^{Q} a_{iq}\theta_{vq} - \beta_i)}{1 + \exp(\sum_{q=1}^{Q} a_{iq}\theta_{vq} - \beta_i)}, \tag{3.22}$$

where θ_v is a Q-dimensional vector with entries θ_{vq} and where the parameters a_{iq} are so-called factor-loadings. Often, the parameters a_{ij} are estimated, but they can also be seen as fixed weights with values chosen on theoretical grounds (see, for instance, Glas, 1997). Further, it is often assumed that θ_v has a Q-variate normal distribution with a covariance matrix $\boldsymbol{\Sigma}_\theta$. Takane & Leeuw (1987) have shown that multidimensional IRT models are equivalent with full-information factor-analysis models (Bock, Gibbons, & Muraki, 1988). Computation of MML estimates is not unproblematic because, as can be seen in Section 3.6.1, it requires the evaluation of a Q-dimensional integral. At this moment, the maximum number of factors is approximately 10 with adaptive quadrature, approximately 5 with nonadaptive quadrature, and approximately 15 with Monte Carlo integration (see, for instance, Bock & Schilling, 1997). In the framework of the two-parameter normal ogive model, an alternative Bayesian procedure using a MCMC algorithm, that is, the Gibbs sampler (Gelman et al., 1995), was suggested by Albert (1992). Recently, the Bayesian approach has been adopted to the estimation of IRT models with multiple raters, multiple item types, missing data (Patz & Junker, 1999b), testlet structures (Bradlow et al., 1999), latent classes (Hoijtink & Molenaar, 1997), models with a multilevel structure on the ability parameters (Fox & Glas, 2001) and the item parameters (Janssen et al., 2000), and multidimensional IRT models (Béguin & Glas, 2001).

In a Bayesian framework, prior distributions are defined for all parameters, and the inferences are based on the posterior distributions of the parameters. An MCMC procedure is used to generate the posterior distributions. These distributions are simulated in an iterative process using the Gibbs sampler (Gelfand & Smith, 1990). To implement the Gibbs sampler, the parameter vector is divided into a number of components, and each successive component is sampled from its conditional distribution given sampled values for all other components. This sampling scheme is repeated until the sampled values form stable posterior distributions. For application of the Gibbs sampler, it is important to create a set of partial posterior distributions that are easy to sample from. This has two consequences. First, it proves convenient that all the components of the model are based on normal distributions. Therefore, the logistic form of the measurement model is replaced by a normal ogive representation. Second, the step from discrete observations to continuous normally distributed variables requires a so-called data augmentation step, that is, the introduction of additional latent variables that lead to a simple set of posterior distributions.

As an example, consider the multidimensional RM given by (3.22). First, the probability of a correct response is replaced by $P(X_{vi} = 1 \mid \boldsymbol{\theta}_v, \beta_i) = \Phi(\eta_{ij})$, where $\Phi(.)$ is the standard normal ogive and $\eta_{vi} = \boldsymbol{\alpha}_i^t \boldsymbol{\theta}_v - \beta_i$. The normal ogive representation and the logistic representation are very close (Lord, 1980) Second, the data augmentation step is derived using a rationale that is analogous to a rationale often used as a justification of the two-parameter normal ogive model (see, for instance, Lord, 1980, Section 3.2). In this motivation, it is assumed that if person v is presented an item i, a latent variable Z_{vi} is drawn from a normal distribution with mean η_{vi} and a variance equal to one. A correct response $x_{vi} = 1$ is given when the drawn value is positive. So the distribution of Z_{ij} is given by

$$Z_{vi} \,|X_{vi} = x_{vi} \sim \begin{cases} N(\eta_{vi}, 1) \text{ truncated at the left by 0} & \text{if } x_{vi} = 1, \\ N(\eta_{vi}, 1) \text{ truncated at the right by 0} & \text{if } x_{vi} = 0. \end{cases} \quad (3.23)$$

In terms of the general model given by (3.1), the aim of the MCMC procedure is to simulate samples from the joint posterior distribution of the parameters θ, β, λ, and ϕ and the augmented data. In the present example λ consists of the mean μ_θ, and covariance matrix Σ_θ of the ability distribution. So the posterior distribution given the data x is given by

$$p(\theta, \beta, \mu_\theta, \Sigma_\theta, z\,|x) = p(z\,|x\,; \beta, \theta,)p(\theta|\mu_\theta, \Sigma_\theta)p(\mu_\theta, \Sigma_\theta)p(\beta), \quad (3.24)$$

where $p(\mu_\theta, \Sigma_\theta)$ and $p(\beta)$ are prior distributions. The prior for μ_θ, and Σ_θ is a normal-inverse-Wishart distribution (see, for instance, Box & Tiao, 1973). In RMs, an uninformative prior usually suffices for the item parameters β.

Although the distribution given by (3.24) has an intractable form, as a result of the data augmentation step, the conditional distributions of $\beta, \theta, \mu_\theta, \Sigma_\theta$ and z are now each tractable and easy to sample from. A draw from the full conditional distribution can be obtained in the following steps:

1. Draw z conditional on θ, β, and x;
2. Draw μ_θ and Σ_θ conditional on θ;
3. Draw θ conditional on z, β, Σ_θ, and μ_θ;
4. Draw β conditional on z and θ.

The first step that maps the discrete responses to a continuous variable amounts to sampling from the distribution defined in (3.23). The next three steps are the standard steps for sampling in the normal model; for details, refer to Gelman et al. (1995).

In the Bayesian framework, model fit can be evaluated using posterior predictive checks (PPC; see, for instance, Gelman et al., 1995, Chapter 6; Hoijtink & Molenaar, 1997; Sinharay & Johnson, 2003). A PPC results in a "posterior predictive p-value," the Bayesian analogue of the significance probability in a frequentist framework. The general idea of a posterior predictive check is to simulate data under the model and compare these data with the observed data. This is done as follows. First the posterior distribution of the parameters, say $p(\xi|x)$, is simulated using an MCMC method. The PPC is based on an index $T(x, \xi)$. When the Markov chain has converged, draws from the posterior distribution can be used to generate model-conforming data x^{rep} and to compute a so-called Bayesian p-value defined by

$$\Pr(T(x^{rep}, \xi) \geq T(x, \xi) \mid x). \quad (3.25)$$

So model fit is evaluated by computing the relative proportion of replications, that is, draws of ξ from $p(\xi|x)$, where the fit index computed using the data,

$T(x, \xi)$, has a smaller value than the analogous index computed using data generated to conform to the IRT model, that is, $T(x^{rep}, \xi)$. So after the burn-in period, the fit index $T(x, \xi)$ is computed using the current draw of the item, person, and population parameters, a new model-conforming response pattern is generated, and a value $T(x^{rep}, \xi)$ is computed. Finally, a Bayesian p-value is computed as the proportion of iterations where $T(x^{rep}, \xi) \geq T(x, \xi)$.

For the evaluation of item fit, $T(x, \xi)$ can be based on test statistics that are defined analogously to the fit statistics for the CML and MML framework. For instance, tests for the appropriateness of the ICCs, DIF, and local independence for the RM can be based on the alternative models defined by (3.13), (3.14), and (3.15), respectively. The alternative models provide the motivation for the indices, that is, they provide the connection between the model violation and $T(x, \xi)$. Then the sufficient statistics for the δ-parameters are derived. For the first two model violations, these are the number of correct scores in the subgroups g, and simultaneous realizations of pairs of items i and k for violation of local independence, respectively. The index $T(x, \xi)$ can then be defined as a Pearson-type statistic, that is, as the squared difference between the sufficient statistics and their expectations given $\boldsymbol{\theta}$ and $\boldsymbol{\beta}$, divided by the standard deviations of the difference. The approach is outlined in detail by Hoijtink (2001) and Sinharay (2003).

One of the advantages of PPCs is that there is no need to derive the distribution of the test statistics under the null model. The distribution is implicitly generated when the MCMC procedure is run. This is also the explanation for the fact that there is no need to implicate a covariance matrix such as the covariance matrix $\mathbf{W}$ in the LM-statistic, where accounting for the dependence between the vectors $\mathbf{d}$ is essential for the derivation of the asymptotic distribution of the statistics. However, as shown above, for item-oriented statistics the definition of test statistics such that the asymptotic distribution is known is not complicated. For person–fit statistics the matter is more complicated. Snijders (2001) derives correction formulas that account for the estimation of θ for a class of person-fit statistics for the RM, but this approach has not yet been generalized to a broader class of models. As an alternative approach, Glas & Meijer (2003) suggest to impute a number of well-known person-fit statistics with an unknown distribution as indices $T(x, \xi)$ in a PPC. As an example pertaining to the RM, they consider the UB-statistic given by (3.6). The correction by Snijders (2001) is needed to derive the asymptotic distribution of UB. To take into account the uncertainty about both the item and ability parameters, Glas & Meijer (2003) propose to use UB as a PPC. So after every replication of the MCMC procedure, UB is computed using the current draw of θ and β, a new response vector is generated and UB is computed for the new response vector, again using the current draw of θ and β. Simulation studies show that the control of Type I error rate is acceptable. However, as for all person-fit indices, the power to detect aberrant persons is not very large. This is, of course, attributable to the fact that for every person, only a very limited number of item responses are available to test person-fit.

3.8 Discussion

In this chapter, it was shown that evaluation of fit to IRT measurement models can be based on residual analyses. It was shown that the residuals can be seen as part of LM statistics. However, acceptance or rejection of a model should not only be based on a strict formal test of model fit but should always also take the sample size, the size of the residuals, and the application into account. For instance, if the sample size is large (say 5,000 students), an average difference of 0.01 across five score levels between the observed proportion correct and the model-based estimate of the probability of a correct response might already result in a significant test of item fit, but for a concrete application, say test equating, this model violation might be of little importance. So tests of model fit should always be interpreted with a sense of reality.

The overview that was given does not have the pretention of being exhaustive. For instance, we did not discuss the use of so-called uniformly most powerful (UMP) tests, which have some interesting connections to LM tests. Also in the UMP approach, a general model and a special case are compared. Ponocny (2000, 2001) proposed UMP item fit tests that have (3.14) and (3.15) as alternatives to the RM, and Klauer (1989) proposed a UMP person-fit test with (3.7) as an alternative model. Since both the RM and these more general alternative models are all exponential family models, a UMP test can be constructed for testing the hypothesis that an parameter additional to the RM, say δ, equals zero (Lehman, 1986, Chapter 3). The test is based on the sufficient statistic for δ, say T. The test is nonparametric: if we condition on the observed values of the sufficient statistics for the item and person parameters, all these parameters vanish from the likelihood. That is, all possible data matrices with these marginals are equally likely given the marginals. Ponocny & Ponocny-Seliger (1999) implemented a Monte Carlo algorithm for generating all matrices with the same marginals. For every generated matrix a value of the sufficient statistic T is computed and the test is then based on the position of the observed value of T in this generated distribution.

Although UMP tests are certainly statistically optimal, the application to more complex response formats, such as the format of polytomously scored items, is hampered by as yet unsolved numerical problems. The LM approach, on the other hand, can be applied to most, if not all, of the commonly used response formats. In fact, M. G. H. Jansen & Glas (2001) show how the test can be applied to detect DIF in Rasch's model for speed tests.

The final remark in this discussion concerns the question what to do if the model does not hold. To make the discussion specific, assume that the RM does not fit a data set consisting of responses to dichotomously scored items. Several approaches to solving the problem are available. The first approach to obtaining model fit is to remove persons or items from the data set that have been flagged as misfits. In some instances this approach is appropriate and well founded. Rasch (1960) (also see Fischer, 1995a) showed that the RM can be derived from a measurement criterion known as specific objectivity.

From that point of view, the RM plays an important role in psychological research, where items can be selected to measure some theoretical construct. In other situations, such as in much educational research, however, items and sampled respondents cannot be discarded without threatening the validity of the inferences made via IRT. This leads to the second approach to obtain model fit: trying to find an IRT model that does fit. Several alternatives to the RM are available. For instance, Glas (1992) and Béguin & Glas (2001) suggest to divide the test into a number of unidimensional subscales and to introduce the assumption that the ability parameters of the subscales have a joint multivariate normal distribution. This is a special case of the model defined by (3.22) in which each item loads on one of the ability dimensions only. Further, the covariance matrix of the multivariate ability distribution models the relation between the subscales. The advantage of this approach is that the covariance between the ability dimensions provides information about the structure of the test. On the other hand, it entails the introduction of an assumption about the distribution of the ability parameters that may in itself be another source of a model violation. Another approach, discussed by Verhelst & Glas (1995), is to retain a unidimensional model but to introduce positive integer scoring weights to the items. The model is a unidimensional special case of the model defined in (3.1) in which the entries in the matrix A consist of positive integers a_i for all items $i = 1, \ldots, k$. So the model has the same functional form as the two-parameter logistic model (see, for instance, Lord, 1980) except that the item-discrimination parameters are confined to be positive integers. As can be verified in Section 3.5 of this chapter, this approach supports CML estimation of the item parameters that do not rely on any assumption about the ability distribution. The bottom line is that several approaches to the choice of an alternative model in case of misfit are open and the choice can best be made with the application in mind.

The Mixed-Coefficients Multinomial Logit Model: A Generalized Form of the Rasch Model

Raymond J. Adams and Margaret L. Wu

University of Melbourne

4.1 Introduction

Since Rasch's introduction of his item response models (Rasch, 1960), there has been a proliferation of extensions and alternatives, each of which has a different name and different matching software package. As Adams, Wilson, & Wang (1997) pointed out, the proliferation of models has, in some ways, been a hindrance to practitioners. This paper presents a generalized item response model that provides a unifying framework for a large class of Rasch-type models. The advantages of a single framework include mathematical elegance, generality in a single software package, and a facilitation of the development, testing, and comparison of new models. The unified model is a multidimensional item response model, the specification of which is achieved through the use of design matrices chosen to represent the parametrization of the model. In the paper we discuss the estimation of the parameters of the model, the testing of model fit, and we illustrate how standard models (such as the simple logistic, the rating scale, and facets models) and alternative user-defined models are specified.

Over the past 30 years, a proliferation of item response models has emerged. In the logistic item response model family, notably, the simple logistic model (Rasch, 1980), the partial-credit model (Masters, 1982), the rating-scale model (Andrich, 1978), the facets model (Linacre, 1989), and the linear logistic model (Fischer, 1973) have all played an important role in the analysis of item response data. Typically, the development of the estimation procedures of parameters for each item response model was specific to the model, as was the development of dedicated software programs for each model. Surveying the family of RMs, Adams & Wilson (1996) developed a unified approach to specifying the models and then consequentially estimating the parameters. There are at least two advantages to developing one single framework to encompass a family of models. First, the development of the estimation procedures and associated software for the implementation of the models can be streamlined within a single framework of models. That is, one needs to develop only one set of estimation procedures and one software program to carry out the estimation of the parameters in the models. Second, a generalized framework provides an opportunity for the development of new models that fit in the framework. This allows for the flexible application of item response models to suit users' requirements.

This paper describes a generalized framework for specifying a family of logistic item response models through the specification of design matrices. The estimation procedures are also described. The idea of the use of design matrices is extended to the construction of a family of goodness-of-fit tests. Flexibility in the construction of fit tests allows the users to target specific hypotheses regarding the fit of the items to the model, such as the violation of local independence between subsets of items.

4.2 The Mixed-Coefficients Multinomial Logit Model

The mixed-coefficients multinomial logit model (MCML) is a categorical response model, and in most applications, the response patterns to a set of test items (the categorical outcomes) are modeled as the dependent variable. Under the model, the response patterns are predicted by logistic regression, where the independent variables are item difficulty and person abilities.[1]

The model is referred to as a mixed-coefficients model because items are described by a fixed set of unknown parameters, ξ, while the student ability (the latent variable), θ, is a random effect.

The model is specified as follows. Assume that there are I items and they are indexed $i = 1, \ldots, I$ with each item admitting $K_i + 1$ response categories indexed $k = 0, 1, \ldots, K_i$. That is, a response to item i by a student can be allocated to one of $K_i + 1$ response categories. The vector-valued random variable $\mathbf{X}_i = (X_{i1}, X_{i2}, \ldots, X_{iK_i})^T$, where for $k = 1, \ldots, K_i$,

$$X_{ik} = \begin{cases} 1 \text{ if response to item } i \text{ is in category } k, \\ 0 \text{ otherwise}, \end{cases} \tag{4.1}$$

is used to indicate the $K_i + 1$ possible responses to item i. A vector of zeros denotes a response in category zero, making the zero category a reference category, which is necessary for model identification. Using this as the reference category is arbitrary, and does not affect the generality of the model.

Each $\mathbf{X}_i$ consists of a sequence of 0's and possibly one 1, indicating the student's response category for that item. For example, if the response category is 0 for an item with four categories (0, 1, 2, 3), then $\mathbf{X}_i^T = (0, 0, 0)$. If the response category is 2, then $\mathbf{X}_i^T = (0, 1, 0)$.

---

[1] Throughout this article the term "ability" is used as a generic placeholder to refer to the latent variable being measured. The term "difficulty" refers to parameters that characterize the items.

The $\mathbf{X}_i$ can also be collected together into the single vector $\mathbf{X}^T = \left(\mathbf{X}_1^T, \mathbf{X}_2^T, \ldots, \mathbf{X}_I^T \right)$, called the response vector. Particular instances of each of these random variables are indicated by their lowercase equivalents, $\mathbf{x}$, $\mathbf{x}_i$, and x_{ik}.

Items are described through a vector $\xi^T = (\xi_1, \xi_2, \ldots, \xi_p)$, of p parameters. Linear combinations of these are used in the response probability model to describe the empirical characteristics of the response categories of each item. These linear combinations are defined by design vectors $\mathbf{a}_{ik}$ $(i = 1, \ldots, I;\ k = 1, \ldots K_i)$, each of length p, which can be collected to form a design matrix $\mathbf{A}^T = (\mathbf{a}_{11}, \mathbf{a}_{12}, \ldots, \mathbf{a}_{1K_1}, \mathbf{a}_{21}, \ldots, \mathbf{a}_{2K_2}, \ldots, \mathbf{a}_{IK_I})$.

The multidimensional form of the model assumes that a set of D traits underlies the individuals' responses. The D latent traits define a D-dimensional latent space. The vector $\boldsymbol{\theta} = (\theta_1, \theta_2, \ldots, \theta_D)^T$ represents an individual's position in the D-dimensional latent space.

The model also introduces a scoring function that allows the specification of the score or performance level assigned to each possible response category to each item. To do so, the notion of a response score b_{ikd} is introduced, which gives the performance level of an observed response in category k, item i, dimension d. The scores across D dimensions can be collected into a column vector $\mathbf{b}_{ik} = (b_{ik1}, b_{ik2}, \ldots, b_{ikD})^T$, and again collected into the scoring submatrix for item i, $\mathbf{B}_i = (\mathbf{b}_{i1}, \mathbf{b}_{i2}, \ldots, \mathbf{b}_{ik_i})^T$ and then into a scoring matrix $\mathbf{B} = \left(\mathbf{B}_1^T, \mathbf{B}_2^T, \ldots, \mathbf{B}_I^T \right)^T$ for the entire test. (The score for a response in the zero category is zero, but other responses may also be scored zero.)

The regression of the response vector on the item and person parameters is

$$f\left(\mathbf{x}; \xi | \theta \right) = \Psi\left(\theta, \xi \right) \exp\left[\mathbf{x}^T \left(\mathbf{B}\theta + \mathbf{A}\xi \right) \right], \tag{4.2}$$

with

$$\Psi\left(\theta, \xi \right) = \left\{ \sum_{\mathbf{z} \in \Omega} \exp\left[\mathbf{z}^T \left(\mathbf{B}\theta + \mathbf{A}\xi \right) \right] \right\}^{-1}, \tag{4.3}$$

where Ω is the set of all possible response vectors.

4.2.1 Simple Logistic Model (SLM) Example

Equations (4.2) and (4.3) can be illustrated with some simple cases. Consider a simple logistic model for dichotomous data. This model would normally be written (in the notation of Wright & Stone, 1979) as

$$\Pr\left(X_{i1} = 1, \delta_i | \theta \right) = \frac{\exp\left(\theta + \delta_i \right)}{1 + \exp\left(\theta + \delta_i \right)}. \tag{4.4}$$

For three dichotomous items, the probability of the response vector, $\mathbf{x}^T = (x_{11}, x_{21}, x_{31})$, is then

$$\Pr\left(\mathbf{X} = \mathbf{x}, \delta_1, \delta_2, \delta_3 | \theta\right) = \prod_{i=1}^{3} \frac{\exp\left\{x_{i1}\left(\theta + \delta_i\right)\right\}}{1 + \exp\left(\theta + \delta_i\right)}$$

$$= \frac{\exp\left\{\sum\limits_{i=1}^{3} x_{i1}\left(\theta + \delta_i\right)\right\}}{\prod\limits_{i=1}^{3}\left\{1 + \exp\left(\theta + \delta_i\right)\right\}} \qquad (4.5)$$

$$= \frac{\exp\left(r\theta + x_{11}\delta_1 + x_{21}\delta_2 + x_{31}\delta_3\right)}{D},$$

where

$$D = 1 + \exp\left(\theta + \delta_1\right) + \exp\left(\theta + \delta_2\right) + \exp\left(\theta + \delta_3\right)$$
$$+ \exp\left(2\theta + \delta_1 + \delta_2\right) + \exp\left(2\theta + \delta_2 + \delta_3\right)$$
$$+ \exp\left(2\theta + \delta_1 + \delta_3\right) + \exp\left(3\theta + \delta_1 + \delta_2 + \delta_3\right),$$

and

$$r = \sum_{i=1}^{3} x_{i1}.$$

To show how (4.2) and (4.5) can be made equivalent, consider the following choices of $\mathbf{A}$, $\mathbf{B}$ and ξ:

$$\mathbf{A} = \begin{bmatrix} 1 & 0 & 0 \\ 0 & 1 & 0 \\ 0 & 0 & 1 \end{bmatrix}, \quad \mathbf{B} = \begin{bmatrix} 1 \\ 1 \\ 1 \end{bmatrix}, \quad \text{and} \quad \xi = \begin{bmatrix} \delta_1 \\ \delta_2 \\ \delta_3 \end{bmatrix}, \qquad (4.6)$$

where the first row of $\mathbf{A}$ corresponds to item one category one; the second row corresponds to item two category one; the third row corresponds to item three category one. The rows of $\mathbf{B}$ correspond to the same item and category as for the rows of $\mathbf{A}$. The elements of ξ correspond to the item difficulty parameters of items one to three respectively. Note that with three dichotomous items there are eight different response patterns.

4.2.2 Partial-Credit Example

As a second example, consider a partial-credit item with three categories: 0, 1, and 2. Using the notation of Wright & Masters (1982), (4.2) and (4.3) can be written as

$$\Pr\left(X_i^T = (0,0); \delta_{i1}, \delta_{i2} | \theta\right) = \Pr\left(\text{category } 0; \mathbf{A}, \mathbf{B}, \xi | \theta\right)$$

$$= \frac{1}{1 + \exp\left(\theta + \delta_{i1}\right) + \exp\left(2\theta + \delta_{i1} + \delta_{i2}\right)},$$

$$\Pr\left(X_i^T = (1,0)\,;\delta_{i1},\delta_{i2}|\theta\right) = \Pr(\text{category } 1; \mathbf{A}, \mathbf{B}, \xi|\theta)$$

$$= \frac{\exp(\theta + \delta_{i1})}{1 + \exp(\theta + \delta_{i1}) + \exp(2\theta + \delta_{i1} + \delta_{i2})}, \quad (4.7)$$

$$\Pr\left(X_i^T = (0,1)\,;\delta_{i1},\delta_{i2}|\theta\right) = \Pr(\text{category } 2; \mathbf{A}, \mathbf{B}, \xi|\theta)$$

$$= \frac{\exp(2\theta + \delta_{i1} + \delta_{i2})}{1 + \exp(\theta + \delta_{i1}) + \exp(2\theta + \delta_{i1} + \delta_{i2})}.$$

For two three-category partial-credit items, the probability of the response vector $\mathbf{x}$ is then

$$\Pr(\mathbf{X} = \mathbf{x}; \delta_{11}, \delta_{12}, \delta_{21}, \delta_{22}|\theta) = \prod_{i=1}^{2} \frac{\exp\left(s_i\theta + \sum_{k=1}^{s_i}\delta_{ik}\right)}{1 + \exp(\theta + \delta_{i1}) + \exp(2\theta + \delta_{i1} + \delta_{i2})}, \quad (4.8)$$

where s_i is the observed response category for item i and $\sum_{i=1}^{0} u \equiv 0$ for all possible values of u.

To show how (4.2) and (4.8) can be made equivalent, consider the following choices of $\mathbf{A}$, $\mathbf{B}$, and ξ:

$$\mathbf{A} = \begin{bmatrix} 1 & 0 & 0 & 0 \\ 1 & 1 & 0 & 0 \\ 0 & 0 & 1 & 0 \\ 0 & 0 & 1 & 1 \end{bmatrix}, \quad \mathbf{B} = \begin{bmatrix} 1 \\ 2 \\ 1 \\ 2 \end{bmatrix}, \quad \text{and} \quad \xi = \begin{bmatrix} \delta_{11} \\ \delta_{12} \\ \delta_{21} \\ \delta_{22} \end{bmatrix}, \quad (4.9)$$

where the first row of $\mathbf{A}$ corresponds to item one category one; the second row corresponds to item one category two; the third row corresponds to item two category one; and the fourth row corresponds to item two category two. The same row referencing applies to the matrix $\mathbf{B}$.

4.2.3 Facet Example

Consider an example of a facets model (Linacre, 1989) in which there are three raters, each rater rating the same two dichotomous items. This is modeled as six *generalized items*. A generalized item is defined for each of the possible combinations of a rater and an actual item. Generalized item one is the response category given by rater one on item one. Generalized item two is the response category given by rater one on item two, and so on. The following choices of $\mathbf{A}$, $\mathbf{B}$, and ξ will give this facets model:

$$\mathbf{A} = \begin{bmatrix} 1 & 0 & 0 & 1 & 0 \\ 1 & 0 & 0 & 0 & 1 \\ 0 & 1 & 0 & 1 & 0 \\ 0 & 1 & 0 & 0 & 1 \\ 0 & 0 & 1 & 1 & 0 \\ 0 & 0 & 1 & 0 & 1 \end{bmatrix}, \quad \mathbf{B} = \begin{bmatrix} 1 \\ 1 \\ 1 \\ 1 \\ 1 \\ 1 \end{bmatrix}, \quad \text{and} \quad \xi = \begin{bmatrix} \rho_1 \\ \rho_2 \\ \rho_3 \\ \delta_1 \\ \delta_2 \end{bmatrix}, \quad (4.10)$$

where the first row of **A** corresponds to category one of generalized item one (rater one, item one); the second row corresponds to category one of generalized item two (rater one, item two); the third row corresponds to category one of generalized item three (rater two, item one); the fourth row corresponds to category one of generalized item four (rater two, item two), and so on. The same row referencing applies to the matrix **B**. The first three elements (ρ_1, ρ_2, ρ_3) of ξ are the severity parameters of raters one to three respectively. The fourth and fifth element, (δ_1, δ_2) of ξ are the item-difficulty parameters for the two dichotomous items.

4.2.4 Multidimensional Examples

Finally, Figure 4.1 shows two possible multidimensional models: a between-item multidimensionality model and a within-item multidimensionality model (Adams, Wilson, & Wang, 1997). In each case, a hypothetical nine-item test is considered. In the between-item multidimensional case (the left-hand side of Figure 4.1), each item is associated with a single dimension, but the collection of items covers three dimensions: three items are associated with each of the three latent dimensions. In the within-item case (the right-hand side of Figure 4.1), some items are associated with more than one dimension. For example, item two is associated with both dimensions one and two.

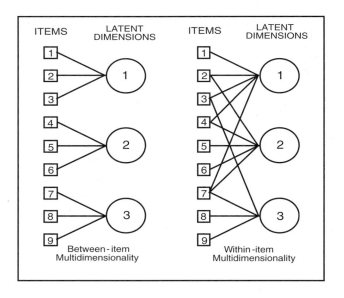

Fig. 4.1. Between- and within-item multidimensionality

If the items shown in Figure 4.1 are all dichotomous, then the matrices $\mathbf{A}$, $\mathbf{B}$, and ξ, as given in (4.11) and (4.12), if substituted into (4.2), will yield the between- and within-item multidimensional models respectively as shown in Figure 4.1.

Note that the only difference between (4.11) and (4.12) is the $\mathbf{B}$ matrix. This matrix is called the score matrix and is used to indicate the scores of the items on each of the three dimensions. Note also that the $\mathbf{B}$ matrices (4.11) and (4.12) have three columns, one for each of the three dimensions that are modeled:

$$\mathbf{A} = \begin{bmatrix} 1\,0\,0\,0\,0\,0\,0\,0\,0 \\ 0\,1\,0\,0\,0\,0\,0\,0\,0 \\ 0\,0\,1\,0\,0\,0\,0\,0\,0 \\ 0\,0\,0\,1\,0\,0\,0\,0\,0 \\ 0\,0\,0\,0\,1\,0\,0\,0\,0 \\ 0\,0\,0\,0\,0\,1\,0\,0\,0 \\ 0\,0\,0\,0\,0\,0\,1\,0\,0 \\ 0\,0\,0\,0\,0\,0\,0\,1\,0 \\ 0\,0\,0\,0\,0\,0\,0\,0\,1 \end{bmatrix}, \quad \mathbf{B} = \begin{bmatrix} 1\,0\,0 \\ 1\,0\,0 \\ 1\,0\,0 \\ 0\,1\,0 \\ 0\,1\,0 \\ 0\,1\,0 \\ 0\,0\,1 \\ 0\,0\,1 \\ 0\,0\,1 \end{bmatrix}, \quad \text{and} \quad \xi = \begin{bmatrix} \delta_1 \\ \delta_2 \\ \delta_3 \\ \delta_4 \\ \delta_5 \\ \delta_6 \\ \delta_7 \\ \delta_8 \\ \delta_9 \end{bmatrix}, \quad (4.11)$$

$$\mathbf{A} = \begin{bmatrix} 1\,0\,0\,0\,0\,0\,0\,0\,0 \\ 0\,1\,0\,0\,0\,0\,0\,0\,0 \\ 0\,0\,1\,0\,0\,0\,0\,0\,0 \\ 0\,0\,0\,1\,0\,0\,0\,0\,0 \\ 0\,0\,0\,0\,1\,0\,0\,0\,0 \\ 0\,0\,0\,0\,0\,1\,0\,0\,0 \\ 0\,0\,0\,0\,0\,0\,1\,0\,0 \\ 0\,0\,0\,0\,0\,0\,0\,1\,0 \\ 0\,0\,0\,0\,0\,0\,0\,0\,1 \end{bmatrix}, \quad \mathbf{B} = \begin{bmatrix} 1\,0\,0 \\ 1\,1\,0 \\ 1\,0\,1 \\ 1\,1\,0 \\ 0\,1\,0 \\ 0\,1\,0 \\ 1\,1\,1 \\ 0\,0\,1 \\ 0\,0\,1 \end{bmatrix}, \quad \text{and} \quad \xi = \begin{bmatrix} \delta_1 \\ \delta_2 \\ \delta_3 \\ \delta_4 \\ \delta_5 \\ \delta_6 \\ \delta_7 \\ \delta_8 \\ \delta_9 \end{bmatrix}. \quad (4.12)$$

4.2.5 The Population Model

The item response model (4.2) is a conditional model, in the sense that it describes the process of generating item responses conditional on the latent variable, $\boldsymbol{\theta}$. The complete definition of the model, therefore, requires the specification of a density, $f_{\boldsymbol{\theta}}(\boldsymbol{\theta};\boldsymbol{\alpha})$, for the latent variable, $\boldsymbol{\theta}$. Let $\boldsymbol{\alpha}$ symbolize a set of parameters that characterize the distribution of θ. The most common practice in specifying unidimensional marginal item response models is to assume that students have been sampled from a normal population with mean μ and variance σ^2. That is,

$$f_{\theta}(\theta;\alpha) \equiv f_{\theta}(\theta;\mu,\sigma^2) = (2\pi\sigma^2)^{-\frac{1}{2}} \exp\left[-\frac{(\theta-\mu)^2}{2\sigma^2}\right], \quad (4.13)$$

or equivalently $\theta = \mu + E$, where $E \sim N(0,\sigma^2)$.

Adams, Wilson, & Wu (1997) discuss how a natural extension of (4.13) is to replace the mean, μ, with the regression model, $\mathbf{Y}_n^T \beta$ where $\mathbf{Y}_n$ is a vector of u fixed and known values for student n, and β is the corresponding vector of regression coefficients. For example, $\mathbf{Y}_n$ could be constituted of student variables such as gender or socioeconomic status. Then the population model for student n becomes,

$$\boldsymbol{\theta}_n = \mathbf{Y}_n^T \beta + E_n, \tag{4.14}$$

where the E_n are assumed to be independently and identically normally distributed with mean zero and variance σ^2, so that (4.13) can be generalized to

$$f_{\boldsymbol{\theta}}\left(\boldsymbol{\theta}_n; \mathbf{Y}_n, \beta, \sigma^2\right) = \left(2\pi\sigma^2\right)^{-\frac{1}{2}} \exp\left[-\frac{1}{2\sigma^2}\left(\boldsymbol{\theta}_n - \mathbf{Y}_n^T\beta\right)^T\left(\boldsymbol{\theta}_n - \mathbf{Y}_n^T\beta\right)\right], \tag{4.15}$$

a normal distribution with mean $\mathbf{Y}_n^T\beta$ and variance σ^2. The generalization needs to be taken one step further to apply it to the vector-valued $\boldsymbol{\theta}$ (of length d) rather than the scalar-valued $\boldsymbol{\theta}$. The extension results in the multivariate population model

$$f_{\boldsymbol{\theta}}\left(\boldsymbol{\theta}_n; \mathbf{W}_n, \gamma, \Sigma\right) = (2\pi)^{-\frac{d}{2}} |\Sigma|^{-\frac{1}{2}} \tag{4.16}$$
$$\exp\left[-\frac{1}{2}\left(\boldsymbol{\theta}_n - \gamma\mathbf{W}_n\right)^T \Sigma^{-1}\left(\boldsymbol{\theta}_n - \gamma\mathbf{W}_n\right)\right],$$

where γ is a $d \times u$ matrix of regression coefficients, a $d \times d$ variance–covariance matrix Σ, and $\mathbf{W}_n$ is a $u \times 1$ vector of fixed variables.

While in most cases, the multivariate normal distribution (4.16) is assumed as the population distribution, other forms of the population distribution can also be considered. For example, Adams, Wilson, & Wang (1997) considered a step distribution defined on a prespecified set of nodes. They argued that this could be used as an opportunity to approximate an arbitrary continuous-trait distribution.

4.2.6 Combined Model

The conditional item response model (4.2) and the population model (4.16) are combined to obtain the unconditional, or marginal, item response model:

$$f_{\mathrm{x}}\left(\mathbf{x}; \xi, \gamma, \Sigma\right) = \int_{\theta} f_{\mathrm{x}}\left(\mathbf{x}; \xi | \theta\right)\, f_{\theta}\left(\theta; \gamma, \Sigma\right)\, d\theta. \tag{4.17}$$

It is important to recognize that under this model, the locations of individuals on the latent variables are not estimated. The parameters of the model are γ, Σ, and ξ, where γ, Σ are the population parameters and ξ are the item parameters.

4.3 Identification

For the purposes of the identification of (4.17), certain constraints must be placed on the design matrices $\mathbf{A}$ and $\mathbf{B}$.[2] Volodin & Adams (1995) show that the following are necessary and sufficient conditions for the identification of (4.17).

Proposition One: If D is the number of latent dimensions, P is the length of the parameter vector ξ, $K_i + 1$ is the number of response categories for item i, and $K = \sum_{i \in \mathbf{I}} K_i$, then model (4.17), if applied to the set of items $\mathbf{I}$, can be identified only if $P + D \leqslant K$.

Proposition Two: If D is the number of latent dimensions and P is the length of the parameter vector ξ, then model (4.17) can only be identified if $\text{rank}(\mathbf{A}) = P$, $\text{rank}(\mathbf{B}) = D$ and $\text{rank}([\mathbf{B}\mathbf{A}]) = P + D$.

Proposition Three: If D is the number of latent dimensions, P is the length of the parameter vector ξ, $K_i + 1$ is the number of response categories for item i, and $K = \sum_{i \in \mathbf{I}} K_i$, then model (4.17), if applied to the set of items I, can be identified only if and only if $\text{rank}([\mathbf{B}\mathbf{A}]) = P + D \leqslant K$.

4.4 Estimation

In the following section, a maximum likelihood approach to estimating the parameters is sketched (Adams, Wilson, & Wu, 1997), and the possibility of using a conditional maximum likelihood (Andersen, 1970) approach is discussed.

4.4.1 Maximum Likelihood

The maximum likelihood approach to estimating the parameters of (4.17) proceeds as follows. Let $\mathbf{x}_n$ be the response pattern of person n and assume independent observations are made for $n = 1, \ldots, N$ persons.[3] It follows that the likelihood for the N sampled students is

$$\Lambda = \prod_{n=1}^{N} f_{\mathbf{x}}(\mathbf{x}_n; \xi, \gamma, \Sigma). \tag{4.18}$$

Differentiating with respect to each of the parameters and defining the marginal posterior as

$$h_\theta(\theta_n; \mathbf{W}_n, \xi, \gamma, \Sigma | \mathbf{x}_n) = \frac{f_{\mathbf{x}}(\mathbf{x}_n; \xi | \theta_n) \; f_\theta(\theta_n; \mathbf{W}_n, \gamma, \Sigma)}{f_{\mathbf{x}}(\mathbf{x}_n; \mathbf{W}_n, \xi, \gamma, \Sigma)}, \tag{4.19}$$

---

[2] In fact, the design matrices as used in the examples do not yield identified models.

[3] For notational convenience, the symbol $\boldsymbol{x}_n$ is used here to denote the full response pattern for person n, and not just the response vector for a particular item as defined in (4.1).

the following system of likelihood equations is derived (see Adams, Wilson, & Wu, 1997):

$$\mathbf{A^T} \sum_{n=1}^{N} \left[\mathbf{x}_n - \int_{\theta_n} E_{\mathbf{z}} (\mathbf{z}|\theta_n) \, h_\theta (\theta_n; \mathbf{Y}_n, \xi, \gamma, \Sigma | \mathbf{x}_n) \, d\theta_n \right] = 0, \qquad (4.20)$$

$$\hat{\gamma} = \left(\sum_{n=1}^{N} \overline{\theta_n} \mathbf{W}_n^T \right) \left(\sum_{n=1}^{N} \mathbf{W}_n \mathbf{W}_n^T \right)^{-1}, \qquad (4.21)$$

$$\hat{\Sigma} = \frac{1}{N} \sum_{n=1}^{N} \int_{\theta_n} (\theta_n - \gamma \mathbf{W}_n)(\theta_n - \gamma \mathbf{W}_n)^T h_\theta (\theta_n; \mathbf{Y}_n, \xi, \gamma, \Sigma | \mathbf{x}_n) d\theta_n, \quad (4.22)$$

where

$$E_{\mathbf{z}} (\mathbf{z}|\theta_n) = \Psi (\theta_n, \xi) \sum_{\mathbf{z} \in \Omega} \mathbf{z} \exp \left[\mathbf{z}^T (\mathbf{b}\theta_n + \mathbf{A}\xi) \right] \qquad (4.23)$$

and

$$\bar{\theta}_n = \int_{\theta_n} \theta_n h_\theta (\theta_n; \mathbf{Y}_n, \xi, \gamma, \Sigma | \mathbf{x}_n) \, d\theta_n. \qquad (4.24)$$

The system of equations is solved using an EM algorithm (Dempster et al., 1977) following the approach of Bock & Aitkin (1981).

Quadrature and Monte Carlo Approximations

The integrals in (4.20) to (4.24) are approximated numerically using either quadrature or Monte Carlo methods. Each case proceeds by defining (Θ_q), $q = 1, \ldots, Q$, a set of Q D-dimensional vectors (referred to as nodes), and for each node defining a corresponding weight $(W_q(\gamma, \Sigma))$. The vector response probability (4.17) is then approximated using

$$f_{\mathbf{x}} (\mathbf{x}; \xi, \gamma, \Sigma) = \sum_{p=1}^{Q} f_{\mathbf{x}} (\mathbf{x}; \xi | \Theta_p) \, W_p (\gamma, \Sigma), \qquad (4.25)$$

and the marginal posterior (4.18) is approximated using

$$h_\Theta (\Theta_q; \mathbf{W}_n, \xi, \gamma, \Sigma | \mathbf{x}_n) = \frac{f_{\mathbf{x}} (\mathbf{x}_n; \xi | \Theta_q) \, W_q (\gamma, \Sigma)}{\sum\limits_{p=1}^{Q} f_{\mathbf{x}} (\mathbf{x}_n; \xi | \Theta_p) \, W_p (\gamma, \Sigma)} \qquad (4.26)$$

for $q=1,\ldots,Q$.

The EM algorithm then proceeds as follows:

Step 1. Prepare a set of nodes and weights depending upon $\gamma^{(t)}$ and $\Sigma^{(t)}$, which are the estimates of γ and Σ at iteration t.

Step 2. Calculate the discrete approximation of the marginal posterior density of θ_n, given $\mathbf{x}_n$ at iteration t, using

$$h_\Theta\left(\Theta_q; \mathbf{W}_n, \xi^{(t)}, \gamma^{(t)}, \Sigma^{(t)}|\mathbf{x}_n\right) = \frac{f_\mathbf{x}\left(\mathbf{x}_n; \xi^{(t)}|\Theta_q\right) W_q\left(\gamma^{(t)}, \Sigma^{(t)}\right)}{\sum\limits_{p=1}^{Q} f_\mathbf{x}\left(\mathbf{x}_n; \xi^{(t)}|\Theta_p\right) W_p\left(\gamma^{(t)}, \Sigma^{(t)}\right)},$$

(4.27)

where $\xi^{(t)}$, $\gamma^{(t)}$, and $\Sigma^{(t)}$ are estimates of $\xi^{(t)}$, $\gamma^{(t)}$, and $\Sigma^{(t)}$ at iteration t.

Step 3. Use the Newton–Raphson method to solve the following to produce estimates of $\hat{\xi}^{(t+1)}$:

$$\mathbf{A}' \sum_{n=1}^{N}\left[\mathbf{x}_n - \sum_{r=1}^{Q} E_\mathbf{z}\left(\mathbf{z}|\Theta_r\right) h_\Theta\left(\Theta_r; \mathbf{W}_n, \xi^{(t)}, \gamma^{(t)}, \Sigma^{(t)}|\mathbf{x}_n\right)\right] = \mathbf{0}\,. \quad (4.28)$$

Step 4. Estimate $\gamma^{(t+1)}$ and $\Sigma^{(t+1)}$, using

$$\hat{\gamma}^{(t+1)} = \left(\sum_{n=1}^{N} \overline{\Theta_n} \mathbf{W}_n^T\right)\left(\sum_{n=1}^{N} \mathbf{W}_n \mathbf{W}_n^T\right)^{-1} \quad (4.29)$$

and

$$\hat{\Sigma}^{(t+1)} = \frac{1}{N} \sum_{n=1}^{N} \sum_{r=1}^{Q}\left(\Theta_r - \gamma^{(t+1)} \mathbf{W}_n\right)$$

$$\left(\Theta_r - \gamma^{(t+1)} \mathbf{W}_n\right)^T h_\Theta\left(\Theta_r; \mathbf{Y}_n, \xi^{(t)}, \gamma^{(t)}, \Sigma^{(t)}|\mathbf{x}_n\right), \quad (4.30)$$

where

$$\bar{\Theta}_n = \sum_{r=1}^{Q} \Theta_r\, h_\Theta\left(\Theta_r; \mathbf{W}_n, \xi^{(t)}, \gamma^{(t)}, \Sigma^{(t)}|\mathbf{x}_n\right)\,. \quad (4.31)$$

Step 5. Return to step 1.

The difference between the quadrature and Monte Carlo methods lies in the way the nodes and weights are prepared. For the quadrature case, begin by choosing a fixed set of Q points, $(Q_{d1}, Q_{d2}, \ldots, Q_{dQ})$, for each latent dimension d and then define a set of Q^D nodes that are indexed $r = 1, \ldots, Q^D$ and are given by the Cartesian coordinates

$$Q_r = (Q_{1j_1}, Q_{2j_2}, \ldots, Q_{dj_d}) \text{ with } j_1 = 1, \ldots, Q; j_2 = 1, \ldots, Q; \ldots; j_d = 1, \ldots, Q.$$

The weights are then chosen to approximate the continuous multivariate latent population density (4.16). That is,

$$W_r = K \left(2\pi\right)^{-d/2} |\Sigma|^{-1/2} \exp\left[-\frac{1}{2}\left(\Theta_r - \gamma \mathbf{W}_n\right)' \Sigma^{-1} \left(\Theta_r - \gamma \mathbf{W}_n\right)\right] , \quad (4.32)$$

where K is a scaling factor to ensure that the sum of the weights is 1.

In the Monte Carlo case, the nodes are drawn at random from the standard multivariate normal distribution; and at each iteration, the nodes are rotated, using standard methods, so that they become random draws from a multivariate normal distribution with mean $\gamma \mathbf{W}_n$ and covariance Σ. In the Monte Carlo case, the weight for all nodes is $1/Q$.

For further information on the quadrature approach to estimating the model, see Adams, Wilson, & Wang (1997); and for further information on the Monte Carlo estimation method, see Volodin & Adams (1995).

4.4.2 Conditional Maximum Likelihood

The first step in the derivation of the conditional maximum likelihood (CML) estimators is to compute the probability of a response pattern conditional on that pattern yielding a specific score. More formally, let $\mathbf{R}$ be a vector-valued random variable that is the vector of scores of a response pattern. Then a realization of this variable is $\mathbf{r} = \mathbf{x}^T \mathbf{B}$, where $\mathbf{x}^T$ and $\mathbf{B}$ are as defined in (4.2), and the probability of a response pattern conditional on $\mathbf{R}$ taking the value $\mathbf{r}$ is given by

$$
\begin{aligned}
f\left(\mathbf{x}; \xi, \gamma, \Sigma | \mathbf{R} = \mathbf{r}\right) &= \frac{f\left(\mathbf{x}; \xi, \gamma, \Sigma, \mathbf{R} = \mathbf{r}\right)}{\sum_{\mathbf{z} \in \Omega_r} f\left(\mathbf{z}; \xi, \gamma, \Sigma, \mathbf{R} = \mathbf{r}\right)} \\[2mm]
&= \frac{\int f_{\mathbf{x}}\left(\mathbf{x}; \xi, \mathbf{R} = \mathbf{r} | \theta\right) f_\theta\left(\theta; \gamma, \Sigma\right) d\theta}{\sum_{\mathbf{z} \in \Omega_r} \int f_{\mathbf{x}}\left(\mathbf{z}; \xi, \mathbf{R} = \mathbf{r} | \theta\right) f_\theta\left(\theta; \gamma, \Sigma\right) d\theta} \quad (4.33) \\[2mm]
&= \frac{\int \Psi\left(\theta, \xi\right) \exp\left(\mathbf{r}\theta + \mathbf{x}^T \mathbf{A}\xi\right) f_\theta\left(\theta; \gamma, \Sigma\right) d\theta}{\sum_{\mathbf{z} \in \Omega_r} \int \Psi\left(\theta, \xi\right) \exp\left(\mathbf{r}\theta + \mathbf{z}^T \mathbf{A}\xi\right) f_\theta\left(\theta; \gamma, \Sigma\right) d\theta} \\[2mm]
&= \frac{\exp\left(\mathbf{x}^T \mathbf{A}\xi\right) \int \Psi\left(\theta, \xi\right) \exp\left(\mathbf{r}\theta\right) f_\theta\left(\theta; \gamma, \Sigma\right) d\theta}{\sum_{\mathbf{z} \in \Omega_r} \exp\left(\mathbf{z}^T \mathbf{A}\xi\right) \int \Psi\left(\theta, \xi\right) \exp\left(\mathbf{r}\theta\right) f_\theta\left(\theta; \gamma, \Sigma\right) d\theta} \\[2mm]
&= \frac{\exp\left(\mathbf{x}^T \mathbf{A}\xi\right)}{\sum_{\mathbf{z} \in \Omega_r} \exp\left(\mathbf{z}^T \mathbf{A}\xi\right)},
\end{aligned}
$$

where Ω_r is the set of response patterns where the vector of scores is $\mathbf{r}$.

Equation (4.33) shows that the probability of a response pattern conditional on $\mathbf{R}$ taking the value $\mathbf{r}$ is not dependent on the ability θ or its distribution. The consequential advantage of the CML approach is that it provides the same estimates for the item parameters regardless of the choice of the population distribution. As such, the CML item parameter estimator is not influenced by any assumption about the population distribution. The disadvantage is that the population parameters are not estimated. If, as is often the case, the population parameters are of interest, they must be estimated in a second step. The second step involves solving the system of equations (4.21) and (4.22) while assuming that the item parameters are known. Apart from underestimating the uncertainty in the population parameter estimates, the consequences of using the CML item-parameter estimates, in this second step, as if they were true values, are not clear.

In contrast, the maximum likelihood approach provides direct estimates of both item parameters and population parameters. However, it suffers from the risk that if the population distributional assumption is incorrect, the item parameters may be biased.

4.4.3 Estimating Standard Errors

Asymptotic standard errors for the parameter estimates are estimated using the observed Fisher's information. For the unidimensional case, a derivation of the formulae for the observed information is provided in Adams, Wilson, & Wu (1997).

The estimation of asymptotic standard errors using the observed information can be very time-consuming. The matrix that is computed is of dimension $p + r + 2$, where p is the number of item parameters and r is the number of regression variables; and the computation of each element requires integration over the posterior distribution of each case. The time taken is therefore quadratic in the number of parameters and linear in the number of cases and nodes. Because the estimation of these errors can take considerable time, the following approximations for the error variances are often used:

$$
\operatorname{var}\left(\hat{\xi}_i\right) = \sum_{n=1}^{N} \left\{ \operatorname{diag}\left[\mathbf{A}' \left(\int_{\theta_n} E_{\mathbf{z}}\left(\mathbf{z}\mathbf{z}'|\theta_n\right) h_\theta\left(\theta_n; \mathbf{Y}_n, \hat{\xi}, \hat{\beta}, \hat{\sigma}^2 | \mathbf{x}_n\right) d\theta_n \right.\right.\right.
$$

$$
\left.\left.\left. - \int_{\theta_n} E_{\mathbf{z}}\left(\mathbf{z}|\theta_n\right) E_{\mathbf{z}}\left(\mathbf{z}'|\theta_n\right) h_\theta\left(\theta_n; \mathbf{Y}_n, \hat{\xi}, \hat{\beta}, \hat{\sigma}^2 | \mathbf{x}_n\right) d\theta_n \right) \mathbf{A} \right]^{-1} \right\},
$$

$$
\tag{4.34}
$$

$$
\operatorname{var}\left(\hat{\beta}_i\right) = \hat{\sigma}^2 \left(\sum_{n=1}^{N} \mathbf{Y}_n \mathbf{Y}_n^T \right)^{-1}, \tag{4.35}
$$

$$\text{var}\left(\hat{\sigma}^2\right) = \frac{2\hat{\sigma}^4}{N}. \tag{4.36}$$

These approximations ignore all of the covariances in the parameter estimates. The approximations of the item parameters will generally underestimate the sampling error, particularly for parameters associated with facets that have few levels for the step parameters in multicategory items. The accuracy of (4.35) and (4.36) depends on the magnitude of the measurement error, since it is reflected in the variances of the individual's posterior distributions.

4.4.4 Latent Ability Estimation and Prediction

The marginal item response model (4.17) does not include parameters for the latent values θ_n; and hence the estimation algorithm does not result in estimates of the latent values for persons. While this may not be of concern when the modeling is undertaken for the purposes of estimating population parameters, that is, the elements of γ and Σ, it does cause inconveniences when there is an interest in estimates of the latent values for individuals.

There are a number of standard approaches that can be applied to provide estimates, or perhaps, more accurately, predictions, of the latent values. Perhaps the most common approach is to use expectation of the posterior distribution of θ_n, the so-called expected a posteriori (EAP) (Bock & Aitkin, 1981). The EAP prediction of the latent quantity for case n is

$$\theta_n^{EAP} = \sum_{r=1}^{Q} \Theta_r \, h_\Theta\left(\Theta_r; \mathbf{W}_n, \hat{\xi}, \hat{\gamma}, \hat{\Sigma} | \mathbf{x}_n\right). \tag{4.37}$$

Variance estimates for these predictions can be estimated using

$$\text{var}\left(\theta_n^{EAP}\right) = \sum_{r=1}^{Q} \left(\Theta_r - \theta_n^{EAP}\right) \left(\Theta_r - \theta_n^{EAP}\right)' h_\Theta\left(\Theta_r; \mathbf{W}_n, \hat{\xi}, \hat{\gamma}, \hat{\Sigma} | \mathbf{x}_n\right). \tag{4.38}$$

An alternative to the EAP is the maximum a posteriori (MAP) (Bock & Aitkin, 1981), which requires finding the modes, rather than the expectations (means), of the posterior distributions.

A maximum likelihood approach to the estimation of the ability estimates can also be used. Following the weighted likelihood approach of Warm (1985, 1989), this is achieved by solving the equations

$$\sum_{i \in \Omega} \left(\left(\mathbf{b}_{ix_{ni}} + \frac{J_{ni}}{2I_{ni}} \right) - \sum_{j=1}^{K_i} \frac{\mathbf{b}_{ij} \exp\left(\mathbf{b}_{ij}\theta_n + \mathbf{a}'_{ij}\hat{\xi}\right)}{\sum\limits_{k=1}^{K_i} \exp\left(\mathbf{b}_{ik}\theta_n + \mathbf{a}'_{ik}\hat{\xi}\right)} \right) = 0 \tag{4.39}$$

for each case, where $\hat{\xi}$ is the vector of item parameter estimates, I_{ni} is the information function evaluated for item i, and J_{ni} is the derivative of I_{ni} with respect to θ_n. These equations can be readily solved using a routine based on the Newton–Raphson method.

Drawing Plausible Values

The model presented in (4.17) provides estimates of the γ and Σ parameters of the population, but of course there are many other characteristics of the population that may be of interest. In most measurement applications, these parameters would be estimated from point estimates of the θ_n parameters. It is well known, however, that the use of point *estimates* such as the EAP, MLE, and WLE in a two-step approach to estimating population parameters is fraught with challenges.

As an alternative to using point estimates, Mislevy (see Mislevy, 1991, and Mislevy, Beaton, et al., 1992) proposed an approach based on the use of random draws from the marginal posterior, (4.19), for each student. These random draws have become widely known as plausible values.

The following describes a method for drawing plausible values from the posterior distributions. Unlike previously described methods for drawing plausible values (Beaton, 1987; Mislevy, Beaton, et al., 1992), the method described here does not assume normality of the marginal posterior distributions. Recall from (4.19) that the marginal posterior is given by

$$h_\theta\left(\theta_n; \mathbf{W}_n, \xi, \gamma, \Sigma | \mathbf{x}_n\right) = \frac{f_{\mathbf{x}}\left(\mathbf{x}_n; \xi | \theta_n\right) \, f_\theta\left(\theta_n; \mathbf{W}_n, \gamma, \Sigma\right)}{\int\limits_\theta f_{\mathbf{x}}\left(\mathbf{x}; \xi | \theta\right) \, f_\theta\left(\theta; \mathbf{W}_n, \gamma, \Sigma\right) d\theta}. \tag{4.40}$$

First draw M vector-valued random deviates, $\{j_{mn}\}_{m=1}^{M}$, from the multivariate normal distribution, $f_\theta\left(\theta_n; \mathbf{W}_n, \gamma, \Sigma\right)$, for each case n. These vectors are used to compute an approximation to the integral in the denominator of (4.40), using the Monte Carlo integration

$$\int\limits_\theta f_{\mathbf{x}}\left(\mathbf{x}; \xi | \theta\right) f_\theta\left(\theta, ; \mathbf{W}_n, \gamma, \Sigma\right) d\theta \approx \frac{1}{M} \sum_{m=1}^{M} f_{\mathbf{x}}(\mathbf{x}; \xi | \varphi_{mn}) \equiv \Im. \tag{4.41}$$

At the same time, the values

$$p_{mn} = f_{\mathbf{x}}\left(\mathbf{x}_n; \xi | \varphi_{mn}\right) \; f_\theta\left(\varphi_{mn}; \mathbf{W}_n, \gamma, \Sigma\right) \tag{4.42}$$

are calculated, and the set of pairs $(\varphi_{mn}, \; {p_{mn}}/{\Im})_{m=1}^{M}$ is obtained. This set of pairs can be used as an approximation of the posterior density (4.34); and the probability that φ_{nj} could be drawn from this density is given by

$$q_{nj} \quad = \quad \frac{p_{mn}}{\sum\limits_{m=1}^{M} p_{mn}}. \tag{4.43}$$

At this point, L uniformly distributed random numbers, $\{\eta_i\}_{i=1}^{L}$, are generated and for each random draw, the vector, φ_{ni_0}, that satisfies the condition

$$\sum_{s=1}^{i_0-1} q_{sn} < \eta_i \leqslant \sum_{s=1}^{i_0} q_{sn} \qquad (4.44)$$

is selected as a plausible vector.

4.5 Generalized Fit Test

A convenient way to assess the fit of the model is to follow the residual-based approach of Wright & Stone (1979) and Wright & Masters (1982). Wu (1997) extended this approach for application with the marginal model used here, and more recently Adams & Wu (2004) generalized the approach so that a range of tests of specific hypotheses could be tested.

If $\mathbf{A}_p$ is used to indicate the pth column of the design matrix $\mathbf{A}$, the Wu fit statistic is based on the standardized residual

$$z_{np}(\theta_n) = \left(\mathbf{A}_p^T \mathbf{x}_n - E_{np}\right) \big/ \sqrt{V_{np}}, \qquad (4.45)$$

where $\mathbf{A}_p^T \mathbf{x}_n$ is the contribution of person n to the sufficient statistic for parameter p, and E_{np} and V_{np} are, respectively, the conditional expectation and the variance of $\mathbf{A}_p^T \mathbf{x}_n$.

To construct an unweighted fit statistic,[4] the square of this residual is averaged over the cases and then integrated over the posterior ability distributions to obtain

$$Fit_{out,p} = \int_{\theta_1} \int_{\theta_2} \cdots \int_{\theta_N} \left[\frac{1}{N} \sum_{n=1}^{N} \hat{z}_{np}^2(\theta_n) \right]$$

$$\prod_{n=1}^{N} h_\theta \left(\theta_n; \mathbf{Y}_n, \hat{x}, \hat{b}, \hat{\sigma}^2 | \mathbf{x}_n \right) d\theta_N d\theta_{N-1} \cdots d\theta_1. \qquad (4.46)$$

For the weighted fit,[5] a weighted average of the squared residuals is used as follows:

$$Fit_{in,p} = \int_{\theta_1} \int_{\theta_2} \cdots \int_{\theta_N} \left[\frac{\sum_{n=1}^{N} \hat{z}_{np}^2(\theta_n) V_{np}(\theta_n)}{\sum_{n=1}^{N} V_{np}(\theta_n)} \right]$$

$$\prod_{n=1}^{N} h_\theta \left(\theta_n; \mathbf{Y}_n, \hat{\xi}, \hat{\beta}, \hat{\sigma}^2 | \mathbf{x}_n \right) d\theta_N d\theta_{N-1} \cdots d\theta_1. \qquad (4.47)$$

---

[4] Often referred to as *outfit*.
[5] Often referred to as *infit*.

It is convenient to use the Monte Carlo method to approximate the integrals in (4.46) and (4.47). Wu (1997) has shown that the statistics produced by (4.46) and (4.47) have approximate scaled chi-squared distributions. These statistics are transformed to approximate normal deviates using the Wilson–Hilferty transformations

$$t_{\mathrm{out},p} = \left(Fit_{\mathrm{out},p}^{1/3} - 1 + 2/(9rN) \right) \Big/ (2/(9rN))^{1/2} \qquad (4.48)$$

and

$$t_{\mathrm{in},p} = \left[Fit_{\mathrm{in},p}^{1/3} - 1 \right] \times \frac{3}{\sqrt{\mathrm{Var}\,(\mathrm{Fit}_{in,p})}} + \frac{\sqrt{\mathrm{Var}\,(\mathrm{Fit}_{in,p})}}{3}, \qquad (4.49)$$

where r is the number of draws used in the Monte Carlo approximation of the integrals in (4.40) and (4.41) and

$$\mathrm{Var}(\mathrm{Fit}_i n, p) = \left(\frac{1}{\sum_n V_{np}} \right)^2 \left(\sum_n \left(E\left((\mathbf{A}_p^T \mathbf{X}_n - E_{np})^4 \right) - V_{np}^2 \right) \right). \qquad (4.50)$$

The derivation and justification for these transformations is given in Wu (1997).

The fit-testing approach described here works at the parameter level; that is, it provides a fit statistic for each of the estimated item parameters. A more general approach was introduced by Adams & Wu (2004), who suggested that the matrix $\mathbf{A}$ that is used in (4.39) could be replaced with an alternative matrix, $\mathbf{F}$ which they called a fit matrix.

Since the derivation of the fit statistics described in the previous section is based on the comparison of a linear combination of item responses, $\mathbf{A}_p^T \mathbf{x}_n$, and its expectation and variance, the fit statistics can be generalized to include any linear combinations of the item responses, and not necessarily be limited to $\mathbf{A}_p^T \mathbf{x}_n$, where $\mathbf{A}_p$ is the design vector for the parameter ξ_p. If $\mathbf{F}_u$ is any vector of the same length as $\mathbf{A}_p$, then $\mathbf{F}_u^T \mathbf{x}_n$ is a linear combination of the item responses of person n. One can compute the expectation and variance of $\mathbf{F}_u^T \mathbf{x}_n$, and construct a fit statistic in exactly the same way as for $\mathbf{A}_p^T \mathbf{x}_n$. The following is an example for constructing user-defined fit tests for a simple dichotomous RM.

Consider a test consisting of 10 dichotomous items; the design matrix, $\mathbf{A}$, for the simple logistic model for such a test would be a 10 by 10 identity matrix.

Using the notation defined earlier, the first column of $\mathbf{A}$ is $\mathbf{A}_1^T = \left(1\,0\,0\,0\,0\,0\,0\,0\,0\,0 \right)$. The product $\mathbf{A}_1^T \mathbf{x}_n$ gives the item response of person n on item 1. This is the contribution of person n to the sufficient statistic for the first item parameter.

Similarly, $\mathbf{A}_2^T = \left(0\,1\,0\,0\,0\,0\,0\,0\,0\,0 \right)$, and $\mathbf{A}_2^T \mathbf{x}_n$ is the contribution of person n to the sufficient statistic for the second item parameter, and so on.

For a user-defined fit test, the design vector $\mathbf{A}_p$ can be replaced by any arbitrary vector $\mathbf{F}_u$. Consider the fit design matrix

$$
\mathbf{F} = \begin{bmatrix} 1 & 0 \\ 1 & 0 \\ 1 & 0 \\ 1 & 0 \\ 1 & 0 \\ 0 & 1 \\ 0 & 1 \\ 0 & 1 \\ 0 & 1 \\ 0 & 1 \end{bmatrix}. \tag{4.51}
$$

If $\mathbf{F}_1$ and $\mathbf{F}_2$ are the first and second columns of $\mathbf{F}$, then the product $\mathbf{F}_1^T \mathbf{x}_n$ gives the total score on the first five items for person n. Similarly, $\mathbf{F}_2^T \mathbf{x}_n$ gives the total score on the last five items for person n.

Adams & Wu (2004) showed how the fit statistics based on $\mathbf{F}_1$ and $\mathbf{F}_2$ worked well as a test of the hypothesis that the first and second five items were tapping into two different latent dimensions, whereas the fit tests given in (4.46) and (4.47) failed to identify the multidimensionality of the test items.

As a second possible set of fit tests, consider the matrix in (4.52). A fit test based on the first column of this matrix tests whether items one and six are both answered correctly as often as would be expected under the model. Similarly, the second column provides a test of whether items two and seven are both answered correctly as often as would be expected under the model. As such, these are tests of the local independence of items one and six, and two and seven respectively.

The third column compares the score on the first five items with its expectation, that is, whether the subtest consisting of the first five items fits with the rest of the items as predicted by the model:

$$
\mathbf{F} = \begin{bmatrix} 1 & 0 & 1 \\ 0 & 1 & 1 \\ 0 & 0 & 1 \\ 0 & 0 & 1 \\ 0 & 0 & 1 \\ 1 & 0 & 0 \\ 0 & 1 & 0 \\ 0 & 0 & 0 \\ 0 & 0 & 0 \\ 0 & 0 & 0 \end{bmatrix}. \tag{4.52}
$$

4.6 Conclusion

This paper has demonstrated the flexibility of using design matrices to specify a family of item response models. Not only can standard item response models such as the partial-credit, the rating-scale, and the facets models be included under one single framework of models, but many other models can be specified through user-defined design matrices.

The estimation procedures described in this paper allow for a joint (or one-step) calibration of both item parameters and population parameters, as opposed to a two-step process in which individual student abilities are first estimated and then aggregated to form population parameter estimates. The advantages of a joint calibration of parameters include more accurate standard errors for the estimates of the population parameters and less bias of some population parameter estimates.

Similarly, user-defined fit-design matrices allow for more focused testing of goodness-of-fit of the data to the model. In many cases, such focused fit tests are statistically more powerful in detecting misfit in the data.

However, the theoretical elegance of the use of design matrices can be overshadowed by the tediousness of the construction of these matrices in practice. A software package, ConQuest (Wu et al., 1997), has been developed in which users can specify various item response models through a command language. The design matrices are then automatically built by ConQuest. ConQuest also allows users to import a design matrix should the need arise. Thus the advantages of a unified framework of item response models can be easily implemented in practice for the analysis of a vast range of data sets.

5

Loglinear Multivariate and Mixture Rasch Models

Henk Kelderman

Vrije Universiteit Amsterdam

5.1 Introduction

In this chapter, Rasch models (RMs) are derived from a stochastic subject model. Fixed-effects RMs are shown to be equivalent to loglinear models with raw-score variables; random-effects RMs are equivalent to loglinear models with latent class variables. Within the larger framework of loglinear models, various extensions of the RM can be formulated. We discuss loglinear RMs for polytomous items, loglinear multidimensional RMs, RMs violating measurement invariance, mixture-distribution RMs, mixture-measurement RMs, RMs in which item responses are conditionally dependent, and RMs with latent responses. We also give some software scripts to compute ML estimates and fit statistics.

In the early eighties, Mellenbergh and Vijn Mellenbergh & Vijn (1981) recognized the connection between the Rasch model (RM) and the loglinear model (LLM). They showed that an LLM for the item × raw-score × item response contingency table yields the same model equations as the RM. The model was later shown to yield unconditional maximum likelihood (UML) estimates for the parameters (Blackwood & Bradley, 1989). However, because the cell entries of the table are not independent, the distribution is not multinomial, so that the usual statistical theory does not hold for this model. Kelderman (1984) removed this dependence by specifying a quasi-independence model for the incomplete item response $1 \times \ldots \times$ item response I × raw-score contingency table and showed that this model yields conditional maximum likelihood (CML) estimates if the raw score is considered fixed.

This fixed-effects RM (FERM) can be extended with a multinomial probability distribution for the raw scores. This random-effects-of-raw-scores RM model is known as the *extended* RM (ERM) (Cressie & Holland, 1983; Duncan, 1984; Duncan & Stenbeck, 1987; Tjur, 1982). However, the model is not necessarily consistent with a model with an underlying latent-trait distribution. For the case of the dichotomous RM, Cressie & Holland (1983) and Hout et al. (1987) have shown that they are equivalent if the raw-score distribution satisfies a complex set of inequality constraints on its moments. These constraints are violated if there are gross differences in the probabilities of consecutive raw-score values. So, to be consistent with an underlying latent trait, the raw-score distribution should be smooth.

The FERM is a fixed-effects model and thus in line with Rasch's original intentions to have a model for individual measurement. However, the (F)ERM has the disadvantage that for complicated RMs, the number of fixed raw-score parameters quickly becomes very large. Models in which the latent trait is assumed to follow a parametric distribution, on the other hand, have many fewer parameters to be estimated. For example, a simple fixed-effects (F)ERM for 40 dichotomous items produces 41 raw-score categories with corresponding fixed parameters, whereas a random-effects RM in which the subjects' latent-trait values are assumed to follow a normal distribution has only two parameters: the mean and the variance. Heinen (1993; 1996) formulated such a random-effects RM as an LLM including discrete latent variables (latent classes). In Heinen's models the continuous latent trait variable is approximated by a latent class variable. If this latent variable approximates a normal distribution, Heinen's method is equivalent to the marginal maximum likelihood estimation method (Bock & Aitkin, 1981; Rigdon & Tsutakawa, 1983; Thissen, 1982).

Unfortunately, in test-construction research, random samples from a well-defined population are rare, and it is not always defensible that the sample comes from some synthetic population that follows a normal distribution. One solution to this problem is to specify a nonparametric distribution for the latent trait. As Follmann (1988) and Leeuw & Verhelst (1986) have shown, such a model is asymptotically equivalent to the ERM. Another solution is to specify a normal mixture distribution for the latent trait. See for example Kreiner's chapter in this volume. The methodology developed by Vermunt is flexible enough to deal with these cases as well.

In what follows we review the theory of LLMs and derive fixed-effects and random-effects RMs as LLMs. The models are then generalized and extended. Because the computer programs LOGIMO or LEM contain algorithms that can handle LLMs for real-sized tests, we have limited our discussion to the type of models that can easily be specified within these programs. The examples are rather small, but the scripts we give can, with some slight modifications, be used for longer tests.

5.2 Loglinear Models

Loglinear models (Agresti, 1990) are models for a set H of discrete variables. A single variable $h \in H$ can take possible values $z_h \in M_{Z_h}$. Similarly, a subset $a \subseteq H$ of variables $h \in a$ can take a vector of values $\mathbf{z}_a \in M_{\mathbf{z}_a}$. The vector $\mathbf{z} \in M$ denotes a joint value of all variables in H. Thus, $M = \{\mathbf{z}\}$ defines the full contingency table with cells $\mathbf{z}$.

For example, if $H = \{1, 2, 3\}$ and $a = \{1, 2\}$, we have $\mathbf{z} = (z_1, z_2, z_3)'$ and $\mathbf{z}_a = (z_1, z_2)'$. If z_1, z_2, and z_3 can each take values $1, 2$, we have $M_{Z_1} = M_{Z_2} = M_{Z_3} = \{1, 2\}$, $M_{\mathbf{z}_a} = \{(1, 1), (1, 2), (2, 1), (2, 2)\}$, and $M = \{(1, 1, 1), (1, 1, 2), (1, 2, 1), (1, 2, 2), (2, 1, 1), (2, 1, 2), (2, 2, 1), (2, 2, 2)\}$.

The counts in the cell $\mathbf{z}$ and in marginal cell $\mathbf{z}_a$ are written as $f_{\mathbf{z}}$ and $f_{\mathbf{z}_a}$ respectively. See Table 5.1 for an example. Marginal counts $f_{\mathbf{z}_a}$ can be obtained by summing the counts in the full contingency table over the variables, $b = H \backslash a$, that are not in the marginal table, that is,

$$f_{\mathbf{z}_a} = \sum_{\mathbf{z}_b \in M_{\mathbf{z}_b}} f_{\mathbf{z}_a, \mathbf{z}_b} = \sum_{\mathbf{z}_b} f_{\mathbf{z}}.$$

The variables in H may be random or fixed. Let $P(\mathbf{z}_a \mid \mathbf{z}_b)$ denote the conditional probability that the random variable $\mathbf{Z}_a$ takes the value $\mathbf{z}_a$ given fixed variables $\mathbf{z}_b$. The expected counts under this probability model are denoted by $F_{\mathbf{z}}$, which, from elementary theory of expectations, are equal to

$$F_{\mathbf{z}} = E(f_{\mathbf{z}}) = f_{\mathbf{z}_b} P(\mathbf{z}_a \mid \mathbf{z}_b). \tag{5.1}$$

Loglinear models further parametrize the logarithm of the expected counts as a sum of a set K of model terms k:

$$\log F_{\mathbf{z}} = \sum_{k \in K} q_k(\mathbf{z}) \phi_k, \tag{5.2}$$

where ϕ_k is a model parameter and $q_k(\mathbf{z})$ the corresponding weight. If $q_k(\mathbf{z})$ depends on one or more random variables, it generates a random variable and its corresponding parameter ϕ_k is random; if not, $q_k(\mathbf{z})$ and ϕ_k are considered fixed. "Fixed" parameters correspond to fixed variables but are functions of the random parameters. They ensure that $f_{\mathbf{z}_b} = F_{\mathbf{z}_b}$ in (5.1). It is easily seen that this is the case, because $P(\mathbf{z}_a \mid \mathbf{z}_b)$ sums to one over $\mathbf{z}_a$ for all $\mathbf{z}_b$. Thus, fixed parameters are related to proportionality constants. Let ϕ_r denote the vector of random parameters in $\phi = (\phi_k; k \in K)$.

If the response vectors $\mathbf{z}_a$ are independently drawn given $\mathbf{z}_b$, the probability of the data is equal to the product of the (conditional) probabilities of each of the observed response vectors. The likelihood function L expresses this probability as a function of the parameters $\phi_r = (\phi_k; k \in r)$:

$$L(\phi_r) = \prod_{\mathbf{z}_b \in M_{\mathbf{z}_b}} \frac{f_{\mathbf{z}_b}!}{\prod_{\mathbf{z}_a \in M_{\mathbf{z}_a}} f_{\mathbf{z}_a, \mathbf{z}_b}!} \prod_{\mathbf{z}_a \in M_{\mathbf{z}_a}} P(\mathbf{z}_a \mid \mathbf{z}_b; \phi_r)^{f_{\mathbf{z}_a, \mathbf{z}_b}}.$$

The kernel of the likelihood is that part of the likelihood that depends on the parameters ϕ. Taking the logarithm, this kernel can be written as

$$\ell = \sum_{\mathbf{z} \in M} f_{\mathbf{z}} \log F_{\mathbf{z}} = \sum_{k \in K} \sum_{\mathbf{z} \in M} f_{\mathbf{z}} q_k(\mathbf{z}) \phi_k = \sum_{k \in K} f^{(k)} \phi_k, \tag{5.3}$$

where $f^{(k)} = \sum_{\mathbf{z} \in M} q_k(\mathbf{z}) f_{\mathbf{z}}$. If all variables are observed, the maximum likelihood estimates $\hat{\phi}_r$ of the parameters can be obtained by solving

$$\max_{\phi_r} \ell$$

and computing the fixed parameters $\hat{\phi}_{K \backslash r}$ from $\hat{\phi}_r$. For (5.3), ℓ has a unique maximum, so we can obtain the maximum likelihood estimates at the point where the likelihood neither increases nor decreases, that is, for

$$\frac{\partial \ell}{\partial \phi_r} = 0, \tag{5.4}$$

from which the equations

$$f^{(k)} = F^{(k)}, \quad k \in K, \tag{5.5}$$

can be derived. Solving (5.5) for ϕ yields the maximum likelihood estimates $\hat{\phi}$ of the loglinear parameters. The solution can be obtained with some numerical algorithm such as iterative proportional fitting (IPF; Deming & Stephan, 1940) or the Newton–Raphson (NERA) algorithm or modifications thereof. Note that the estimation equations (5.5) are the same whether the parameters are fixed or random. Therefore, the maximum likelihood estimates of the random parameters are not affected by the probability model. However, it does affect their variances.

The parameter estimates $\hat{\phi}_r$ have an asymptotic normal distribution with mean ϕ_r and covariance matrix equal to the negative expectation of the matrix of second derivatives,

$$-E \left(\frac{\partial^2 \ell}{\partial \phi_r \partial \phi_r^T} \right),$$

of which an estimate can be obtained using $\hat{\phi}_r$ for ϕ_r.

Overall goodness-of-fit tests for this model are the Pearson statistic

$$X^2 = \sum_{\mathbf{z} \in M} \frac{(f_{\mathbf{z}} - \hat{F}_{\mathbf{z}})^2}{\hat{F}_{\mathbf{z}}} \tag{5.6}$$

and the likelihood ratio statistic

$$G^2 = 2 \sum_{\mathbf{z} \in M} f_{\mathbf{z}} \log \frac{f_{\mathbf{z}}}{\hat{F}_{\mathbf{z}}}. \tag{5.7}$$

Both statistics are asymptotically distributed as chi square (χ^2), with degrees of freedom equal to the difference between the number of cells, $\#(M)$, and the number of estimable parameters. The approximation of X^2 and G^2 to χ^2 tends to become bad if one or more $\hat{F}_{\mathbf{z}}$ are close to zero. In that case it is better obtain an estimate of the distribution of the statistic through parametric bootstrapping. That is, the distribution of X^2 and G^2 is obtained by repeatedly drawing data from the probability distribution $\hat{P}(\mathbf{z}_a \mid \mathbf{z}_b)$ of the estimated model.

The likelihood-ratio statistic can be used to compare two models. If one model, say Model a, is a special case of another model, say Model b, Model a can be tested against Model b by the statistic

$$\triangle G^2 = G_a^2 - G_b^2 = -2(\ell_a - \ell_b).$$

Under model b, $\triangle G^2$ converges to the χ^2-distribution if N becomes large.

To compare the fit of two models with the same probability space but where one model is not a special case of the other or the larger model does not fit, the Akaike information criterion (AIC) and the Bayesian information criterion (BIC) are particularly useful. The AIC (Akaike, 1981, 1983) and BIC statistics (Schwarz, 1978) are model-selection criteria that take into account both the model fit and the number of parameters that are used to achieve that fit. The criteria take the form of the penalized likelihood functions

$$AIC = -2\ell + 2 \times \text{npar} \tag{5.8}$$

and

$$BIC = -2\ell + \text{npar} \times \log N, \tag{5.9}$$

where npar denotes the number of independent parameters. The model with the smallest value is chosen as the best-fitting model. The BIC statistic imposes a heavier penalty on the number of parameters than AIC for $\log N > 2$. Consequently, BIC tends to favor more restrictive models. Note that these fit statistics are unaffected by the probability model as the likelihood equations (5.5) are.

5.2.1 Loglinear Models with Nominal Effects

As an example of an LLM with nominal effects, consider three variables, $z_1 = 1, 2, 3$, $z_2 = 1, 2$, and $z_3 = 1, 2$ from $H = \{1, 2, 3\}$, where $\{2, 3\}$ are random and $\{1\}$ is fixed. Define functions l such that

$$z_1 = \begin{cases} 0 & : & l_{z_1}^{(1)} = 0, \quad l_{z_1}^{(2)} = 0, \\ 1 & : & l_{z_1}^{(1)} = 1, \quad l_{z_1}^{(2)} = 0, \\ 2 & : & l_{z_1}^{(1)} = 0, \quad l_{z_1}^{(2)} = 1, \end{cases}$$

$l_{z_2} = z_2 - 1$, and $l_{z_3} = z_3 - 1$. Suppose we have

$$q_1(\mathbf{z}) = 1, \qquad q_2(\mathbf{z}) = l_{z_1}^{(1)}, \qquad q_3(\mathbf{z}) = l_{z_1}^{(2)}, \qquad q_4(\mathbf{z}) = l_{z_2},$$
$$q_5(\mathbf{z}) = l_{z_3}, \qquad q_6(\mathbf{z}) = l_{z_1}^{(1)} l_{z_2}, \qquad q_7(\mathbf{z}) = l_{z_1}^{(2)} l_{z_2},$$
$$q_8(\mathbf{z}) = l_{z_1}^{(1)} l_{z_3}, \qquad q_9(\mathbf{z}) = l_{z_1}^{(2)} l_{z_3},$$

so that (5.2) becomes

$$\log F_{\mathbf{z_1 z_2 l_{z_3}}} = \phi_1 + \phi_2 l_{z_1}^{(1)} + \phi_3 l_{z_1}^{(2)} + \phi_4 l_{z_2} + \phi_5 l_{z_3} + \phi_6 l_{z_1}^{(1)} l_{z_2} \quad (5.10)$$
$$+ \phi_7 l_{z_1}^{(2)} l_{z_2} + \phi_8 l_{z_1}^{(1)} l_{z_3} + \phi_9 l_{z_1}^{(2)} l_{z_3}.$$

Applying (5.3), the log-likelihood of this model becomes

$$\ell = \sum_{k \in K} \sum_{\mathbf{z} \in M} f_{\mathbf{z}} q_k(\mathbf{z}) \phi_k \quad (5.11)$$
$$= \phi_1 N + \phi_2 f_{z_1=2} + \phi_3 f_{z_1=3} + \phi_4 f_{z_2=2} + \phi_5 f_{z_3=2}$$
$$+ \phi_6 f_{z_1=2, z_2=2} + \phi_7 f_{z_1=3, z_2=2} + \phi_8 f_{z_1=2, z_3=2} + \phi_9 f_{z_1=3, z_3=2}$$
$$= \sum_{k \in K} f^{(k)} \phi_k.$$

In (5.11), only ϕ_4 through ϕ_9 are random parameters because only the functions q_4 through q_9 are functions of random variables. Note that the marginal frequency tables $\{f_{z_1 z_2}\}$ and $\{f_{z_1, z_3}\}$ suffice to estimate the parameters. Thus, to estimate an LLM, one does not need to deal with the full table $\{f_{\mathbf{z}}\}$.

If the effects are nominal, it is customary to write model (5.10) as

$$\log F_{\mathbf{z_1 z_2 z_3}} = \lambda + \lambda_{z_1}^{Z_1} + \lambda_{z_2}^{Z_2} + \lambda_{z_3}^{Z_3} + \lambda_{z_1 z_2}^{Z_1 Z_2} + \lambda_{z_1 z_3}^{Z_1 Z_3}, \quad (5.12)$$

where the terms' superscripts denote the variables involved and the subscripts their values. Note that there is an indeterminacy in this model. Adding a constant to one model term and subtracting it from another does not change the model. To remove this indeterminacy the λ parameters are constrained to be zero if one or more of the indices are at their lowest values so that in this case the nonzero parameters of model (5.12) are exactly equal to the ϕ parameters in model (5.10). That is,

$$\phi_1 = \lambda, \quad \phi_2 = \lambda_2^{Z_1}, \quad \phi_3 = \lambda_3^{Z_1}, \quad \phi_4 = \lambda_2^{Z_2},$$

$$\phi_5 = \lambda_2^{Z_3}, \quad \phi_6 = \lambda_{22}^{Z_1 Z_2}, \quad \phi_7 = \lambda_{32}^{Z_1 Z_2}, \quad \phi_8 = \lambda_{22}^{Z_1 Z_3},$$

$$\text{and} \qquad \phi_9 = \lambda_{32}^{Z_1 Z_3}.$$

The nominal-effects model (5.12) is a hierarchical LLM. In hierarchical models, effects are defined as deviations from lower-order effects. Thus, in these models it is assumed that once an interaction term is in the model, all lower-order (interaction) terms are also in the model. Because of this property, hierarchical models can simply be denoted by the sets of variables that define their highest-order effects. For example, model (5.12) can be written as

$$\log F_{\mathbf{z_1 z_2 z_3}} = \Lambda_{z_1 z_2}^{Z_1 Z_2} + \Lambda_{z_1 z_3}^{Z_1 Z_3}, \quad (5.13)$$

where the Λ-parameters denote the sums of the corresponding lower-order terms that precede them and that are not already absorbed by previous higher-order terms. Note that it does not matter how the parameters that constitute

$\Lambda_{z_1 z_2}^{Z_1 Z_2}$ are constrained; one might as well leave it at estimating $\Lambda_{z_1 z_2}^{Z_1 Z_2}$ if the lower-order terms are not of interest. A convenient syntax for the specification of a nominal linear model is proposed by Wilkinson & Rogers (1973). For model (5.13) it is $z_1.z_2 + z_1.z_3$, where the dot denotes an interaction. This notation is especially useful if the number of variables is high and/or there are complicated higher-order terms. For example, the model $z_1 + z_2 + \cdots + z_{19} + z_{20}.z_{21}.z_{22}$ would be hard to represent in the form (5.12). We will also use this notation to write the interaction structure of models with metric effects.

5.2.2 Loglinear Models with Metric Effects

In the previous section, the q-functions are used to designate response categories of nominal z-variables. If one or more of the z variables, say z_1 is assumed to have metric scale properties, one can use this property to restrict the interaction with other variables accordingly (Haberman, 1978a). For example, if z_1 is measured on an interval scale we can take $l_{z_1} = z_1 - 1$ and write

$$\log F_{z_1 z_2 z_3} = \phi_1 + \phi_2 l_{z_1}^{(1)} + \phi_3 l_{z_1}^{(2)} + \phi_4 l_{z_2} + \phi_5 l_{z_3} + \phi_6 l_{z_1} l_{z_2} \quad (5.14)$$
$$+ \phi_7 l_{z_1} l_{z_3}.$$

In standard loglinear notation this becomes

$$\log F_{z_1 z_2 z_3} = \lambda + \lambda_{z_1}^{Z_1} + \lambda_{z_2}^{Z_2} + \lambda_{z_3}^{Z_3} + l_{z_1} \lambda_{z_2}^{Z_1 Z_2} + l_{z_1} \lambda_{z_3}^{Z_1 Z_3}, \quad (5.15)$$

where, as before, the parameters are constrained to be zero if one of its indices is zero. In model (5.15) the parameter $\lambda_2^{Z_1 Z_2}$ can be interpreted as the effect of a change of one point on the variable z_1 given that $z_2 = 2$ and $\lambda_1^{Z_1 Z_2}$ is set to zero.

If two variables in an interaction have metric properties, we have the log-bilinear model (Goodman, 1979, 1991; Clogg & Goodman, 1984; Xie, 1992):

$$\log F_{z_1 z_2 z_3} = \lambda + \lambda_{z_1}^{Z_1} + \lambda_{z_2}^{Z_2} + \lambda_{z_3}^{Z_3} + l_{z_1} \lambda_{z_2}^{Z_1 Z_2} + l_{z_1} l_{z_3} \lambda^{Z_1 Z_3}, \quad (5.16)$$

where $\lambda^{Z_1 Z_3}$ is a parameter describing the strength of the interaction between z_1 and z_3. Note that in this example, models (5.16) and (5.15) are equivalent since z_3 is dichotomous.

5.2.3 Loglinear Models with Latent Variables

Loglinear models with discrete latent variables are described by Haberman (1979). In fact, they are generalizations of latent class models (Lazarsfeld & Henry, 1968), where each latent class corresponds to the value of a vector of latent variables. Latent class models, in turn, can be seen as an example of nonnormal mixtures (McLachlan & Peel, 2000, p. 166).

If u (o) denotes the set of unobserved (observed) variables, with $u \cup o = H$ $(u \cap o = \emptyset)$, the observed table is $f_{\mathbf{z}_o} = \sum_{\mathbf{z}_u} f_{\mathbf{z}}$ and the expected observed table is $F_{\mathbf{z}_o} = \sum_{\mathbf{z}_u} F_{\mathbf{z}}$, so that the kernel of the observed data likelihood becomes

$$\ell_o = \sum_{\mathbf{z}_o \in M_{\mathbf{z}_o}} f_{\mathbf{z}_o} \log F_{\mathbf{z}_o}.$$

One way to estimate the model parameters if one or more of the variables is unobserved is to use the EM algorithm (Dempster et al., 1977). The EM algorithm can help find a solution to problems that can be cast as a missing-data problem. Starting with a guess $\tilde{\phi}$ of ϕ, the algorithm maximizes ℓ_o by repeatedly applying an E-step (expectation step),

$$\tilde{f}_{\mathbf{z}} = E(f_{\mathbf{z}} \mid f_{\mathbf{z}_o}, \tilde{\phi}) = f_{\mathbf{z}_o}\tilde{P}(\mathbf{z}_u \mid \mathbf{z}_o) = f_{\mathbf{z}_o}\frac{\tilde{P}(\mathbf{z})}{\tilde{P}(\mathbf{z}_o)} = f_{\mathbf{z}_o}\frac{\tilde{F}_{\mathbf{z}}}{\tilde{F}_{\mathbf{z}_o}}, \tag{5.17}$$

and, using $\tilde{f}_{\mathbf{z}}$, an M-step (maximization step),

$$\max_{\phi_r} \tilde{\ell}, \tag{5.18}$$

using (5.5), to compute a new $\tilde{\phi}$. The E and M steps are alternated until $\tilde{\phi}$ converges to an estimate $\check{\phi}$. In (5.17), $\tilde{F}_{\mathbf{z}}$ denotes the expected frequencies computed from (5.2) using $\tilde{\phi}$. In (5.18), $\tilde{\ell}$ denotes the log-likelihood, where the estimated frequencies $\tilde{f}_{\mathbf{z}}$ of the full table are used in (5.3). Since for loglinear models with unobserved variables, ℓ_o does not necessarily have a unique maximum, the EM algorithm must be repeated a sufficient number of times until the set of distinct estimates $\{\check{\phi}\}$ does not become larger. The estimate $\hat{\phi} \in \{\check{\phi}\}$ for which ℓ_o is largest is then taken as the maximum likelihood estimate. In general, $\#\{\check{\phi}\}$ as well as the number of EM steps needed to obtain each $\check{\phi}$ tends to increase if the number of latent variables become large relative to the number of observed variables.

Note that the E-step does not require the full observed contingency table. Equation (5.17) need be applied only if $f_{\mathbf{z}_o} > 0$ and $\#\{f_{\mathbf{z}_o} > 0\} \leq N$. A similar reduction in computations can be achieved for the fit statistics (5.6) through (5.9), or, for loglinear models with latent variables, (5.6) through (5.9), where $f_{\mathbf{z}}$ is replaced by $f_{\mathbf{z}_o}$.

Finally, note that one can approximate the continuous distribution to any degree of precision by taking more-discrete categories, and there is no need to take more categories than the number of moments of the distribution of the observed variables, which is at most $\#M$ for discrete data (Stroud & Sechrest, 1966). For RMs, however, their number is usually much less. For example for a 61-item dichotomously-scored test, the RM requires at most 30 support points to describe the latent trait distribution (Follmann, 1988).

5.3 The Rasch Model as a Loglinear Model

Let $x = 1, \ldots, m_i$ denote nominal item response categories and let s_{ix} denote a score that is assigned to response x of item i. If the number of response categories is $m_i = 2$, and $s_{ix} = x - 1$, we have the dichotomous RM Rasch (1960):

$$P(x_i \mid \theta, \beta_i) = \frac{\exp[s_{ix_i}(\theta - \beta_i)]}{\sum_{x=1}^{m_i} \exp[s_{ix}(\theta - \beta_i)]}. \tag{5.19}$$

For arbitrary discrete category scores s_{ix} this model was studied by Verhelst & Glas (1995) and implemented in their computer program OPLM.

For $m_i > 2$ and $s_{ix} = x - 1$, we have a unidimensional RM for polytomously scored items

$$P(x_i \mid \theta, \boldsymbol{\beta}_i) = \frac{\exp[s_{ix_i}(\theta - \beta_{ix_i})]}{\sum_{x=1}^{m_i} \exp[s_{ix}(\theta - \beta_{ix})]} = \frac{\exp[\sum_{x=2}^{x_i}(\theta - \beta_{ix})]}{1 + \sum_{x=2}^{m_i} \exp[\sum_{k=2}^{x}(\theta - \beta_{ik})]}, \tag{5.20}$$

where $\beta_{i1} = 0$. The second equation of (5.20) is known as the partial-credit model (Andrich, 1988; Masters, 1982). Note that the formulation in the first equation of (5.20) is more general because it allows the category scores s_{ix} to be arbitrary functions of x. An alternative interpretation of the category scores s_{ix} is to consider them as fixed discrimination parameters, that is, a parameter that describes the degree to which the item response probability varies with θ.

Note that there is an indeterminacy in these models. Adding a constant to both θ and β does not change the model. Usually a linear restriction is imposed on the β's to fix the location of the θ scale.

The RM must be valid for all subjects in the population Π to which it is to be applied. The fit of the RM is studied for a sample of subjects $Q \subseteq \Pi$. Although Q should be representative of Π, it need not be an independent random sample of Π; Q can be an arbitrary ensemble of subjects. The RM is a *stochastic subject model* (Holland, 1990b), that is, it describes the probability that a fixed subject gives the response x_i rather than the probability that a subject with response x_i is randomly drawn from a population. The RM states that these response probabilities are the same for all subjects in Π with a latent trait value θ. Thus, the response probabilities depend only on θ, that is, given θ, each item response is independent of all other variables. In particular, it does not depend on responses to other items $(x_1, \ldots, x_{i-1}, x_{i+1}, \ldots, x_I)$ nor on any covariates $(y_1, \ldots, y_J)$ (Lord & Novick, 1968, p. 538):

$$P(x_i \mid \theta, \beta_i) = P(x_i \mid \theta, \beta_i, x_1, \ldots, x_{i-1}, x_{i+1}, \ldots, x_I, y_1, \ldots, y_J). \tag{5.21}$$

From elementary probability calculus it follows from (5.21) that

$$P(x_1, \ldots, x_I \mid \theta, \beta_1, \ldots, \beta_I, y_1, \ldots, y_J) = \prod_{i=1}^{I} P(x_i \mid \theta, \beta_i, y_1, \ldots, y_J), \tag{5.22}$$

which is the assumption of *local independence*, and also

$$P\left(x_i \mid \theta, \beta_i, y_1, \ldots, y_J\right) = P\left(x_i \mid \theta, \beta_i\right), \qquad (5.23)$$

which is the assumption of *measurement invariance* (Mellenbergh, 1989; Mill-sap, 1997). Denoting $(x_1, \ldots, x_I)$ by $\mathbf{x}$, $(\beta_1, \ldots, \beta_I)$ by $\boldsymbol{\beta}$, and $(y_1, \ldots, y_J)$ by $\mathbf{y}$ and substituting (5.19) in (5.23) and the result in (5.22), we have

$$P\left(\mathbf{x} \mid \theta, \boldsymbol{\beta}, \mathbf{y}\right) = P\left(\mathbf{x} \mid \theta, \boldsymbol{\beta}\right) = c(\theta, \boldsymbol{\beta})^{-1} \exp\left(\theta r - \sum_{i=1}^{I} s_{ix}\beta_i\right), \quad (5.24)$$

where $r = \sum_{i=1}^{I} s_{ix}$ is the raw score corresponding to response pattern $\mathbf{x}$ and

$$c(\theta, \boldsymbol{\beta}) = \prod_{i=1}^{I} \sum_{x=1}^{m_i} \exp[s_{ix}(\theta - \beta_i)].$$

Maximizing the likelihood of model (5.24) for $(\theta, \boldsymbol{\beta})$ gives the unconditional maximum likelihood (UML) estimates. Unfortunately, the UML estimates tend to be inconsistent because the number of subject parameters grows with the number of subjects in the sample (Andersen, 1973b). However, there are alternative estimation methods that provide better estimates of the item parameters. All these methods are based on models that are slightly different from the original RM, and they can all be formulated as LLMs.

5.3.1 Fixed Effects

A feature that distinguishes the RM from other item response models is that the category scores s_{ix} are known in advance. As a result, r is function of observed data only. The first approach depends on a defining property of the RM, the sufficiency of the raw score for the subject parameter (Andersen, 1973b; Fischer, 1974). It means that the raw score contains all information about θ that is in the data. As a result, the RM can be written as

$$P\left(\mathbf{x} \mid \theta, \boldsymbol{\beta}\right) = P\left(\mathbf{x} \mid r; \boldsymbol{\beta}\right) P\left(r \mid \theta, \boldsymbol{\beta}\right), \qquad (5.25)$$

where, from (5.24),

$$P\left(r \mid \theta, \boldsymbol{\beta}\right) = \exp(\theta r)c(\theta, \boldsymbol{\beta})^{-1}\gamma_r$$

and

$$P\left(\mathbf{x} \mid r; \theta, \boldsymbol{\beta}\right) = \gamma_r^{-1} \exp\left(-\sum_{i=1}^{I} s_{ix}\beta_i\right) = P\left(\mathbf{x} \mid r; \boldsymbol{\beta}\right), \qquad (5.26)$$

with

$$\gamma_r = \sum_{\mathbf{x} \in M_{\mathbf{x}.r}} \exp\left(-\sum_{i=1}^{I} s_{ix}\beta_i\right),$$

Table 5.1. Lazarsfeld & Stouffer data: observed and expected frequencies

					Model						
Response					(F)ERM	EDRM4	EDRM3	EDRM2	NDRM	MNDRM2a	Indep.
x_1 x_2 x_3 x_4				$f_\mathbf{x}$	Estimated expected frequencies ($\hat{F}_\mathbf{x}$)						
1 1 1 1				299	299.00	299.00	297.10	296.46	286.66	298.98	153.14
1 1 1 2				16	20.67	20.67	21.22	21.49	23.15	20.68	47.67
1 1 2 1				25	27.95	27.95	28.67	28.84	31.67	27.96	59.67
1 1 2 2				10	6.42	6.42	6.22	6.14	6.44	6.41	18.57
1 2 1 1				52	43.76	43.76	44.97	45.07	49.94	43.78	82.29
1 2 1 2				8	10.05	10.05	9.75	9.59	10.15	10.04	25.62
1 2 2 1				16	13.59	13.59	13.18	12.87	13.89	13.58	32.06
1 2 2 2				3	7.56	7.56	7.88	8.54	7.11	7.57	9.98
2 1 1 1				199	199.60	199.62	203.41	203.29	214.36	199.72	228.82
2 1 1 2				45	45.85	45.85	44.12	43.25	43.58	45.80	71.23
2 1 2 1				60	62.01	62.01	59.61	58.05	59.62	61.94	89.15
2 1 2 2				42	34.48	34.48	35.67	38.50	30.53	34.52	27.75
2 2 1 1				96	97.07	97.08	93.50	90.70	94.02	96.97	122.96
2 2 1 2				55	53.97	53.97	55.94	60.16	48.14	54.04	38.27
2 2 2 1				69	72.99	72.99	75.58	80.74	65.85	73.08	47.91
2 2 2 2				75	75.00	75.00	73.19	66.32	84.90	74.93	14.91
					Fit statistics						
X^2					10.48	10.48	11.05	14.19	17.14	10.48	515.28
p					0.23	0.16	0.20	0.12	0.07	0.23	0.00
G^2					10.93	10.93	11.66	15.12	17.48	10.93	388.88
p					0.21	0.14	0.17	0.09	0.06	0.21	0.00
df					8	7	8	9	10	8	11
BIC					−44.87	−37.90	−44.14	−47.66	−52.27	−44.87	312.15
AIC					−5.07	−3.07	−4.34	−2.88	−2.52	−5.07	366.88

wherein $M_{\mathbf{X}.r}$ is the set of response patters $\mathbf{x}$ consistent with r. For example, for $I = 3$ dichotomous item responses $x=1, 2$, scored $s_{ix} = x - 1$, we have for $r = 1$, $M_{\mathbf{X}.1} = \{(2, 1, 1), (1, 2, 1), (1, 1, 2)\}$. Note that γ_r is the proportionality constant of $P(\mathbf{x} \mid r; \theta, \boldsymbol{\beta})$ and from (5.26) that this conditional probability does not depend on θ.

This RM is equivalent to the nominal-effects LLM (Section 5.2.1)

$$\log F_\mathbf{x} = \lambda + \lambda_r^R + \sum_{i=1}^I \lambda_{x_i}^{X_i}, \qquad (5.27)$$

where for the FERM we have $\log F_\mathbf{x} = f_r P(\mathbf{x} \mid r; \theta, \boldsymbol{\beta})$, so that

$$\lambda + \lambda_r^R = \log f_r - \log \gamma(r) \quad \text{(fixed)} \quad \text{and} \quad \lambda_{x_i}^{X_i} = -s_{ix}\beta_i \quad \text{(random)},$$

and for the ERM we have $\log F_\mathbf{x} = NP(\mathbf{x}r \mid \theta, \boldsymbol{\beta})$, so that

$$\lambda = \log N \quad \text{(fixed)} \quad \lambda_r^R = \log \pi_r^R - \log \gamma(r) \quad \lambda_{x_i}^{X_i} = -s_{ix}\beta_i \quad \text{(random)},$$

where $\{\pi_r^R\}$ is the probability distribution of r. Note again that whether r is considered random or fixed does not affect the fit of the model nor the point estimates of the parameters (Section 5.2).

In (5.27) there is an overparametrization resulting from the linear dependence of the item responses and the score: adding a constant to each of the item parameters $\lambda_2^{X_i}$ and subtracting it from $\Lambda_r^R = \lambda + \lambda_r^R$ does not change the model. To eliminate the indeterminacy we can set a linear constraint on the item parameters, e.g., $\lambda_2^{X_1} = 0$. The number of degrees of freedom is equal to $\#(M)$ minus the number of Λ_r^R-parameters, $I + 1$, minus the number of estimable $\lambda_2^{X_i}$-parameters, $I - 1$, which equals $\#(M) - 2I$. For example, if there are four dichotomous items we have $\#(M) = 2^4 = 16$ cells and $2I = 8$ parameters, resulting in eight degrees of freedom. The shorthand notation for this model is (F)ERM$(X_1 + \cdots + X_I + R)$. This model yields conditional maximum likelihood (CML) estimates of the parameters.

Table 5.1 shows the observed frequencies of response patterns by noncommissioned officers responding to four dichotomous items on attitudes toward the army (Lazarsfeld, 1950a). The next column shows the estimated expected frequencies under the (F)ERM (5.27). Table 5.2 gives the LOGIMO script for this model. LOGIMO (keyword NORM) automatically determines the rank of

Table 5.2. LOGIMO script for ERM

```
TITLE Data from Lazarsfeld & Stouffer (1950);
DATAFILE LASTOU.DAT; NINPVAR 4; WEIGHT 3;
    COMMENT free format data file with three-digit  frequency
    followed by the response pattern;
POSITIONS 1 4 5 6 7; MODEL 5 [1][2][3][4][5];
    COMMENT LOGIMO wants to know the number of model terms.
    Main effects are default and need not be specified;
NSCORVAR 1; SCORING [1..4] 5 [2] 1;
    COMMENT defines the
    score r as the fifth variable. Default value is 0.
    For each response 2 the value 1 is added to the score r;
IPF STOPCRIT 0.00001000; MAXITER 5000 NORM;
    COMMENT Iterative Proportional Fitting until convergence;
NERA STOPCRIT 0.00001000; MAXITER 10 FIT;
    COMMENT Finally, Newton Raphson iterations;
FINISH
```

the model and aliases parameters that are functions of previous parameters. This ensures that the solution is unique and degrees of freedom are correct. So this LOGIMO script restricts $\lambda_2^{X_i}(i = 1, 2, 3)$ as well as $\lambda_x^{X_4}$ to zero. Table 5.1 gives the fit statistics for various models. The (F)ERM fits the data quite well.

5.3.2 Random Effects

If the subjects, Q, are independently drawn from population Π, the fixed subject-effect parameter θ can be treated as a random variable T taking values $t \in M_T$. Bock & Aitkin (1981) and Mislevy (1984) suggested estimating the distribution of T by estimating the probability histogram for a fixed set of values of t. In this section we formulate this random-effects RM as an LLM model with discrete latent variables for t (Section 5.2.3).

Let $M_{T^\circ} = \{t^\circ\}$ be a sufficiently large bounded set of known discrete values of t°. Let $\{t^*\}$ be an equally large set with $t^* = a + bt^\circ$, where $a > 0$ and $b > 0$ are unknown. Furthermore, let $\pi_{t^\circ}^{T^\circ}$ denote the probability that a randomly selected subject from Π has latent trait score t closest to t° ($M_{T^\circ} \subset M_T$). Note that since $t^* = a + bt^\circ$ is a one-to-one transformation, we have $\{\pi_{t^*}^{T^*}\} = \{\pi_{t^\circ}^{T^\circ}\}$. Replacing θ by t^* in (5.24) , we can derive

$$P\left(\mathbf{x}, t^* \mid \boldsymbol{\beta}, \{\pi_{t^*}^{T^*}\}\right) = P\left(\mathbf{x} \mid t^*; \boldsymbol{\beta}\right) P\left(t^* \mid \{\pi_{t^*}^{T^*}\}\right) \qquad (5.28)$$

$$= \pi_{t^*}^{T^*} c(t^*, \boldsymbol{\beta})^{-1} \exp\left(t^* r - \sum_{i=1}^{I} s_{ix}\beta_i\right)$$

$$= \pi_{t^\circ}^{T^\circ} c(t^\circ, a, b, \boldsymbol{\beta})^{-1} \exp\left(ar + bt^\circ r - \sum_{i=1}^{I} s_{ix}\beta_i\right),$$

where $c(t^\circ, a, b, \boldsymbol{\beta}) = c(a + bt^\circ, \boldsymbol{\beta}) = c(t^*, \boldsymbol{\beta})$. The model can be seen as a finite mixture of joint-RMs models (5.24), where the probabilities $\{\pi_{t^*}^{T^*}\} = \{\pi_{t^\circ}^{T^\circ}\}$ are the mixture weights (McLachlan & Peel, 2000).

The expected frequencies under this model are

$$F_{\mathbf{x}, t^*} = NP(\mathbf{x}, t^* \mid \boldsymbol{\beta}, \{\pi_{t^*}^{T^*}\})$$

(Section 5.2). Model (5.28) is equivalent to a metric-effects LLM for $(x_1, \ldots, x_I, t^*)$, where t^* is unobserved (Section 5.2.3). To see this let

$$\lambda_2^X = \lambda^R = a, \qquad \lambda_2^{XT^\circ} = \lambda^{RT^\circ} = b, \qquad \lambda_1^X = \lambda_1^{XT^\circ} = 0,$$

so that we have

$$\log F_{\mathbf{x}, t^*} = \lambda + \lambda_{t^\circ}^{T^\circ} + r\lambda^R + rt^\circ \lambda^{RT^\circ} + \sum_{i=1}^{I} \lambda_{x_i}^{X_i} \qquad (5.29)$$

$$= \lambda + \lambda_{t^\circ}^{T^\circ} + \sum_{i=1}^{I} s_{ix_i}\lambda^R + \sum_{i=1}^{I} s_{ix_i}t^\circ \lambda^{RT^\circ} + \sum_{i=1}^{I} \lambda_{x_i}^{X_i}$$

$$= \lambda + \lambda_{t^\circ}^{T^\circ} + \sum_{i=1}^{I} \left(\lambda_{x_i}^{X} + t^\circ \lambda_{x_i}^{T^\circ X} + \lambda_{x_i}^{X_i}\right),$$

where

$$\lambda = \log N,$$
$$\lambda_{t^\circ}^{T^\circ} = \log \pi_{t^\circ}^{T^\circ} - \log c(t^\circ, a, b, \boldsymbol{\beta}), \quad \text{and}$$
$$\lambda_{x_i}^{X_i} = -s_{ix}\beta_i.$$

Note that the first equation of (5.29) is a log-bilinear model (Section 5.2.2) and the last equation an ordinary loglinear model.

To remove the indeterminacy between item parameters, $\lambda_2^{X_i}$, and the location of the latent trait scale, $\lambda_1^X (= a)$, one of the item parameters, say $\lambda_{x_1}^{X_1}$, can be set to zero. We will call model (5.29) the empirical distribution random-effects RM (EDRM). The shorthand notation for an EDRM with $\#(M_{T^*}) = 3$ is EDRM3$(X_1 T + \cdots + X_I T)$.

For the dichotomous RM, Leeuw & Verhelst (1986) and Follmann (1988) have shown that, under an EDRM with at most $(I + 2)/2$ support points, the ERM (5.27) and the EDRM model are asymptotically equivalent (see also Section 5.2.3).

Table 5.3 gives the LEM script for an EDRM with $\#(M_{T^\circ}) = 4$. In Table 5.1 it is seen that the (F)ERM fits better than EDRM2 and EDRM3. Furthermore, for EDRM4 the χ^2-statistics and expected frequencies are the same as for (F)ERM, but EDRM4 has one degree of freedom fewer than (F)ERM. As a result, BIC and AIC favor (F)ERM. The EDRM2 fits worse than the other EDRMs except on BIC, which favors parsimonious models (Section 5.2).

Table 5.3. LEM script for the EDRM4 estimation

```
* Data from Lazarsfeld & Stouffer (1950)
latent_variables 1;  manifest_variables 4
dimensions 4 2 2 2 2;  labels T X1 X2 X3 X4
model  {T,X2,X3,X4}
all {special(T.X1,T.X2,T.X3,T.X4,1b),      * a
     special(X1,X2,X3,X4,1b)}              * b
dummy 1 1 1 1 1
data [299 016 025 010 052 008 016 003 199
          045 060 042 096 055 069 075]
```

If one is willing to assume a parametric distribution for the latent trait, $\pi_{t^*}^{T^*}$ may be restricted to be consistent with such a distribution. If $\#(M_{T^*})$ is chosen large enough, the continuous normal distribution $P(t) = N(0, 1)$ can be approximated to any degree of precision by $\pi_{t^*}^{T^*}$. Gain in precision is obtained using Gauss–Hermite quadrature (Bock & Aitkin, 1981). The t^*-points are then chosen not as equidistant, but as quadrature points with corresponding quadrature weights $\pi_{t^*}^{T^*}$ (Stroud & Sechrest, 1966). This normal distribution

RM (NDRM) yields estimates that are known as marginal maximum likelihood (MML) estimates. The difference with EDRM is that in NDRM the probabilities $\pi_{t^*}^{T^*}$ are known in advance. The shorthand notation for this model is NDRM($X_1 T + \cdots + X_I T$). Note that if π_{t° is chosen such that t° is approximately distributed as $N(0, 1)$, the distribution of t^* approximates $N(a, b^2)$. Thus, estimates of the loglinear parameters λ_2^X and $|\lambda_2^{XT^\circ}|$ are estimates of the mean and standard deviation of the latent trait distribution. The absolute value of $\lambda_2^{XT^\circ}$ should be taken because its sign depends on the direction of the latent scale, which is essentially indeterminate. Table 5.4 gives the LEM script for the NDRM. Table 5.1 gives the estimated expected frequencies under the

Table 5.4. LEM script for the NDRM

```
* Data from Lazarsfeld & Stouffer (1950)
latent_variables 1;  manifest_variables 4
dimensions 21 2 2 2 2;  labels T X1 X2 X3 X4
model  {weighted(T),X2,X3,X4}
all {special(X1,X2,X3,X4,1b),               * a
     special(T.X1,T.X2,T.X3,T.X4,1b)}       * b
dummy 1 1 1 1
starting_values weight(T) normal_distribution(1,10)
* starting_values fixes pi_t to follow a standard
* normal distribution which range from -10 to 10
* approximated via re-scaled densities
data [...]
```

NDRM. Comparing the X^2 and G^2 statistics with their degrees of freedom, the NDRM, like the (F)ERM, cannot be rejected. The information statistics show an inconsistent picture in which BIC favors the more-restrictive NDRM and AIC the least-restrictive (F)ERM. Under NDRM, the latent-trait variance is estimated as 0.23, suggesting that the RM fits because of near independence of the item responses, which is equivalent to small variance of θ (Wood, 1978). However, Table 5.1 shows that the independence model fits very badly.

One way to relax the normality assumption of the latent trait is to assume a mixture of normal distributions. To do this, we extend the model with an unobserved random grouping variable C taking values c. It is then assumed that the parameters a and b depend on c, that is, we have a_c and b_c. For example, for $M_C = 2$ the distribution of t is a mixture of two normal distributions, $N(a_1, b_1^2)$ and $N(a_2, b_2^2)$. The model can be formulated as a mixture of NDRMs in which the probabilities $\{\pi_c^C\}$ can be seen as the mixture weights (McLachlan & Peel, 2000):

$$F_{\mathbf{x},t^*,c} = \pi_c^C \exp\left(\lambda + \lambda_{t^\circ}^{T^\circ} + r\lambda_c^{RC} + rt^\circ \lambda_c^{RT^\circ C} + \sum_{i=1}^{I} \lambda_{x_i}^{X_i} \right).$$

In its loglinear form it becomes a metric log-bilinear (Section 5.2.2) or loglinear model with latent variables (Anderson & Vermunt, 2000), Section 5.2.3)

$$\log F_{\mathbf{x},t^*,c} = \lambda + \lambda_{t^\circ}^{T^\circ} + \lambda_c^C + r\lambda_c^{RC} + rt^\circ\lambda_c^{RT^\circ C} + \sum_{i=1}^{I} \lambda_{x_i}^{X_i} \qquad (5.30)$$

$$= \lambda + \lambda_{t^\circ}^{T^\circ} + \lambda_c^C + \sum_{i=1}^{I}(\lambda_{x_i c}^{XC} + t^\circ\lambda_{x_i c}^{XT^\circ C} + \lambda_{x_i}^{X_i}),$$

where

$$\lambda_1^C = 0, \quad \lambda_{2c}^{XC} = \lambda_c^{RC} = a_c, \quad \lambda_{2c}^{XT^\circ C} = \lambda_c^{RT^\circ C} = b_c, \quad \lambda_{1c}^{XC} = \lambda_{1c}^{XT^\circ C} = 0.$$

The shorthand notation for this model is $\text{MNDRM}(CT + X_1T + \cdots + X_IT)$. The LEM script obtains by replacing the specials in Table 5.4 by

```
all {special(X1,X2,X3,X4,1b,C,c),           * for 'a_c'
     special(T.X1,T.X2,T.X3,T.X4,1b,C,c)}   * for 'b_c'
* 'C,c' means that the (equal) interactions may vary over C.
```

For two mixture components, the MNDRM, say MNDRM-2, has three parameters more than the NDRM. We have λ_2^C, λ_{21}^{XC}, λ_{22}^{XC}, $\lambda_{21}^{XT^\circ C}$, and $\lambda_{22}^{XT^\circ C}$, rather than λ_2^X and $t^\circ\lambda_2^{T^\circ X}$, so we have $10 - 3 = 7$ degrees of freedom, which is the same as for the EDRM4. For the Lazarsfeld & Stouffer data, the model has the same fit as the EDRM4 but was almost underidentified for this small example. To restrict the variances b_c^2 to be equal over mixture components we replace $\lambda_{x_i c}^{XT^\circ C}$ by $\lambda_{x_i}^{XT^\circ}$ in model (5.30) and specify

```
special(T.X1,T.X2,T.X3,T.X4,1b)  * for 'b'.
```

This model, say MNDRM2a, has eight degrees of freedom and has the same fit as the EDRM4. The parameter estimates of MNDRM2a along with those of NDRM and EDRM4 are shown in Table 5.5. The lack of fit of NDRM, the difference between the locations of the mixture components on the t scale, $\hat{\lambda}_{21}^{XC} = 1.75$ of MNDRM2a as well as the distribution $\{\hat{\pi}_{t^\circ}^{T^\circ}\}$ of EDRM suggests that the latent-trait distribution is bimodal. It is seen that item-parameter estimates of the misfitting NDRM are different from the well-fitting models, MNDRM2a and EDRM4. The item parameters of the (F)ERM, not shown here, have the same values.

5.3.3 Speeding Up Computations

If the number of items is large, the number of cells in the full contingency table becomes unmanageable. There are two ways to avoid this.

Firstly, Kelderman (1992) describes modified versions of the iterative proportional fitting and Newton–Raphson algorithms for (F)ERMs that work on the minimal sufficient statistics rather than on the counts in the full contingency table. In the case of the (F)ERM these can be obtained from the

Table 5.5. Parameter estimates for the EDRM4, MNDRM2a, and NDRM

EDRM4			MNDRM2a			NDRM		
Param.	Est.	(s.e.)	Param.	Est.	(s.e.)	Param.	Est.	(s.e.)
λ	3.00		λ	1.02		λ	2.96	
$\lambda_2^{X_2}$	−1.52	(0.12)	$\lambda_2^{X_2}$	−1.52	(0.12)	$\lambda_2^{X_2}$	−1.46	(0.12)
$\lambda_2^{X_3}$	−1.97	(0.12)	$\lambda_2^{X_3}$	−1.97	(0.12)	$\lambda_2^{X_3}$	−1.91	(0.12)
$\lambda_2^{X_4}$	−2.27	(0.13)	$\lambda_2^{X_4}$	−2.27	(0.13)	$\lambda_2^{X_4}$	−2.23	(0.13)
λ_2^{X}	0.92	(1.49)	λ_2^{X}	0.67	(0.32)	λ_2^{X}	1.09	(0.78)
$\lambda_2^{XT^\circ}$	1.42	(0.82)	$\lambda_2^{XT^\circ}$	0.72	(0.23)	$\lambda_2^{XT^\circ}$	0.48	(1.57)
$\pi_{t_1^\circ}^{T^\circ}$	0.12		λ_2^{C}	1.88	(1.61)			
$\pi_{t_2^\circ}^{T^\circ}$	0.36		λ_{21}^{XC}	1.75	(0.38)			
$\pi_{t_3^\circ}^{T^\circ}$	0.20							
$\pi_{t_4^\circ}^{T^\circ}$	0.31 $(t_1^\circ < \cdots < t_4^\circ)$							

one-variable marginal tables for each item and for a vector or raw scores that are arbitrary functions of the item responses onto the natural numbers. To calculate the expected sufficient statistics and other expected marginal sums of the table, a method is implemented that avoids summing large numbers of elementary cell frequencies by formulating them as sums of products of multiplicative model parameters and applying the distributive law of multiplication over summation. In this algorithm, the raw-score functions are handled dynamically. This algorithm is implemented in LOGIMO (Kelderman & Steen, 1993).

Secondly, random-effects latent-variable models often have the advantage that the full probability can be collapsed into a product of a series of conditional probabilities. For example, suppressing the model parameters, (5.29) can be written as

$$P(\mathbf{x}, t^*) = \prod_{i=1}^{I} P(x_i \mid t^*) P(t^*). \tag{5.31}$$

Vermunt (1997b) describes an expectation-maximization (EM) algorithm in which each conditional probability satisfies a (restrictive) loglinear or log-bilinear model. To obtain this for (5.29), the model formula script in Table 5.4 should be replaced by

```
model T {weight(T)} X1|T {} X2|T {X2} X3|T {X3} X4|T {X4},
```

where the loglinear model specification is between braces. The algorithm has been implemented in the program LEM (Vermunt, 1997b,a). With Vermunt's work the estimation problem has largely been solved for random-effects models.

5.4 Other Loglinear Rasch Models

5.4.1 Loglinear Rasch Models for Polytomous Items

It is easily seen that the LLRMs described above are also valid for polytomous arbitrary category scores (Kelderman, 1996). Consider the following example, in which van Kuyk (1988) collected data in an observation program for 4- to 6.5-year-old children. The aim of the program was to test skills that are prerequisite for arithmetic abilities. The subtest analyzed here measures the application of size concepts such as long–short, high–low, thick–thin, wide–narrow, etc. Answers are rated correct if the right size concept (e.g., long–short) is given and is correctly applied (e.g. short(er) rather than long(er)). Children may be unable to produce the correct specific concept (e.g. long–short), but use the general size concept "big–small" instead. If "big–small" is correctly applied (e.g., the skirt is small(er)), the answer is rated partially correct.

Suppose we expect these three responses ($x_i = 1, 2, 3$) to be related to a single latent trait and score the responses as $s_{ix} = x - 1$. For these scores the LLM (5.27) is equivalent to the partial-credit model (5.20), where $\lambda_x^{X_i} = -\beta_{ix}$ (Kelderman, 1996). The LOGIMO script differs but little from that in Table 5.2. The main difference is that the scoring keywords now become

```
SCORING [1..5] 6 [2] 1
SCORING [1..5] 6 [3] 2
```

where 6 is the variable number of the latent trait and category score [2] gets the score 1 and so on. In Table 5.6 it is seen that $(F)ERM(R + X_1 + \cdots + X_4)$ does not fit very well compared to other models. The model specifications of the random-effect version of the partial-credit model are identical to those of the dichotomous RM except that the interactions with x_i become metric. For brevity we limit ourselves mainly to the (F)ERM case.

Table 5.6. Fit statistics for van Kuyk data

(F)ERM Model	G^2	df	AIC	BIC
$R_1.R_2 + X_1 + \cdots + X_4$	256.52	36.00	184.52	55.92
$R + X_1 + \cdots + X_4$	274.99	46.00	182.99	18.67
$Z.R_1.R_2 + Z.X_1 + \cdots + Z.X_4$	225.25	185.00	-144.75	-805.60
$Z.R_1.R_2 + X_1 + \cdots + X_4$	256.52	198.00	-139.48	-846.77
$Z.R + Z.X_1 + \cdots + Z.X_4$	293.05	199.00	-104.95	-815.81
$Z.R + X_1 + \cdots + X_4$	383.79	213.00	-42.21	-803.08

5.4.2 Loglinear Multidimensional Rasch Models

If it is expected that giving the correct specific concept requires a different latent trait than giving the general concept, we may define multiple latent-trait variables. The loglinear multidimensional RM can be obtained by generalizing (5.27) and (5.29). Denote the multidimensional scoring functions and raw scores by

$$\mathbf{s}_{ix} = (s_{1ix}, \ldots, s_{dix}, \ldots, s_{Dix})' \qquad \text{and} \qquad \mathbf{r} = (r_1, \ldots, r_d, \ldots, r_D)'$$

and similarly for $\boldsymbol{\beta}_{ix}, \boldsymbol{\theta}, \mathbf{t}, \mathbf{a},$ and $\mathbf{b}$. For some t_d° we have $t_d^* = a_d + b_d t_d^\circ$ and

$$P(\mathbf{x}, \mathbf{t}^*) = \pi_{\mathbf{t}^\circ} c(\mathbf{t}^\circ, \mathbf{a}, \mathbf{b}, \boldsymbol{\beta})^{-1} \exp\left[\sum_{d=1}^{D}(a_d r_d + b_d t_d^\circ r_d - \sum_{i=1}^{I}\beta_{dix})\right], \quad (5.32)$$

where β_{dix} is the parameter of response x on item i with respect to dimension d and $\{\pi_{\mathbf{t}^\circ}\}$ is a D-dimensional histogram. Note that the β_{dix} are not identifiable if an item response x_i pertains to two or more dimensions. Therefore, without loss of generality, we sum these parameters over dimensions. In loglinear notation this model becomes

$$\log F_{\mathbf{x}, \mathbf{t}^\circ} = \lambda + \lambda_{\mathbf{t}}^\circ + \sum_{d=1}^{D} r_d \lambda^{R_d} + \sum_{d=1}^{D} r_d t_d^\circ \lambda^{R_d T_d^\circ} + \sum_{i=1}^{I} \lambda_{x_i}^{X_i}. \quad (5.33)$$

The loglinear formulation of the multidimensional NDRM is obtained by taking $\pi_{\mathbf{t}^*}$ so that the distribution of $\mathbf{t}^*$ approximates $N(\mathbf{0}, \mathbf{I})$ and linear transformations $\mathbf{t}^* = \mathbf{a} + \mathbf{b}\mathbf{t}^\circ$. This model can more easily be specified in LOGIMO, so we return to the (F)ERM case.

Suppose that we have

$$\mathbf{r} = (r_1, r_2) = \left(\sum_{i=1}^{I} s_{1ix_i}, \sum_{i=1}^{I} s_{2ix_i}\right),$$

where

$$x_i = \begin{cases} 1 & : \quad s_{1ix_i} = 0, \quad s_{2ix_i} = 0, \\ 2 & : \quad s_{1ix_i} = 1, \quad s_{2ix_i} = 0, \\ 3 & : \quad s_{1ix_i} = 0, \quad s_{2ix_i} = 1. \end{cases}$$

In fact, this LLRM is the multidimensional RM described by Andersen (1973b). In LOGIMO this model is easily specified. The LOGIMO specification for $(F)ERM(R_1.R2 + X_1 + \cdots + X_I)$ now changes by

```
NSCORVAR 2
SCORING [1..5] 6 [2] 1
SCORING [1..5] 7 [3] 1
```

The AIC and BIC statistics in Table 5.6 indicate that the one-dimensional fixed-effects model $R + X_1 + \cdots + X_4$ fits somewhat better than the two-dimensional model $R_1.R_2 + X_1 + \cdots + X_4$, although the overall fit of neither model seems very good. Note that if we want the correct answer $x = 3$ to pertain to the general size concept as well, we must specify

```
SCORING [1..5] 6 [2,3] 1,
```

which is the multidimensional partial credit model (Kelderman, 1996).

5.4.3 Rasch Models Violating Measurement Invariance

Models that violate the assumption of measurement invariance are easily specified by adding one or more interactions between a grouping variable and an item response. For a fixed-effects model, uniform bias is specified as $C.T+C.X_1+X_2+\cdots+X_I$ and nonuniform bias as $C.T+C.T.X_1+X_2+\cdots+X_I$. In this case ordinary nominal interaction parameters are added. For random effects we have for uniform bias $C.T+C.X_1+X_1.T+\ldots+X_I.T$, where $[CT]$ denotes the addition of C terms as in model (5.30). For nonuniform bias we have in this case $C.T+C.X_1+CX_1.T+\cdots+X_I.T$, where $[CX_1T]$ denotes the addition of a nominal interaction term $\lambda_{x_1c}^{X_1C}$ and a metric interaction term $t^\circ \lambda_{x_1c}^{X_1T^\circ C}$ to the model. In fact, the parameter $\lambda_{x_1c}^{X_1T^\circ C}$ specifies a different slope of the item characteristic curve in each subgroup c. If all items are biased with respect to C, we have the mixture RM (Gitomer & Yamamoto, 1991; Kelderman & Macready, 1990; Mislevy & Verhelst, 1990; Rost, 1990, 1991; Rost et al., 1997; Wilson, 1989).

Models with an observed grouping variable are specified by replacing C by Z. In van Kuyk's testing program, the children's ages were known with $z = 1$ (ages 4 to 5), 2 (ages 5 to 5.5), 3 (ages 5.5 to 6). From the AIC and BIC statistics in Table 5.6 it can be seen that two-dimensional fixed-effects model, where the raw score distributions are different in each age group, $Z.R_1.R_2+X_1+\cdots+X_4$, fits markedly better than the one-dimensional model $Z.R + X_1 + \cdots + X_4$. To see whether the first item in this two-dimensional model deviates from measurement invariance, we compare the fit of model $Z.R_1.R_2 + X_1 + \cdots + X_4$ with that of model $Z.R_1.R_2 + Z.X_1 + \cdots + Z.X_4$. From Table 5.6 it is seen that the AIC and BIC statistics give contradictory results. The likelihood ratio statistic indicates that, given $Z.R_1.R_2 + Z.X_1 + \cdots + Z.X_4$, the hypothesis that the item1×age interaction are zero must be rejected ($\triangle G_3^2 = 31.27, p = 0.00$).

5.4.4 Locally Dependent Rasch Models

Locally dependent RM are easily specified by adding an item interaction effect $\lambda_{x_ix_{i'}}^{X_iX_{i'}}$ ($i \neq i$) to the model. For example, suppose we specify model (F)ERM($X_1X_4 + X_2 + X_3 + R$). We must replace the LOGIMO model specification in Table 5.2 by

```
MODEL 4
[1,4][2][3][5].
```

For the Lazarsfeld & Stouffer data, adding this interaction to the (F)ERM gives a very good fit indeed ($X_7^2= 8.63$, p=0.32, $L_7^2= 8.21$, p=0.30), but there is no significant difference with the (F)ERM ($\triangle L_1^2=2.72$, p=0.10). Its information statistics give an inconsistent picture ($BIC = -40.62, AIC = -5.79$), where AIC favors this model as the best fitting (see Table 5.1). A similar result was obtained for other interactions.

Note that in the LEM specification the interaction should be specified between items whose parameters are not fixed to zero. So in the case of $NDRM(X_1X_2 + X_1T + \cdots + X_4T)$ models we must set another item-main-effect parameter to zero to fix the scale. The model is specified by replacing the first line of the model specification by

```
model
{weighted(T),X1,X3,X4,X1.X4}.
```

Allowing Items 1 and 4 to interact improves the χ^2 fit of the NDRM somewhat ($X_9^2 = 13.86$, p=0.12, $L_9^2 = 13.25$, p=0.15). However, the difference between both models is not significant ($\triangle L_1^2 = 17.48\text{-}13.86 = 3.62$, p=0.06) and the AIC and BIC statistics of both models are identical.

5.4.5 Rasch Models with Latent Responses

The RM assumes that the probability of a positive (correct, agree) response approaches zero if the latent trait decreases. However, educational and psychological tests often contain multiple-choice items in which it is possible that the subject obtains a positive answer through guessing. Similarly, a negative response may accidentally be given by a subject that has a high latent-trait value. To account for these response errors the RMs discussed above may be modified to describe such effects.

Let x_i be the observed response on item i and let this response depend on a latent response u_i that satisfies an RM. The shorthand notation of this part of the model is $X_1.U_1 + \cdots + X_I.U_I$. The complete model is specified by adding this to an RM where the X's are replaced by U's. For example, $Z.R_1.R_2 + X_1 + \cdots + X_4$ becomes $X_1.U_1 + \cdots + X_4.U_4 + Z.R_1.R_2$. For the Lazarsfeld & Stouffer data we specify a latent response RM in which item difficulties are assumed to be equal. The fit of the model is quite bad ($X_3^2 = 511.48$, p=0.00, $L_3^2 = 496.48$, p = 0.00). A more realistic example of latent response RMs can be found in Chapter 20.

5.5 Discussion

In this section the basics of loglinear Rasch modeling are discussed as well as some possible generalizations based on the LLRM. One advantage of formulating the RM as an LLM is that the estimation equations and other statistical properties need not be derived separately for each new model. Furthermore, existing programs can be used for computations.

Some easy generalizations that go beyond the actual RM have been left undiscussed. One that falls beyond the scope of this book is the estimation of discrimination parameters such as in the Birnbaum model and Bock's nominal response model (Birnbaum, 1968; Bock, 1972). This can be done by relaxing the assumption of $\lambda_x^{XT^{\circ}}$ that the item trait associations are the same across items (Smit et al., 2000, 2003).

6

Mixture-Distribution and HYBRID Rasch Models

Matthias von Davier and Kentaro Yamamoto

Educational Testing Service

6.1 Introduction

This chapter provides an overview of mixture-distribution Rasch models (RMs) and HYBRID RMs and their extensions. Discrete mixture-distribution IRT models assume that the observed data were drawn from an unobservable mixture of populations. Within each of these populations, a different item response model may hold (HYBRID models), or models with different sets of item parameters and different ability distributions may hold (mixture Rasch models, or more generally, mixture IRT models). A rationale for these models, drawing on the introductory chapters in this volume, will be given. Among other things, mixture IRT models can be regarded as a tool to test ordinary IRT models for parameter invariance across populations.

Early work on the HYBRID model (Yamamoto, 1989) as well as the mixed RM (Rost, 1990, von Davier & Rost, 1995) are reviewed in this chapter, as well as more recent work that incorporates covariates (Smit et al., 2000) and research that generalizes the treatment of missing grouping variables (von Davier & Yamamoto, 2004b). Relationships to discrete mixture models using other IRT models (see Mislevy & Verhelst, 1990, and Kelderman & Macready, 1990) are outlined. Finally, extensions of multidimensional Rasch-type IRT models, sometimes referred to as diagnostic models (von Davier & Yamamoto, 2004a; von Davier, 2005), to mixture-distribution models are discussed.

6.2 Mixture-Distribution Rasch Models

Haberman (1979) and Kelderman (1984) laid out important building blocks for loglinear models with unobserved (latent) variables and loglinear RMs. This research was used by Kelderman & Macready (1990) in order to extend Rasch-type loglinear models by employing an unobserved discrete variable. IRT models with both a continuous ability variable and a discrete "strategy" or "skill" variable were developed in the late eighties and independently published by a number of researchers in 1990 (Kelderman & Macready, 1990; Mislevy & Verhelst, 1990; Rost, 1990). Rost (1990) integrated RMs into latent class analysis (LCA) (Lazarsfeld & Henry, 1968) and derived the mixed Rasch model. Mislevy & Verhelst (1990) derived a mixture IRT model extending previous work of Yamamoto (1987, 1989).

mixture-distribution RMs are a special case of discrete mixture-distribution models (McLachlan & Basford, 1988; McLachlan & Peel, 2000) with multivariate, categorical observed variables. The following section (6.2.1) describes discrete mixture distributions in general terms. Section 6.2.2 gives an overview of the dichotomous mixed RM, and Section 6.2.3 describes polytomous mixed RMs.

6.2.1 Discrete Mixture Distributions

The underlying concept of discrete mixture distributions is that an I-dimensional vector of random variables $\boldsymbol{x} = (x_1, \dots, x_I) \in \Omega$ may be viewed as a projection of an $(I + 1)$-dimensional random vector $(x_1, \dots, x_I, c)$, with discrete random variable c, and a marginal density

$$f(\boldsymbol{x}) = \sum_{c=1}^{C} \pi_c f(\boldsymbol{x} \mid c) = \sum_{c=1}^{C} f(\boldsymbol{x}, c), \qquad (6.1)$$

where the $\pi_c = P(c)$ denote the relative class sizes or mixing proportions, and $f(\boldsymbol{x} \mid c)$ is the conditional distribution of $\boldsymbol{x}$ given c.

More specifically, assume that $(x_{v1}, \dots, x_{vI})$ are the observed variables for each of $v = 1, \dots, N$ examinees, and that there is an unobserved classification $c = c(v)$ with $c(v) \in \{1, \dots, C\}$. The different discrete values c takes on are referred to as latent classes, subpopulations, or mixing components. The individual outcomes $c_v = c(v)$ will be referred to as class-membership outcomes throughout this chapter, since many initial developments concerning mixture Rasch and more generally mixture IRT models were made in the context of extensions of latent class analysis. If the values c_v are observed for all examinees v in the sample, discrete mixture models do not pose any additional estimation problem, since this case can be treated as a multigroup analysis, a common type of analysis in IRT.

If we use discrete mixture distributions for modeling item response data, we may assume that $\boldsymbol{x}$ is an I-dimensional vector of binary or polytomous variables x_i for $i = 1, \dots, I$. Below, we will assume that an item response model such as the RM will be used to model the conditional distributions $f(\boldsymbol{x} \mid c)$, while the mixture distribution will be defined as given in Equation 6.1. However, there is a less-complex alternative for modeling item response data with a mixture-distribution approach. We may assume that item responses are locally independent given the outcome of the mixing variable c, without assuming an additional continuous person variable θ. Then we have

$$f(\boldsymbol{x}) = \sum_{c=1}^{C} \pi_c \prod_{i=1}^{I} p(x_i \mid c) \tag{6.2}$$

with probabilities $p(c) = \pi_c$ representing the class sizes, sometimes also referred to as mixing proportions.

Equation 6.2 is the model equation for LCA. Local independence given unobserved latent traits (the classification c in LCA, the ability θ in the RM and more general IRT models) is an important defining feature of many latent-trait models. Therefore, LCA can be viewed as a latent-trait model with a nominal latent-trait variable c.

Figure 6.1 presents a graph of fictitious conditional probabilities for a model that contains three latent classes $C \in \{1, 2, 3\}$ based on data from six dichotomous items.

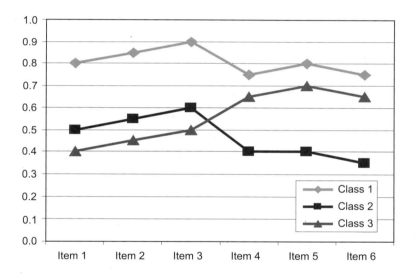

Fig. 6.1. Profiles of conditional probabilities in three latent classes for six dichotomous items

In most of the cases treated in this chapter, the c_v will be unobserved for all examinees, and thus have to be inferred using model assumptions and calculations involving some form of assigning classifications to individual response vectors, often involving the application of Bayes's theorem. These assumptions impose restrictions on the conditional distributions $f(x \mid c)$ and in some cases introduce covariates z and additional assumptions to derive an expression for determining the posterior distribution $p(c \mid \boldsymbol{x}, z)$. The posterior distribution can be determined using the assumption that all functional dependency in the item response functions is mediated through the person variable, either a discrete classification variable c or a continuous latent-trait variable θ, and item parameters. More formally, item response models assume

$$f(\boldsymbol{x}|\theta, z) = f(\boldsymbol{x}|\theta, z') = p(\boldsymbol{x}|\theta)$$

for all z, z', so that the distribution of the observed responses $\boldsymbol{x}$ depends on the latent-trait θ only, while the distribution of θ depends on z, that is,

$$p(\theta|z) \neq p(\theta|z') \quad \text{for} \quad z \neq z'.$$

The impact of the covariates z can be assumed to operate only through a conditional distribution $p(\theta|z)$, or $p(c|z)$ in the discrete case.

Putting these building blocks together results in a general expression that subsumes many of the models treated in this and some other chapters of this volume. We then have

$$f(\boldsymbol{x}|z) = \sum_{c=1}^{C} p(c \mid z) f(\boldsymbol{x} \mid c) \tag{6.3}$$

with observed variables $\boldsymbol{x}$, and covariates z of the classification variable c. If no covariates are available, the expression reduces to the original definition of the mixture distribution given in (6.2). For continuous variables θ instead of a discrete classification c, this expression becomes

$$f(\boldsymbol{x}|z) = \int_{\theta} h(\theta \mid z) f(\boldsymbol{x} \mid \theta) d\theta.$$

This marginalization is very common in latent-trait models with covariates. It is also found in Chapter 4 in this volume on latent regression models as well as in models using covariates and multiparameter IRT models (Mislevy, 1985, 1991).

6.2.2 Dichotomous Mixed Rasch Models

Discrete mixtures of RMs (Rost, 1990) assume a more complex structure within each mixing component than does LCA. More specifically, in addition to the discrete classification variable c, the complete data also include a continuous latent variable θ. Then the complete data becomes a concatenation of observed variables $\boldsymbol{x}$, the classification variable c, and the continuous latent-trait variable θ, that is, (x, c, θ).

In order to extend the RM to a mixture-distribution model, the model equation of the ordinary RM needs to be modified. The RM contains the continuous latent variable θ_v, reflecting the ability of examinee v, and an item difficulty parameter β_i, which reflects the location of the item characteristic curve for item i. Missing is a representation of the discrete mixture assumption, the dependency on a discrete unobserved classification variable c. In the case of a latent variable (θ, c) and without assuming any specific functional form we have

$$f(x) = \sum_{c=1}^{C} \pi_c \int_\theta h(\theta \mid c) P(x \mid \theta, c) d\theta,$$

where $h(\theta \mid c)$ denotes the conditional density of θ given c, which may be of a specific parametric form such as the normal density or some more flexible parametric family of densities.

The assumptions governing the conditional probabilities $P(x \mid \theta, c)$ of the observed variable x given latent variable (θ, c) are yet to be specified. The dichotomous mixed RM defines this as

$$p(x \mid \theta, c) = \prod_{i=1}^{I} \frac{\exp(x_i(\theta - \beta_{ic}))}{1 + \exp(\theta - \beta_{ic})}, \tag{6.4}$$

where the item parameters are denoted by β_{ic} and therefore depend on the discrete class variable c. Restrictions to remove the indeterminacy of the scale are applied conditionally by class, i.e., $\sum_i \beta_{ic} = 0$ for all c.

The dichotomous mixed RM was described by Rost (1990) and Rost & von Davier (1993, 1995). This model can be viewed as an extension of the RM that relaxes item-parameter invariance and allows different ability distributions in different subpopulations. The subpopulations need not be known and are identified during the course of parameter estimation. The mixed RM contains LCA, the RM, and the saltus model (compare Chapter 7 in this volume) for dichotomous data as special cases. Therefore, one obvious application of the mixed RM is testing the fit of the ordinary (nonmixed) RM (Rost & von Davier, 1995).

6.2.3 Polytomous Mixed Rasch Models

A straightforward extension of the dichotomous mixed RM allows one to specify a mixture RM for polytomous data (Rost, 1991). The model equation for a response vector $\boldsymbol{x} = (x_1, \ldots, x_I)$ with $x_i \in \{0, \ldots, m_i\}$ is

$$p(\boldsymbol{x} \mid \theta, c) = \prod_{i=1}^{I} \frac{\exp(x_i \theta - \beta_{ix_ic})}{1 + \sum_{y=1}^{X_i} \exp(y\theta - \beta_{iyc})},$$

where $\beta_{ixc} = \sum_{y=1}^{x} \alpha_{iyc}$ are the class-dependent cumulative item parameters. Without the classification index c, this model is equivalent to the partial-credit model (Masters, 1982).

The development of estimation equations and algorithms for the necessary calculations of symmetric functions in conditional maximum likelihood (CML) estimation for polytomous (mixed) RMs with and without constraints on the α parameters is outlined in von Davier & Rost (1995). This allows one to estimate more parsimonious models than the partial-credit mixed RM, such as mixture-distribution versions of Andrich's rating-scale model (Andrich, 1978) and Rost's successive-intervals model (Rost, 1988) originally formulated for LCA for ordinal data.

Note that each latent class $c = 1, \ldots, C$ has its unique set of item parameters in the unconstrained mixed RM. This means that the number of parameters to be estimated in these models grows linearly with the number of latent classes C.

As an example, the number of item parameters for ten items with four response categories each is equal to 30 for the partial-credit model, since the four response categories $x \in \{0, \ldots, 3\}$ require three threshold parameters β_{ix} for $x = 1, 2, 3$ in this model. If the mixed partial-credit model is assumed to hold in a discrete mixture RM with four latent classes, this increases the number to a total of 120 item parameters that have to be estimated. Note that, in addition to these item parameters, mixture-distribution models also model the joint distribution of the unobserved (θ, c), for which additional parameters have to be estimated for each outcome $c = 1, \ldots, C$. This means that the sample size required for an unconstrained mixture model to be estimable with the same accuracy as a one-population model should at least be multiplied by the number of classes C in the model. Note that this does not mean that the model parameter cannot be estimated with smaller samples, but the standard errors of parameter estimates will increase when the number of classes is increased, since the same number of observations are distributed across more classes, and hence class-specific parameter estimates rely on fewer observations in each class c.

However, for moderate numbers of classes and appropriate sample sizes, mixed RMs for dichotomous and polytomous data can be estimated efficiently with the EM-algorithm (von Davier, 1994, 2001). Parsimonious ways to constrain the conditional ability distributions using a two-parameter loglinear smoothing were developed that can be used to save parameters (von Davier, 1994). These smoothed score distributions are described in the next section together with the conditional maximum likelihood (CML) framework for mixture-distribution RMs.

6.2.4 Conditional Mixed Rasch Models and Latent Score Distributions

Rewriting the RM in its conditional form is useful both for estimation as well as for studying similarities with other models. The conditional form of the RM makes use of the fact that the total score $r = \sum_i x_i$ is a sufficient statistic for the person parameter θ.

The Conditional Framework for Rasch Models

The conditional form of the RM has been mentioned in the introduction to this volume as well as in other chapters. Here, we state the mixed RM in conditional form, which allows us to rewrite the conditional probabilities of a response vector $\boldsymbol{x}$ given class membership c and observed total score r as

$$p(\boldsymbol{x} \mid \theta, c, r) = \frac{p(\boldsymbol{x}, r \mid \theta, c)}{p(r \mid \theta, c)} = \frac{\exp(-\sum \beta_{ix_ic})}{\sum_{\boldsymbol{y}|r} \exp(-\sum \beta_{iy_ic})},$$

since the term $r\theta$ can be eliminated in this fraction. The sum in the denominator includes all possible response vectors $\boldsymbol{y}$ with the same raw score $r(\boldsymbol{y}) = r(\boldsymbol{x}) = \sum_i x_i$.

The denominator $\gamma_{rc}(\beta_{..}) = \sum_{\boldsymbol{y}|r} \exp(-\sum \beta_{iy_ic})$ is the class-c-specific form of an expression that is commonly referred to as a symmetric function of order r in the context of the conditional RM. These symmetric functions exist for each of the possible raw scores $r = 0, \ldots, R_{\max}$ where $R_{\max} = \sum_i m_i$ is the maximum raw score for the set of items under consideration. Andersen (1972) and Gustafsson (1980) present accurate and fast summation algorithms to compute the symmetric functions for the RM, and von Davier & Rost (1995) provide an efficient algorithm for calculating these functions for a variety of constrained and unconstrained polytomous RMs and polytomous mixture RMs.

Let $\pi_{r|c}$ denote the probability of raw score r in class c. Then we may write

$$p(\boldsymbol{x} \mid c) = p(\boldsymbol{x}, r \mid c) = \pi_{r|c} \frac{\exp(-\sum \beta_{ix_ic})}{\gamma_{rc}(\beta_{..})}, \qquad (6.5)$$

since $p(\boldsymbol{x}, r(\boldsymbol{x})) = p(\boldsymbol{x})$ and $p(\boldsymbol{x}, s) = 0$ if $s \neq r(\boldsymbol{x})$. The above expression does not contain the person parameter θ. Eliminating the θ parameter using the conditional formulation of the RM enables one to estimate the item parameters without having to jointly estimate the N person parameters. One of the advantages of conditional estimation is that it avoids a problem encountered when the number of parameters increases with sample size (see Kiefer & Wolfowitz, 1956; Neyman & Scott, 1948). By eliminating the "nuisance" parameters θ_v, which increase with sample size N, the consistency of item-parameter estimates can be ensured.

Rost & von Davier (1995) outlined the conditional estimation of the dichotomous mixed Rasch model using the EM algorithm. In von Davier & Rost (1995), estimation equations are developed for the conditional estimation of polytomous mixed RMs, i.e., the conditional mixed partial-credit model and other ordinal RMs for polytomous data such as the rating-scale model (Andrich, 1978).

Kelderman (1984, 1995) described loglinear (mixed) RMs; see also Chapter 5 in this volume. The conditional RM is closely related to a loglinear model $\log n_{x_1,\ldots,x_I,r} = \lambda + \lambda_r - \sum_i \beta_{x_i}$ that incorporates a term λ_r for the raw score $r = \sum_i x_i$ into the model (Kelderman & Macready, 1990). The reader is referred to Chapter 5 for information and examples of how to estimate extended RMs with general loglinear modeling software, for example, the LEM software (Vermunt, 1997a).

Latent Score Distributions

In the ordinary RM, the raw-score probabilities π_r may be written without the index c, since there is only one population and since no latent class index is required. Then, these proportions may be directly estimated by

$$\hat{\pi}_r = \frac{n(r)}{N},$$

where $n(r)$ refers to the observed sample frequency of score r and N is the total sample size.

In the mixed RM, the estimation of $\pi_{r|c}$ cannot be carried out in the same direct manner, since the frequency of score r in class c is not directly observable. Let $n(r \mid c)$ denote this frequency in the following equations. The $\pi_{r|c}$ for $r = 0, \dots, R_{\max}$ have to be treated as latent score distributions in each class c and need to be replaced by estimates. For example, in the EM algorithm the $\hat{\pi}_{r|c}$ are aggregated as a part of the generation of expected counts in the E-step.

The $\pi_{r|c}$ quickly amount to a large number of parameters (depending on the number of classes C and the maximum total score $R_{\max}$), which have to be estimated in addition to the item parameters β_{ixc}. This is especially true if mixed RMs for polytomous data are considered. For $r \in \{0, \dots, R_{\max}\}$ there are $R_{\max}$ independent $\pi_{r|c}$'s. The maximum raw score is given by $R_{\max} = \sum_i m_i$ assuming that m_i is the maximum category for item i and $x_i \in \{0, \dots, m_i\}$. As an example, for ten items with four categories $(0, 1, 2, 3)$ each, there are $R_{\max} = 30 = 10 \times 3$ parameters necessary for estimating the latent score distribution, that is, 30 in each latent class.

A simple loglinear smoothing approach is used by von Davier (1994), and described in more detail in Rost & von Davier (1995), to parametrize the $\pi_{r|c}$ more parsimoniously. In this model for the latent score distributions, it is assumed that

$$\hat{\pi}_{r|c} = \frac{\exp\left(\tau_c \times \frac{r}{R_{\max}} + \delta_c \times g(r, R_{\max})\right)}{\sum_s \exp\left(\tau_c \times \frac{s}{R_{\max}} + \delta_c \times g(s, R_{\max})\right)} \tag{6.6}$$

holds with $g(r, R_{\max}) = \frac{4r(R_{\max} - r)}{R_{\max}^2}$ with location parameter τ_c and dispersion parameter δ_c.

Obviously, this can be also written as a loglinear model

$$\ln \frac{\pi_{r|c}}{\pi_{0|c}} = \tau_c \times \frac{r}{R_{\max}} + \delta_c \times g(r, R_{\max})$$

of the log-odds ratio of π_r against π_0. This approach utilizes only 2 instead of $R_{\max}$ parameters to model the latent score distributions by introducing a parametric family of discrete distributions. Holland & Thayer (2000) demonstrated the use of loglinear models for discrete score distributions in the context of presmoothing for test-equating purposes (Moses et al., 2004).

The most striking advantage of using loglinear smoothing of score distributions lies in the fact that the number of score-distribution parameters can be greatly reduced. This is especially true if there are multiple score distributions that are indirectly observed, as is the case in mixture RMs. In these cases, this loglinear restriction enables one to use a parametric family of discrete score distributions that is quite flexible in fitting a variety of shapes, and in many cases adds a positive side effect of making parameter estimation more stable. This is partly due to the fact that unobserved score distributions in multiple populations may contain very small counts (especially for the smaller latent classes), and a loglinear smoothing like the one introduced earlier ensures that the counts stay positive and ensures that the model avoids zero counts. As with all smoothing techniques, the main drawback is that the observed marginal distribution of raw scores is not fitted perfectly. When using this approach with mixture RMs, however, the marginal raw score distribution is fitted by a mixture of loglinear smoothed distributions, which makes for a rather flexible family of distributions.

6.3 HYBRID Mixture Rasch Models

The HYBRID model (Yamamoto, 1989) represents a discrete mixture-distribution model that allows different item response models to hold in the different components of the mixture. This is a deviation from the population homogeneity assumption that goes somewhat further than assuming that different parameter sets may hold in different subpopulations. In this sense, the HYBRID model is unlike most mixture-distribution models treated in the literature. This is one way to look at HYBRID models, but in this generality, the previous statement seems true and false at the same time, since concrete realizations of the HYBRID model can often be expressed in the following way: HYBRID models may more accurately be represented as discrete mixture models for item response data with mixture components that contain different degrees of constraints in the different mixture components. As an example, consider a model that combines a latent-class-type component and a Rasch-type mixture component. These two mixture components may be represented either as two different models, or as a mixture of two Rasch-type classes, where one of the classes is constrained such that there is no ability variation in that class.

More formally, a HYBRID model may be written as

$$P(\boldsymbol{x} = x_1, \ldots, x_I) = \sum_{c=1}^{C} \pi_c P_{Mo(c)}(\boldsymbol{x}|c),$$

where $P_{Mo(c)}$ represents the notion that different mixture components may include different parameter constraints representing the qualitatively different ways members of the respective classes are responding to the items.

A typical application of the HYBRID model is to fit data where one portion of the respondents are assumed to respond in "random" mode, maybe due to a lack of motivation, whereas another portion of the sample are assumed to respond in a way that can be modeled using an RM. This "Rasch" portion may be viewed as the sample that follows the instructions and tries to respond to the test items according to their ability.

In a case like this, the HYBRID RM for dichotomous data assumes that

$$P(x) = \pi_{rasch}\pi_{r|rasch}\frac{\exp(-\sum \beta_{ix_i})}{\gamma_r(\beta_{..})} + \pi_{lca}\prod_{i=1}^{I}p(x_i \mid lca),$$

where the $\pi_{rasch} = 1 - \pi_{lca}$ denotes the proportion of the subpopulation conforming to the RM, and π_{lca} is the relative size of the latent class type subpopulation.

The question whether a model with a HYBRID structure is appropriate to fit a data set can be answered only in connection with a substantive research hypothesis. If there is indeed a very specific hypothesis for why a certain subsample might respond completely randomly to all items, the HYBRID model proves to be a useful tool in identifying this portion of the sample (Yamamoto, 1989). If noncognitive factors are considered to play a role, assuming that one part of the sample may in fact drop out from responding systematically seems quite plausible. Measures of goodness-of-fit allow one to check the need for assuming additional random-response classes, so that models employing a potentially unnecessary high level of complexity can be identified.

6.3.1 Extensions of HYBRID Rasch Models

The HYBRID model was extended to a model for polytomous data, where mixtures of Rasch models and latent-class models with more than one component in each model category as well as with different polytomous RMs may be combined (von Davier, 1994, 1996). Moreover, the different RM mixture components may differ with respect to their parameter restrictions both in the latent-class components and the RM components.

Applications of polytomous HYBRID RMs and polytomous mixed RMs are presented in von Davier (1997) and Rost et al. (1997). Eid & Rauber (2000) identify a small set of random responders in organizational surveys using mixtures of RMs.

6.3.2 The Speededness Model

Yamamoto & Everson (1997) described the speededness model, a HYBRID model (Yamamoto, 1989) with a complex set of constraints that describe the switch from an ability-driven response behavior to a series of random responses under speeded testing conditions. For recent extensions and applications of this model, see Chapter 9 in this volume.

The speededness model assumes that each observation may be classified according to a switching point, where response behavior is no longer guided by the person's ability and may no longer be described by an IRT model with a quantitative ability variable. Beyond this switching point, response behavior follows a random process, which is assumed to be independent of the person's ability parameter and to be sufficiently described by item-specific response probabilities, independent of latent ability level or class membership. For small and moderately sized samples, the speededness model may be estimated using MCMC (Gilks et al., 1996). Bolt et al. (2002) as well as Boughton & Yamamoto (2004) estimated the model using the general MCMC software WINBUGS (Spiegelhalter et al., 2003). For larger samples, computationally more efficient algorithms should be considered.

Yamamoto & Everson (1997) (see Chapter 9 in this volume) use an EM algorithm based on the HYBIL software (Yamamoto, 1987) to estimate the speededness model. This implementation has been used to detect and model speededness for data sets from operational large-scale testing programs.

6.4 Borrowing Information About the Mixture

Borrowing information about the latent ability distribution from background data is a useful technique if information from the item responses is insufficient. This is, for example, the case in large-scale educational survey assessments, where individual ability estimates are not the focus of inference (Mislevy, 1987). In such cases, individual item response vectors are often very sparse, since each student responds to one of a number of test booklets that contain only a small selection of items. However, additional noncognitive variables on the student level may be available in abundance through school databases and background questionnaires that do not impose high cognitive demands on students.

The general idea is straightforward: The conditional distribution of the latent cognitive proficiency variable can be assumed to be more concentrated (e.g., of smaller variance in the case of normally distributed, continuous ability variables) given the different levels of student background data than the marginal distribution across all students. This holds if student background data are related to the proficiency variable. Examples may include background variables such as socioeconomic status (SES) of students' parents as well as number of hours spent in front of the TV. More specifically, if an IRT model distinguishes between groups defined by a background variable (example: three levels of SES) that correlates with the proficiency variable, the conditional proficiency distributions defined by the grouping variable can be expected to be less variable than the marginal distribution across the different levels of the background data. This observation can then be used to define a more appropriate prior distribution of student proficiency in order to improve estimation of subgroup proficiency averages and variances. Methods drawing on similar arguments are in operational use in several national and international educational surveys such as the National Assessment of Educational Progress (NAEP), the Programme for International Student Assessment (PISA), and the Trends in Mathematics and Science Study (TIMSS). See Chapter 4 in this volume for details on how an approach using covariates to determine conditional ability distributions is implemented in large-scale survey assessments.

The same idea of conditioning on available background data may be applied to a categorical latent variable, in our case a variable that represents latent-class memberships in a mixture model. Given one or more conditioning background variables, the multinomial distribution of the class variable will be more concentrated around certain latent classes as compared to the overall distribution, assuming that class membership and background variables are not independently distributed.

More formally, assume we have a latent categorical variable C and a covariate Z with $P(c) = \sum_z P(z)P(c \mid z)$. Let $\boldsymbol{x}$ denote the item responses as before. If Z and C and not independent, we have $P(c \cap z) \neq P(c)P(z)$ for at least some pairs (c, z) and it follows that

$$P(c \mid \boldsymbol{x}, z) = \frac{p(\boldsymbol{x} \mid c)p(c \mid z)}{\sum_{c'} p(\boldsymbol{x} \mid c')p(c' \mid z)} \neq P(c \mid \boldsymbol{x}).$$

In which cases do we expect that this inequality can be utilized for our purpose of predicting the class membership c more appropriately? Obviously, we gain accuracy if the true class membership is c, where $p(c \mid \boldsymbol{x}, z) > p(c \mid \boldsymbol{x})$ for this c and $p(c \mid \boldsymbol{x}, z) > p(c' \mid \boldsymbol{x}, z)$ for all $c' \neq c$. In plain words, the posterior distribution given $(\boldsymbol{x}, z)$ should be more concentrated than given $\boldsymbol{x}$ alone. In this case, we actually improve accuracy when predicting the class membership using both $\boldsymbol{x}$ and z as compared to using $\boldsymbol{x}$ alone.

6.4.1 Covariates of Mixture Components and Partial Knowledge of Class Membership

In order to increase the precision of posterior classification probabilities, Smit and colleagues (Smit et al., 1999) used collateral background information together with item responses to estimate class memberships. Smit et al. (1999) and Smit et al. (2000) developed a dichotomous mixture IRT model in which the posterior probabilities of class membership are calculated using background variables. They showed that the knowledge about background variables can substantially improve correct classification rates in cases in which class membership and background data are correlated.

von Davier & Yamamoto (2004b) developed a mixture-distribution generalized partial-credit model (GPCM; Muraki, 1992) and extended the estimation of mixture IRT models by developing a general method for incorporating class or group membership into these models. In latent-class models, class membership is treated as an unobserved variable, whereas multiple-group models treat class or group membership as observed without error.

The approach developed by von Davier & Yamamoto (2004b) allows one to treat class membership as a random variable with partially missing observations, or observed with error. Technically, this is handled by assuming different prior distributions for each observation, one that is based on the class sizes π_c for observations with unknown class membership and another one that is deterministic, i.e., $\pi_c^* = 1$ if the class membership g is known and equals c and $\pi_{c'}^* = 0$ for $c' \neq g$.

This approach provides a general way of incorporating covariate information on the classification variables. Instead of defining only two distinct priors, this allows one to use covariate information to define examinee-level prior distributions for the classification into the mixture components.

6.4.2 Mixtures of Diagnostic Rasch Models

von Davier & Yamamoto (2004a) and von Davier (2005) developed a framework for a general diagnostic model (GDM) that allows one to test hypotheses about skill requirements or item attributes using a design matrix.

The central building block of most, if not all, diagnostic models is a design matrix that is often referred to as a Q-matrix (Tatsuoka, 1983), an $I \times K$ matrix that relates the I items to K skills/attributes/dimensions. The entries q_{ik} are integers in most cases, often $q_{ik} \in \{0, 1\}$. The Q-matrix can be understood as the structural component of the model defining a hypothesis as to which items require which combination of skills.

von Davier (2005) presented a general diagnostic model that utilizes a multidimensional discrete version of the (mixture) generalized partial-credit model. This model, pGDM, is suitable for dichotomous and ordinal responses $x \in \{0, 1, 2, \ldots, m_i\}$. The model equation for a mixture Rasch version of the pGDM is

$$P(X = x \mid \beta_{i..}, a_., q_{i.}, c) = \frac{\exp\left[\beta_{xic} + \sum_{k=1}^{K} x\gamma_k q_{ik} a_k\right]}{1 + \sum_{y=1}^{m_i} \exp\left[\beta_{yic} + \sum_{k=1}^{K} y\gamma_k q_{ik} a_k\right]} \quad (6.7)$$

with K attributes (discrete latent traits) $a = (a_1, \ldots, a_K)$, latent class c and a design Q-matrix $(q_{ik})_{i=1,\ldots,I, k=1,\ldots,K}$. The β_{ixc} are difficulty parameters, the γ_k are skill or attribute specific slope parameters. This parametrization makes use of the fact that the RM can be viewed as a two-parameter IRT model with one common slope parameter for all items. The GDM allows one common slope per skill, so that it coincides with the RM if only one skill variable with a limited set of ordinal levels is assumed (see Chapter 11 by Formann in this volume). The a_k are discrete scores determined before estimation and can be chosen by the user. These scores are used to assign real numbers to the skill levels, for example $a(0) = -1.0$ and $a(1) = +1.0$ may be chosen for dichotomous skills. For ordinal skills with s_k levels, the a_k may be defined using $a(x) = x$ for $x = 0, \ldots, (s_k - 1)$ or $a(0) = -s_k/2, \ldots, a(s_k - 1) = s_k/2$.

The RM variant of the GDM does not estimate slope parameters for each item by skill combination, and treats the Q matrix as fixed and known. The mixture-distribution version of this constrained Rasch GDM already contains LCA, the mixed RM, as well as multiple-classification latent-class models (Maris, 1999) as special cases. This class of constrained GDMs can be viewed as discrete multidimensional mixture IRT models. The estimation algorithm used in *mdltm* was validated in a parameter recovery study using simulated data and through a comparison of diagnostic modeling approaches based on real data (von Davier, 2005). Xu & von Davier (2006) apply the GDM to sparse-matrix samples of item responses, and have presented a successful parameter-recovery study for such data. In that study, the GDM was used to analyze data from the National Assessment of Educational Progress (NAEP), and the authors described how to aggregate results for policy-relevant subgroups using this diagnostic mixture model. von Davier et al., 2006 present a shortlist of models for cognitive diagnosis ranging from the rule space methodology (Tatsuoka, 1983) to current research and applications of the GDM.

The GDM as implemented in the *mdltm* software (von Davier, 2005) can be used to estimate mixture versions of the RM and the partial-credit model, as well multidimensional mixture versions of this model.

6.5 Estimation

For conditional and marginal maximum likelihood (CML and MML) estimation, the estimation maximization (EM) algorithm (Bock & Aitkin, 1981) has proven to be very useful in the context of estimating RMs and mixture RMs. Markov-chain Monte Carlo (MCMC) estimation of IRT models has been suggested (Patz & Junker, 1999b,a) as an alternative to ML techniques. MCMC methods claim to allow estimation of more complex extensions of IRT models, since the implementation of models using MCMC does not require finding roots of likelihood functions and implementing estimation equations. Bolt et al. (2001, 2002) have used MCMC methods as implemented in BUGS or Win-BUGS (Spiegelhalter et al., 1996, 2003) for estimating mixed RMs (Rost, 1990) and variants of the HYBRID model (Yamamoto, 1989; Yamamoto & Everson, 1995). The downside of using MCMC is computational cost, since MCMC calculations to estimate parameters for models using moderately sized data structures (tens of items and a few thousands of examinees) may take hours even on modern computer hardware as compared to minutes or seconds using customary methods like the EM algorithm.

Recently, ways of estimating RMs and extensions of RMs, as well as more general IRT models with general-purpose statistical software packages such as STATA, SAS, as well as R and SPLUS, have been explored (De Boeck & Wilson, 2004; Skrondal & Rabe-Hesketh, 2004). This approach is a useful line of research, for example in cases in which several different versions of models are experimented with or analysis output needs to be embedded or reintegrated into a larger database using standard software for statistical analysis.

Estimating multivariate or mixture-distribution latent-variable models with standard statistical software and/or MCMC methods is a useful way to prototype new models or to try out extensions of existing models, but operational needs may require the implementation of computationally more efficient estimation methods once the different components of the model extensions are understood.

The mixed RMs can be estimated using conditional maximum likelihood techniques with WINMIRA 2001 (von Davier, 2001). HYBRID IRT models can be estimated using HYBIL II (Yamamoto, 1993) and HYBRID RMs can be estimated using WINMIRA 2001. Log-linear (mixed) RMs can be estimated using LOGIMO (Kelderman & Steen, 1993) and LEM (Vermunt, 1997a). Mixture versions of the general diagnostic RM (GDM) can be estimated using marginal maximum likelihood as implemented in the *mdltm* software (von Davier, 2005).

6.6 Areas of Applications and Outlook

Examples of the use of Rasch-type mixture models are given in the applications chapters of this volume. The reader is referred to these chapters for details on these applications. Here, domains of application, rather than examples in which the mixed RM has a proven record of utility, will be surveyed. These domains include goodness of fit, assessment of strategy differences and strategy shifts, testing for multidimensionality, and a general approach to assess differential item functioning (DIF) for single items or groups of items.

Goodness-of-Fit Testing: Rost & von Davier (1995) suggested testing the ordinary RM versus the 2-class mixture RM. This procedure allows one to check whether the sample for which the RM is assumed can be viewed as homogeneous, or whether subgroups with different sets of item parameters need to be distinguished. Based on work by Efron (1979) on bootstrap resimulation methods and applications of these methods by Langeheine et al. (1996), von Davier (1997) developed a framework for testing mixture-distribution item response models using resimulation methods. Testing ordinary item response theory models by means of comparisons with mixture IRT models can be viewed as a generalized approach for testing for differential item functioning (DIF; Holland & Wainer, 1993). Discrete mixtures of IRT models do not require the formation of focus and comparison groups, since mixture models optimize the group allocations by finding maximally homogeneous subpopulations for a given number of mixture components.

Strategy Differences and Strategy Shifts: The application of different strategies by different subpopulations in solving a set of cognitive items may be viewed as the foundational example for mixture IRT models and mixed RMs. In 1990, three independently published papers addressed the problem of observing differential profiles of item difficulties given certain strategy differences in solving items. Rost (1990), Mislevy & Verhelst (1990), and Kelderman & Macready (1990) all addressed this issue by devising mixture-distribution versions of commonly used models for item response data. Prior to that, Yamamoto (1987) developed a model that combined an IRT mixture component for students who solve the items using their skills with an independence class for examinees who show a random response pattern instead of using a more promising strategy to solve the items. Since then, many applications of mixture Rasch and IRT models have been used to model and identify differences in response behavior that may be attributed to strategy differences. See Chapter 20 in this volume for further examples.

Multidimensionality: Modeling response processes involves decisions about where to attribute response variance. Common questions involve whether different testing modes or situational effects lead to systematic differences in responses or whether more than one skill or ability is involved in producing differences in response probabilities that cannot be explained by a unidimensional variable. The underlying question is whether within-item multidimensionality of abilities or population heterogeneity with respect to item difficulties (or a combination of both) is the reason for observed deviations from unidimensionality. In multidimensional IRT (MIRT), the conditional probability of an item response depends on more than one continuous person (ability) variable. In most mixture IRT models, the conditional probabilities depend on one continuous person (ability) variable, along with a categorical person (type or strategy) variable. In diagnostic mixture IRT models (von Davier, 2005) such distinctions become somewhat obsolete, since the general diagnostic model allows much greater flexibility in defining categorical, located, ordinal, and (pseudo) continuous person variables. Nevertheless, observing the need for a categorical mixing variable may be viewed as a discrete realization of multidimensionality, since the different outcomes of the mixing variable moderate the conditional response variable in addition to one or more continuous person variables.

Mixture-distribution models for item response data range from LCA to mixture versions of diagnostic item response models with multiple skill variables. RMs play an important part in defining the model that holds within all or some of the mixture components. Common to all mixture-distribution item response models is the assumption that the observed data stem from a composite population with an unknown number of mixture components. The aim of mixture IRT models is therefore twofold: to identify homogeneous (sub-)populations in which the class-specific model assumptions are met, and to unmix the sample into these unobserved homogeneous components of the population.

The increasing complexity of models that are available within the mixing component may counteract the necessity for mixtures to some extent. For example, the mixed RM accounts for ability differences within the mixture components, whereas LCA assumes no differences in conditional response probabilities within each class. A multiparameter IRT model such as the 2PL will allow even more flexibility and may remove the need for more than one mixture component at the cost of losing some of the unique mathematical properties of RMs. This may be desirable from the perspective of flexibility, but it may prove less desirable from the perspective of model selection, and from the perspective of studying how different examinees solve the items using different strategies, or using no strategies at all. The reasoning attributed to Ben Wright, "The items are not guessing, the examinees are," illustrates this dilemma. It may seem useful to model guessing in terms of a more flexible item-characteristic curve, but it does not allow for the identification of those examinees who actually are guessing on the majority of the items. In contrast, applying the HYBRID model allows exactly this by assuming a comparably more constrained item response function in the Rasch mixing component, and assuming complete random responses for the guessing class. This enables one to estimate the proportion in the sample that produces responses indistinguishable from a random process.

While a greater flexibility in choosing among different model assumptions can be viewed as desirable, the reality is that substantive research seldom provides hypotheses that are specific enough to suggest which model is most appropriate. Therefore, many different alternatives may be chosen, estimated, and checked. Among these, several models may provide comparable model–data fit and thus challenge the researcher in making a final choice. Parsimony and the requirements of the specific application provide some guidance here, so that the number of models that will actually be carried to the next level of consideration will hopefully be small. Measures of model–data fit can only guide one so far, since a comparison based on observed and expected responses relies only on comparisons within the set of observed variables on which the models are based. Advisable are comparisons using cross validation or external validation techniques, so that predictions based on more- or less-complex models are compared with respect to their utility in predicting behavior outside of the testing situation or at least outside of the sample used for parameter estimation and model selection.

Part II

Generalized Models—Specific Research Questions

Application of the Saltus Model to Stagelike Data: Some Applications and Current Developments

Karen Draney and Mark Wilson

University of California, Berkeley

7.1 Background of the Saltus Model

The saltus model was developed in dichotomous form by Wilson (1989), and expanded to polytomous form by Draney (1996) as a method for detecting and analyzing discontinuities in performance that are hypothesized to occur as a result of rapidly occurring person growth (e.g.,Fischer, Pipp, & Bullock, 1984). Such discontinuities are often theorized to occur as the result of progression through developmental stages or levels. The most influential such theory was developed by Jean Piaget (e.g., Piaget, 1950; Inhelder & Piaget, 1958). Although Piagetian theory has been somewhat controversial of late (e.g., Lourenço & Machado, 1996), there is still a strong interest in stagelike development in a number of areas, including moral and ethical reasoning (e.g., Dawson, 2002; Kohlberg & Candee, 1984), evaluative reasoning (e.g., Dawson-Tunik, 2002; Armon, 1984), adult development (e.g., Commons et al., 1998; Fischer, Hand, & Russel, 1984), and cognitive development (e.g., Bond, 1995b,a; Bond & Bunting, 1995; Demetriou & Efklides, 1989, 1994; Hiele, 1986).

The work of Piaget describes the cognitive developmental stages through which children progress as they grow. In particular, school-age children progress from the preoperational stage, through the concrete operational stage, to the formal operational stage. In the preoperational stage, children are able for the first time to produce mental representations of objects and events, but unable to consistently perform logical mental operations with these representations. In the concrete operational stage, children are able to perform logical operations, but only on representations of concrete objects. In the formal operational stage, which starts to occur around the beginning of adolescence, children are able to perform abstract operations on abstractions as well as concrete objects.

According to Piaget, progress from stage to stage is characterized by more than simple linear growth in reasoning ability. The transition from one stage to another involves a major reorganization of the thinking processes used by children to solve various sorts of problems. Theories with similar structure, but perhaps different substantive focus, are described by the many neo-Piagetian researchers, and by other researchers who use stage-based theories.

Researchers in the Piagetian tradition are using increasingly complex statistical and psychometric models to analyze their data. Béland & Mislevy (1996) analyze proportional reasoning tasks using Bayesian inference networks. Noelting et al. (1995) discuss the advantages of Rasch scaling for the understanding of Piagetian tasks. Bond (1995b,a) discusses the implications of RMs for Piagetian theory and philosophy.

In addition, researchers in psychometrics have begun wrestling with the problem of developing and applying models with sufficient complexity to address such substantive issues. For example, the three-parameter model has been used diagnostically by researchers such as Yen (1985). She describes patterns of problematic item fit that are sometimes observed in analyzing complex data and asserts that these may be indicators for increasing item complexity. Differences in item complexity such as she describes could potentially be indicative of a set of items that represent more than one developmental stage.

Another approach to the problem of incorporating different response patterns and their associations with classes is given by latent-class modeling. For example, Dayton & Macready (1976) applied this approach to behavioral hierarchies of the type often seen in developmental theories. In this approach, each underlying class is represented by a set of response probabilities to the items in question. Whereas Yen's (1985) research might be considered exploratory, latent-class theory can be used in a more confirmatory way. Additional examples of such models and their uses are given in Rijmen & De Boeck (2003), Formann (1992), and Croon (1990),

However, Rost (1988) states that the defining feature of latent-class models is the characteristic that all persons within a latent class have the same probabilities of answering a set of items correctly, and thus (if considered in an educational context) the same ability or proficiency. It is plausible that children within a given developmental stage might vary in overall proficiency within that stage.

The saltus model was developed to combine the advantages of the RM, including varying person proficiency, and latent-class modeling, including differing patterns of response probability across different latent subgroups of persons. In this way, it is similar in its origins to the HYBRID model (Yamamoto, 1989; compare also Chapter 4 in this volume), a latent-class model that included as one of the classes a "catch-all" latent-trait model for those persons who did not fit well into one of the other classes. However, unlike the HYBRID model, the saltus model provides a latent-trait model within each of the latent classes identified.

7.2 The Saltus Model

The saltus model is based on the assumption that there are C classes, representing developmental stages or levels. Each level is represented by a set of items, which are constructed such that only persons at or above the developmental stage represented by those items are fully equipped to answer them correctly, and once persons enter that developmental stage, they should gain a substantial advantage in answering those items.

In the discussion to follow, the terms "person class" and "item group" will be used. This is merely a device used for clarity when it is necessary to differentiate between classes of persons and groups of items, and does not have any particular substantive significance.

The saltus model assumes that all persons in class c answer all items in a manner consistent with membership in that class. However, persons within a class may differ by proficiency. In a Piagetian context, this means that a child in, say, the concrete operational stage is always in that stage, and answers all items accordingly. The child does not show formal operational development for some items and concrete operational development for others. However, some concrete operational children may be more proficient at answering items than are other concrete operational children.

In the saltus model, two parameters describe a person v: a unidimensional proficiency parameter θ_v, and an indicator vector for class membership ϕ_v. If there are C latent person classes, then $\phi_v = (\phi_{v1}, \ldots, \phi_{vC})$, where ϕ_{vc} takes the value of 1 if person v is in class c and 0 if not. Note that only one ϕ_{vc} is theoretically nonzero; however, since it is a latent parameter, it must in practice be estimated.

Just as persons are members of only one class, items are associated with one and only one group. In a developmental context, an item's group would be said to be the first developmental stage at which a child would have all of the skills necessary to perform that item correctly. It is, of course, possible for children at lower developmental stages to perform items correctly from time to time; however, this usually occurs because of guessing or a poorly developed strategy that happens to produce the correct answer in some cases. Unlike person-class membership, however, which is unknown and must be estimated, item-group membership is known a priori, based on the theory that was used to produce the items. It will be useful to denote item-group membership by the indicator vector $\mathbf{b}_i$. As with person classes indicated by the ϕ_v, we assume that there are C item groups, and each item is member of exactly one group, i.e., $\mathbf{b}_i = (b_{i1}, \ldots, b_{iC})$, when b_{ic} takes the value of 1 if item i belongs to item class k, and 0 otherwise. The set of all $\mathbf{b}_i$ is denoted by $\mathbf{b}$.

The equation

$$P\left(X_{vij} = j|\theta_v, \phi_{vc} = 1, \beta_i, \tau_{ck}\right) = \frac{\exp \sum\limits_{s=0}^{j} (\theta v - \beta_{is} + \tau_{ck})}{\sum\limits_{t=0}^{m_i} \exp \sum\limits_{s=0}^{t} (\theta_v - \beta_{is} + \tau_{ck})} \qquad (7.1)$$

defines the probability of response j to item i, with step difficulty β_{ij}. This defines a polytomous item response model that has been augmented by the introduction of the saltus parameter τ_{ck} as an additive element of the logistic argument. The saltus parameter describes the additive effect—positive or negative—for people in class c on the item parameters of all items in group k. Typically, in developmental contexts involving stages, this has taken the form of an increase in probability of success at higher levels as the person achieves the stage at which an item is located, indicated by $\tau_{ck} > 0$ when $c \geq k$ (although this need not be the case). The saltus parameters can be represented as a C x C matrix $\mathbf{T}$.

The probability that a person with parameters ϕ_v and θ_v will respond in category j to item i is given by

$$P\left(X_{vij} = j|\theta_v, \phi_v, b_i, \beta_i, T\right) = \prod_h \prod_k P(X_{vij} = j|\theta_v, \phi_{nh} = 1, b_i, \tau_{hk})^{\phi_{vh} b_{ik}}.$$

$$(7.2)$$

Note that for only one combination of c and k do the product terms have a nonzero exponent $\phi_{vc} b_{ik}$. Since item responses are assumed to be independent given θ_v, ϕ_v, and all of the item and saltus parameters, the model-based probability of a response vector is

$$P\left(X_v =_v |\theta_v, f_v, b_i, \beta_i, T\right) = \prod_h \prod_k \prod_i P(X_{vij} = x_{ij}|\theta_v, \phi_{vh} = 1, b_i, \tau_{hk})^{\phi_{vh} b_{ik}}.$$

$$(7.3)$$

The saltus model requires a number of constraints on the parameters. For item-step parameters, we use two traditional constraints: first, $\beta_{i0} = 0$ for every item, and second, the sum of all the β_{ij} across all items is set equal to zero. Some constraints are also necessary on the saltus parameters. This could be accomplished in several ways, but once parameters have been estimated with one set of restrictions, they can be translated to corresponding values under another set. The set of constraints we have chosen is the same as that used by Mislevy & Wilson (1996), and will allow us to interpret the saltus parameters as changes relative to the first (lowest) developmental stage. Two sets of constraints are used. First $\tau_{c1} = 0$; thus, the difficulty of the first (lowest) group of items is held constant for all person classes; changes in the difficulty of groups of items for $k > 1$ are interpreted with respect to this first group of items for all person classes. Also $\tau_{1k} = 0$; thus, items as seen by person classes with $c > 1$ will be interpreted relative to the difficulty of those items as seen by person class 1.

The saltus model is a special case of the more general *mixed RM* described by Rost (1990, compare also Chapter 6 in this volume). The estimation of polytomous mixed RMs with and without constraints using conditional maximum likelihood methods is discussed in von Davier & Rost (1995). This model is itself a member of the class of finite mixture-distribution models (e.g.,Titterington et al., 1985; Everitt & Hand, 1981). Perhaps the most general of such models to have been discussed in an educational context is the mixture multidimensional random coefficients multinomial logit (M^2RCML) model described by Pirolli & Wilson (1998).

7.3 An Example Application

An example of the application of the saltus model will be based on a set of responses to Noelting's (1980a; 1980b) orange juice mixtures test for assessing proportional reasoning. The items in this test consist of pictures of a certain number of glasses of juice and glasses of water, representing a mixture. In each item, the child is shown two such mixtures and asked which would taste more strongly of juice, or if they would taste the same. A representation of such an item is shown in Figure 7.1.

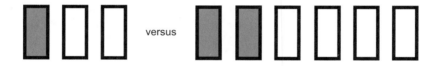

Fig. 7.1. Representation of Noelting juice mixture item. Dark indicates juice, light indicates water.

Noelting postulates a Piagetian stage hierarchy consisting of three stages— the intuitive, the concrete operational, and the formal operational—for persons solving these items. Noelting develops juice mixture problems to represent the skills that differentiate between each developmental stage.

In the intuitive stage, the child can additively compare the relative quantity of an attribute (e.g., more glasses of juice or more glasses of water), but tends to pay attention only to one attribute or the other. In the concrete operational stage, the child begins to learn the concept of ratio and proportionality. Rather than simply comparing the number of glasses of juice or water between the two mixtures, the child is able to recognize the concept of "one glass of juice for every glass of water" or "twice as much juice as water." In the formal operational stage, the child learns to deal formally with fractions, ratios, and percentages. Here, the child begins to master the formal mathematical rules for comparing two arbitrary mixtures. For this example, we will consider the items developed for the first two stages (the intuitive and the concrete operational).

Noelting postulates three problem types (representing ordered substages) within a stage and develops between one and four replications of each of these substage problem types. These problem types and replications are described in Table 7.1. The items were administered to a sample of 460 subjects ranging in age from 5 to 17 years. The number of persons at each age is given in Table 7.2.

Table 7.1. Noelting items

Item	Stage	Mixture 1	Mixture 2
1	intuitive	4 Juice, 1 Water	1 Juice, 4 Water
2	intuitive	1 Juice, 2 Water	2 Juice, 1 Water
3	intuitive	1 Juice, 0 Water	1 Juice, 1 Water
4	intuitive	1 Juice, 2 Water	1 Juice, 3 Water
5	intuitive	2 Juice, 3 Water	1 Juice, 1 Water
6	intuitive	2 Juice, 1 Water	3 Juice, 4 Water
7	concrete	1 Juice, 1 Water	2 Juice, 2 Water
8	concrete	2 Juice, 2 Water	3 Juice, 3 Water
9	concrete	1 Juice, 2 Water	2 Juice, 4 Water
10	concrete	2 Juice, 4 Water	3 Juice, 6 Water
11	concrete	4 Juice, 3 Water	8 Juice, 6 Water
12	concrete	3 Juice, 1 Water	6 Juice, 2 Water
13	formal	3 Juice, 1 Water	5 Juice, 2 Water
14	formal	8 Juice, 3 Water	3 Juice, 1 Water
15	formal	5 Juice, 2 Water	7 Juice, 3 Water
16	formal	3 Juice, 5 Water	5 Juice, 8 Water
17	formal	1 40 %, 0 10 %, 1 Water	0 40 %, 2 10 %, 0 Water
18	formal	0 40 %, 2 10 %, 1 Water	2 40 %, 0 10 %, 4 Water
19	formal	1 40 %, 1 10 %, 1 Water	1 40 %, 0 10 %, 2 Water
20	formal	1 40 %, 1 10 %, 1 Water	2 40 %, 1 10 %, 2 Water

The saltus model to be fit to these data will be a two-stage model, comparing the intuitive and the concrete items. In this model, saltus class 1 should include the youngest children in the intuitive stage, saltus class 2 should include middle-aged children in the concrete operational stage, as well as the oldest children in the formal operational stage. In this model, there will be one between-class saltus parameter, for the older children taking the concrete operational items. This parameter is expected to be positive.

Parameter estimates and standard errors for this model are given in Table 7.3. Approximately 60% of the sample is classified into saltus class 1, and 40% into class 2. Class 1 is lower in mean proficiency than class 2. This is not surprising, since older children are in general higher in proficiency on the

Table 7.2. Ages of subjects in the Noelting sample

Age	Frequency	Percent
5	3	0,01
6	26	0,06
7	40	0,09
8	53	0,12
9	45	0,10
10	51	0,11
11	60	0,13
12	40	0,09
13	48	0,10
14	26	0,06
15	29	0,06
16	28	0,06
17	11	0,02
	Total 460	

intuitive items (i.e., less prone to errors) than are younger children, in addition to having the skills necessary to solve developmentally more complex groups of items. Also as predicted, the saltus parameter τ_{22} is statistically different from zero (with magnitude more than twice its standard error), indicating that there is some systematic effect of class membership on item performance for concrete operational items.

Recall that item difficulties as shown in Table 7.3 are interpreted relative to the lowest person class. The following is an example of how the τ parameter may be interpreted. For the lowest person class, intuitive item 1 has difficulty parameter -7.08, while concrete item 1 has difficulty parameters 1.89. For person class 2, intuitive item 1 retains the same difficulty parameter (although the mean proficiency of person class 2 is higher than for class 1, and thus the probability of correct responses to the intuitive items is higher for person class 2). However, the difficulty parameter for concrete item 1 is adjusted by τ when seen by person class 2, and thus becomes $1.89 - 5.66 = -3.77$. Not only are persons in class 2 more likely to answer items correctly than are persons in class 1 (because of the higher average proficiency of class 2), the difference between the difficulties of intuitive and concrete items is greater for persons in class 1 than it is for persons in class 2. In probability terms, this means that an average person in class 1 has a .10 probability of scoring 1 on concrete item 1. If τ had been zero (and the difficulties of concrete items had been the same for person class 2 as for person class 1), an average person in class 2 would have scored 1 with a probability of approximately .58. However, because of the size of τ, the average person scores 2 on this item with a probability greater than .99.

The interpretation of item difficulties and mean abilities for classes is often easier when these parameters are displayed in a graphical form sometimes referred to as a Wright map (Wilson, 2005) in honor of its creator, Benjamin

Table 7.3. Parameter estimates and standard errors

Parameter	Estimate	S. E.
β_1	−7.08	0.532
β_2	−6.61	0.446
β_3	−4.10	0.232
β_4	−3.75	0.218
β_5	−1.97	0.168
β_6	−2.38	0.177
β_7	1.89	0.183
β_8	1.49	0.179
β_9	5.30	0.181
β_{10}	5.89	0.164
β_{11}	5.66	0.171
β_{12}	5.66	0.171
τ_{22}	5.66	0.131
μ_1	−0.26	
σ_1	2.61	
π_1	0.59	
μ_2	2.21	
σ_2	1.72	
π_2	0.41	

D. Wright, of the University of Chicago. Maps have long been used with RMs such as the partial-credit and rating-scale models, and are incorporated into many estimation software packages for these models. These maps are not meant to decide whether a particular model fits the item response data, but they are very useful in describing which persons (here which classes) and which groups of items are close when comparing (average) ability estimate and item difficulty.

A Wright map of the mean class abilities and the item difficulties as seen by each class is given in Figure 7.2. In this figure, the units of the logit scale (the scale in which parameters for this model are estimated) are shown on the extreme left side of the page. The column to the right of this contains the mean abilities of the person classes, with a range of one standard deviation on either side of each class mean. The mean of each class is represented by the letter M followed by the class number (e.g., M1 for the mean of class 1). Similarly, the upper and lower limits of the standard deviation range are represented by the letter S and the class number; these limits are connected by dashed lines to the class mean.

The difficulty levels for the various item steps as seen by each class are shown in the remaining columns. The difficulty levels for the items as seen by class 1 are shown in the column labeled "Item difficulty," under the heading

```
                   Group 1                      Group 2
       ────────────────────────────  ──────────────────────────
Logits  proficiency  item difficulty  proficiency  item difficulty
  6.5
  6.0                     C4
  5.5                C3, C5, C6
  5.0
  4.5
  4.0                                      S2
  3.5                                       |
  3.0                                       |
  2.5                                       |
  2.0       S1           C1                 M2
  1.5        |           C2                  |
  1.0        |                               |
  0.5        |                               |            C4
  0.0        |                               S2       C3, C5, C6
 -0.5       M1
 -1.0        |
 -1.5        |
 -2.0        |           I5                              I5
 -2.5        |           I6                              I6
 -3.0       S1
 -3.5                    I4                             I4,C1
 -4.0                    I3                            I3, C2
 -4.5
 -5.0
 -5.5
 -6.0
 -6.5                    I2                              I2
 -7.0                    I1                              I1
 -7.5
```

Fig. 7.2. Wright map of person distributions and item difficulties for two groups

for class 1, and similarly for class 2. More-difficult item steps and more able persons are toward the top of the page, and less-difficult item steps and less able persons are toward the bottom of the page.

The effect of the saltus parameters can be seen quite clearly in this figure: The gap between the difficulties of the intuitive items and the concrete items is substantial for class 1. While the difficulty of the intuitive items is held fixed for both classes, the difficulty of the concrete items drops for class 2, such that the easier of the concrete items are nearly identical in difficulty to the harder intuitive items for this class.

Model-based response probabilities by a person whose proficiency was equal to the mean of each class, using the estimated parameter values, are given in Table 7.4. For the intuitive items, both classes are most likely to score 1. Response probabilities for the concrete items are quite different for the two classes, with Class 1 most likely to answer incorrectly to all of the items, while Class 2 is most likely to answer correctly. Even class 2, however, has about a 10% chance of answering all but the first two concrete items incorrectly.

Table 7.4. Item difficulty and probability of correct response by item for the average ability level of two saltus groups

	Group 1		Group 2	
Item	Difficulty	$P(X = 1)$	Difficulty	$P(X = 1)$
I1	−7.08	1.00	−7.08	1.00
I2	−6.61	1.00	−6.61	1.00
I3	−4.10	0.98	−4.10	1.00
I4	−3.75	0.97	−3.75	1.00
I5	−1.97	0.85	−1.97	0.98
I6	−2.38	0.89	−2.38	0.99
C1	1.89	0.10	−3.77	1.00
C2	1.49	0.15	−4.17	1.00
C3	5.30	0.00	−0.36	0.93
C4	5.89	0.00	0.23	0.88
C5	5.66	0.00	0.00	0.90
C6	5.66	0.00	0.00	0.90

An example set of person-response vectors, classification probabilities, ability estimates, and standard errors is given in Table 7.5. Classification probabilities are in fact estimates of the person-class-indicator parameters ϕ_c, which range from zero to one, and which sum to one for c = 1, ..., C, and thus are interpretable as probabilities. Persons such as A and B, who respond correctly only to intuitive items, are classified solidly into class 1. Even persons such as C and D, who respond correctly to all of the intuitive items, and one or two of the easier concrete items, are still most likely to be in class 1, although person D has a small probability of being in class 2. Persons such as G and H, who respond correctly to all of the intuitive items and most of the concrete items, including some of the most difficult of these, are classified into class 2, although person G, who misses two of the concrete items, still has nearly a 1 in 5 probability of being in class 1.

Persons such as E and F are more difficult to classify. These persons answer some but not all of the concrete items, including some of the more difficult ones. In addition, person F misses one of the intuitive items. These persons

Table 7.5. Example person-response strings with proficiency and classification

			Group 1			Group 2	
Person	Responses	Probability	Ability	SE	Probability	Ability	SE
A	111000 000000	1.00	−3.60	.99	.00	−3.50	.76
B	111111 000000	1.00	−0.15	1.17	.00	−1.78	.76
C	111111 010000	1.00	1.23	1.17	.00	−1.19	.77
D	111111 110000	.93	2.56	.08	.08	− .59	.79
E	111111 010101	.58	3.76	1.04	.43	0.06	.82
F	110111 000110	.43	1.23	1.17	.57	−1.19	.77
G	111111 110011	.18	4.67	.64	.82	.79	.90
H	111111 111110	.03	5.24	.65	.97	1.74	1.06

have probabilities between .4 and .6 of being in either of the two classes; essentially, they do not fall clearly into either class.[1]

The response vectors given in this table are typical of most of the response vectors in the data set; in particular, most of the persons classified as intuitive responded either like person B (responding correctly to all of the intuitive items and to none of the concrete items), or by missing only one or two of the intuitive items and still missing all of the concrete items—a total of 136 persons, or about 30%. Most of the persons classified as concrete responded like persons F and G, responding correctly to all of the intuitive and all or nearly all of the concrete items. Such persons accounted for 170, or about 37%. Relatively few persons (19 in all, or 4%) missed one or more of the intuitive items while responding correctly to some of the concrete items—persons such as F. The remaining persons either solved all of the intuitive, and one to three of the concrete items, correctly (99, or about 22% of the data set), or solved only a small number of the intuitive, and none of the concrete, items correctly (36, or about 7% of the data set).

7.4 Discussion

The use of the saltus model has allowed us to learn some interesting things about the example data set. For instance, it would seem that the saltus model is more suitable for use with these data than a latent-class model. Latent-class models are similar to mixture IRT models such as the saltus model and the mixed RM, in that they assume that the observed population is composed of latent subpopulations; however, in contrast to the latter, latent-class models include no quantitative person parameters. In latent-class models;

---

[1] In order to determine whether persons such as E and F can be fitted by the model appropriately, fit diagnostics (Molenaar, 1983) such as person-fit statistics may be used. von Davier & Molenaar (2003) present person-fit statistics that can be used with latent-class and discrete-mixture RMs.

class membership accounts for all explained variation between persons, and within-class variation is considered random variation. However, as seen in Table 7.3, person classes have relatively large standard deviations (between 1.7 and 2.6 logits), indicating that there is substantial and more importantly, systematic, within-class variability in these data.

Various types of fit analysis might prove useful. For example, it might be useful to develop a saltus-like model with variable item slopes, since models with equal slopes for all items are often too restrictive to fit well. In addition, it might be the case that models that included saltus parameters indexed by individual item (and perhaps by step in polytomous items), rather than simply associating saltus parameters with items as a whole, and estimating a single parameter across all items within an item class, might yield interesting differences by item and/or step.

One promising method for estimating parameters for such models is through their expression as generalized nonlinear mixed models. Statistical software packages are being developed that can estimate a wide variety of such models. An example of how this could be done using SAS was given by Fieuws et al. (2004); other software packages could also be used.

The saltus model has shown potential for aiding researchers, especially in the fields of cognitive science and Piagetian or neo-Piagetian theory, as do other extended models able to reflect the complexities of polytomous data and latent classes. For example, Commons and his colleagues have begun investigating the use of the saltus model for Commons's general stage theory of development (see, for example, Dawson et al., 1997). Other promising applications should follow as researchers in psychometrics continue their collaboration with educational and psychological researchers.

8

Determination of Diagnostic Cut-Points Using Stochastically Ordered Mixed Rasch Models

Svend Kreiner

Department of Biostatistics, University of Copenhagen

8.1 Introduction

Diagnostic tests aim to discriminate between clinically normal and clinically abnormal cases. When raw scores summarizing responses to items in psychiatric or health related scales are used for diagnostic purposes, it is required that measurements are both valid and reliable. Diagnostic tests are also supposed to be simple to use with either markedly higher or lower scores among persons with the specific target disorder than among normal individuals. When diagnostic tests are used for screening in large populations, the requirement of simplicity is of course of utmost importance.

One very useful way to address a diagnostic classification problem is to treat it as a latent-class problem. In particularly simple cases, the latent classes of normal and abnormal cases may in particularly simple cases define a mixed distribution of the latent trait being measured. In most cases, it is reasonable to assume that response behavior differs qualitatively between normal and abnormal cases. Mixed IRT models, and in particular mixed RMs (Rost, 1990; Rost & von Davier, 1995), are natural modeling frameworks for this kind of analysis.

If we adopt the mixed Rasch model (RM) for these purposes, it follows that conventional definitions of validity and reliability have to be extended to fit the notion of this type of mixture distribution model. Diagnostic construct validity should insist that item responses fit a mixed IRT and preferably a mixed RM with two latent classes. Diagnostic criterion validity becomes a question of whether the estimate of the latent class to which a person belongs is associated with the presence of the target disorder and all variables known to depend on the disorder. Finally, diagnostic reliability is a question of satisfactory sensitivity and specificity of the diagnoses.

Simplicity and feasibility are other requirements of diagnostic procedures. A natural diagnostic procedure based on mixed RMs use estimates of the posterior conditional distribution of the latent-class variable given the vector of item responses. Although such a procedure is definitely feasible using results provided by WINMIRA (von Davier, 1994), it can hardly be described as a simple procedure when the diagnostic test contains a large or even moderate number of items. Diagnoses by item response vectors will therefore not be practical in most applications.

If the latent class of patients with the target disorder is characterized not only by qualitatively different response behavior and correspondingly different item parameters, but also by extremely low or high test scores, we have a case of a stochastically ordered (to be defined in section 3 below) mixed RM where a simple diagnostic procedure comparing scores to an appropriately chosen cut-point may suffice. Analysis of local homogeneity in stochastically ordered mixed RMs were introduced by Kreiner et al. (1990) and further discussed and developed in Kreiner et al. (2006). An analysis of local homogeneity comparing item parameter estimates in pairs of score groups will both identify the appropriate cut-points and—together with conventional analyses by mixed RMs—provide additional evidence for or against diagnostic validity as described above.

The Mini-Mental State Examination (MMSE) developed by Folstein et al. (1975) is one of the most widely used screening scales for detection of cognitive impairment. It contains 14 dichotomous and 5 polytomous items. The summated rating scale counts the number of correct responses leading to a score of 30 when all items have been correctly responded. A cut-point equal to 24 has generally been accepted as a practical cut-point for MMSE. Scores less than 24 indicate cognitive impairment, while scores greater than or equal to 24 indicate normal cognitive function. Many studies report moderate to high degree of both sensitivity and specificity for this cut-point. Several studies raise questions concerning the construct validity of MMSE because items and factor analyses suggest that the assumption of unidimensionality has been violated. A recent Danish study of 1189 elderly (Schultz-Larsen et al., 2005a,b) comes to the same conclusion but also reports disturbingly low sensitivity. This finding motivated renewed analyses aimed at determining cut-points with a higher sensitivity than those conventionally used. The complete analysis is documented in Schultz-Larsen et al. (2005a,b), which contains additional MMSE related references. In this chapter, we illustrate the analysis by stochastically ordered mixed RMs by analysis of responses to a subset of nine dichotomized MMSE items.

Section 8.2 describes some key properties required of diagnostic tests. Sections 8.3 and 8.4 summarize the definition of stochastically ordered mixed RMs and analysis of local homogeneity. Section 8.5 discusses a few technical issues connected with analysis by stochastically ordered mixed RMs. Finally, the MMSE items are analyzed in Section 8.6.

8.2 Properties of Diagnostic Tests

The required properties of diagnostic tests are described by Streiner (2003). Suppose that D is a variable indicating whether a specific disorder is present and that T is the outcome of a diagnostic procedure for the disease. Table 8.1 illustrates the situation classifying results from a hypothetical study where it has been possible to compare the diagnosis, T, with the gold standard, D. Both variables are coded 0 for absent and 1 for present

Table 8.1. Classification of different results of comparison of the diagnostic results with a gold standard

	Gold Standard	
Result of diagnosis	Target disorder is absent	Target disorder is present
Negative	True negative	False negative
Positive	False positive	True positive

The quality of a diagnostic procedure is usually described by a number of conditional probabilities. The sensitivity is the probability $P(T = 1|D = 1)$ of a true positive result. The specificity is the probability $P(T = 0|D = 0)$ of a true negative result. The positive predictive value (PPP) is the probability, $P(D = 1|T = 1)$, that a person with a positive diagnosis has the disease in question. The negative predictive value (NPP) is the probability, $P(D = 0|T = 0)$, that a person with a negative diagnosis does not have the disease. PPP and NPP depend on the prevalence $P(D = 1)$ of the disease in the population, whereas sensitivity and prevalence are not influenced by the prevalence.

All four diagnostic criteria should be as high as possible, but deciding on a specific diagnostic procedure often requires some kind of trade-off between sensitivity and PPP on one hand and specificity and NPP on the other. In connection with large-scale population screening, economic considerations will always insist that specificity has to be very high, in which case the evaluation of the diagnostic procedure becomes a question of whether a satisfactory sensitivity is obtainable.

8.3 Mixed RMs with Stochastically Ordered Classes

Here, we only consider RMs for dichotomous items. Everything extends, however, to RMs for polytomous ordinal items without problems.

8.3.1 Conventional Mixed Rasch Models

A mixed RM adds a latent-class variable, K, to a conventional RM and assumes that item parameters depend on K,

$$P(Y_1 = y_1, \ldots, Y_k = y_k | \Theta = \theta, \mathrm{K} = \kappa, X = x) = \frac{\exp(s\theta - \sum_i y_i \beta_{\kappa,i})}{\prod_i (1 + \exp(\theta - \beta_{\kappa,i}))} \tag{8.1}$$

where $Y = (Y_1, \ldots, Y_k)$ are items and X is a vector of exogenous covariates. Mixed RMs usually assume that the effect of K is more than just a question of differential functioning of a few items; in other words, that item responses are fundamentally heterogeneous across the latent classes. One consequence of this is that comparisons of scores across groups are meaningless because they depend on qualitatively different types of latent traits; the two latent classes define two different frames of reference for measurement. X is added to the model to remind the reader that disregarding K will lead to evidence of differential item functioning relative to all exogenous variables statistically associated with K.

In addition to the conditional probabilities (8.1), a mixed RM also contains marginal probabilities —class sizes— π_κ, and conditional densities of the latent trait in each class, $f(\theta | \kappa)$.

Rost & von Davier (1995) give details on item analysis by mixed RMs. Inference in these models is conditional in the sense that item parameters are estimated from the conditional distribution of item responses given the raw score,

$$P(Y_1 = y_1, \ldots, Y_k = y_k | S = s, \kappa) = \frac{\exp(\sum_i y_i \beta_{\kappa,i})}{\gamma_s(\kappa)} \tag{8.2}$$

where $(\gamma_s(\kappa))_{s=0,\ldots,k}$ are the symmetrical functions of the parameters in the κ'th class. Instead of imposing assumptions on the latent trait distribution in each class, Rost & von Davier (1995) use a smooth two-parameter power series model for the conditional distributions of the score in each class. This model is equivalent to a model first discussed by Leunbach (1976). The probability of a specific score is given by

$$P(S = s | \kappa) = \frac{\exp(\tau_\kappa s + \delta_\kappa s^2)}{\mathrm{K}(\tau_\kappa, \delta_\kappa)} \tag{8.3}$$

where $\mathrm{K}(\tau_\kappa, \delta_\kappa)$ is a normalizing constant needed to insure that probabilities add up to 1.

Item parameters, class sizes π_κ, and score distribution parameters, τ_κ and δ_κ, can be estimated by an extended EM algorithm implemented by von Davier (1994). The classification problem of assigning persons to latent classes is best approached using Bayes's theorem. Given estimates of class sizes, item parameters and parameters of the conditional score distributions, posterior class probabilities can be estimated by

$$\begin{aligned} P(\kappa | Y_1 = y_1, \ldots, Y_k = y_k) &= \frac{P(Y_1 = y_1, \ldots, Y_k = y_k | \kappa) \pi_\kappa}{P(Y_1 = y_1, \ldots, Y_k = y_k)} \\ &= \frac{P(Y_1 = y_1, \ldots, Y_k = y_k | S = s, \kappa) P(S = s | \kappa) \pi_\kappa}{P(Y_1 = y_1, \ldots, Y_k = y_k)} \end{aligned} \tag{8.4}$$

The posterior class probabilities depend on the marginal distribution $P(Y_1=y_1,\ldots, Y_k=y_k)$. Posterior probabilities are needed if one wishes to estimate the latent class to which a specific person belongs. For this purpose, the denominator of (8.4) can be disregarded. We estimate κ by the class with the largest posterior probability given an observed vector of item responses, that is by the class, λ, satisfying

$$P(Y_1 = y_1,\ldots,Y_k = y_k|S = s, \lambda)P(S = s|\lambda)\pi_\lambda >$$
$$P(Y_1 = y_1,\ldots,Y_k = y_k|S = s, \kappa)P(S = s|\kappa)\pi_\kappa$$

$$\Leftrightarrow \quad \frac{P(Y_1 = y_1,\ldots,Y_k = y_k|S = s,\kappa)P(S = s|\kappa)}{P(Y_1 = y_1,\ldots,Y_k = y_k|S = s,\lambda)P(S = s|\lambda)} < \frac{\pi_\lambda}{\pi_\kappa} \tag{8.5}$$

for all $\kappa \neq \lambda$.

Equation (8.5) shows that the Bayesian posterior estimate of latent classes depends on both the distribution of scores and on the conditional distribution of item responses given scores in the different latent classes. $P(Y_1,\ldots,Y_k \mid S, \kappa)$ does not depend on the latent trait, Φ, but the distribution of Φ has an effect on posterior estimates through the conditional score distribution.

A simple diagnostic procedure requires that we estimate the latent class using nothing but the raw scores. The posterior estimates would in this case be

$$P(\kappa|S = s) = \frac{P(S = s, \kappa)}{P(S = s)} = \frac{P(S = s|\kappa)\pi_\kappa}{P(S = s)} \tag{8.6}$$

with the estimate, λ, of the latent class satisfying

$$\frac{P(S = s|\kappa)}{P(S = s|\lambda)} < \frac{\pi_\lambda}{\pi_\kappa} \tag{8.7}$$

for all $\kappa \neq \lambda$.

From a practical point of view, (8.7) is a more attractive estimate than (8.5) because it does not require estimates of the conditional probabilities, $P(Y_1 = y_1,\ldots,Y_k = y_k|S = s)$. In general (8.7) will, however, be an inferior estimate with too high a risk of misclassification and therefore not worthy of serious consideration. The one exception to this rule may be the case of stochastically ordered classes, where comparison of scores across groups is reintroduced.

8.3.2 Stochastically Ordered Classes

Suppose that items in a test require a specific type of performance, that one class, κ_1, consists of persons who for some reason are not able to perform, and that the second class, κ_2, contains persons who function well. This is similar to the situation that inspired Yamamoto (1987) to develop the HY-BRID model, in which one class is unable to perform the tasks and produces essentially random responses, and the other class of examinees functions as intended by the test authors. If this is the case, and the members of the "not able to perform" class have very low success probabilities, the two classes will be stochastically ordered in the sense that expected scores are relatively low in the first class and relatively higher in the second. The following definition of stochastically ordered classes where $P_1(s) = P(S=s|\kappa_1)$ and $P_2(s) = P(S=s|\kappa_2)$ are the probabilities of the score distributions in the two latent classes formalizes this situation.

Definition 1. The two classes are stochastically ordered if $\omega(s) = P_2(s)/P_1(s)$ is an increasing function of s.

Let $\pi_{2|s}$ be the posterior probability that a person belongs to κ_2 given an observed score equal to s. It follows from Definition 1 and Bayes's theorem that $\pi_{2|s}$ is an increasing function of s if, and only if, the two classes are stochastically ordered, because $\pi_{2|s}$ depends on the marginal class sizes π_1 and π_2 in the following way,

$$\pi_{2|s} = \frac{P_2(s)\pi_2}{P_1(s)\pi_1 + P_2(s)\pi_2} = \frac{\omega(s)\left(\frac{\pi_2}{\pi_1}\right)}{1 + \omega(s)\left(\frac{\pi_2}{\pi_1}\right)} \tag{8.8}$$

When latent classes of mixed RMs are stochastically ordered, diagnosis by cut-points becomes promising. Cut-points are usually defined by studies where both test scores and gold standards are available. In studies where gold standards are not available, cut-points can be identified by the probabilities of the joint distribution, P(S,K), of the test score and the latent-class variable obtained during analysis by mixed RMs where the latent-class variable adopts the role of the missing gold standard.

There are (at least[1]) two different ways to select the diagnostic cut-point, s_d, so that a score satisfying $S \leq s_d$ indicates that the target disorder is present. The likelihood principle (Royall, 1997) would select the largest score as the cut-point for which $\omega(s) = P_2(s)/P_1(s)$ is less than one. From a Bayesian point of view, the cut-point should be the largest score for which $\pi_{2|s}$ is less than one.

Both cut-points are uniquely identifiable if the two classes are stochastically ordered according to Definition 1, but the two cut-points need not agree. The Bayesian cut-point depends on the prevalence of the disorder, whereas the likelihood cut-point is independent of the prevalence. Both cut-points may be determined from the estimates of $P(S, K)$ obtained during analysis by mixed RMs.

---

[1] A more complex loss function could be defined that accounts for differential risks associated with assigning a class at different score points or regions.

8.4 Analysis of Local Homogeneity

Equation (8.8) shows that negatively skewed score distributions in κ_2 together with strong positive skewness in κ_1 will generate data where persons with high scores almost exclusively will consist of persons from κ_2, while persons with low scores belong to κ_1. On the other hand, extreme class sizes will tend to generate data where persons at one end of the score range consist of persons from one class, while persons at the other end will tend to be a mixture of persons of both classes. This means, as long as one only compares score groups belonging to the same end of the score range, that one may expect little or no evidence against homogeneity of item parameters estimated in score groups at one or maybe both extreme ends of the score range. This motivates the following definitions of local homogeneity and the simple procedure for identification of score groups suggested by Kreiner et al. (1990).

Definition 2. Let $[1, s_1]$, $[s_1 + 1, s_2]$, $\ldots$, $[s_{r-1} + 1, k - 1]$ be a partitioning of the range of the score of k dichotomous items into r score intervals. We assume that at least one score interval contains more than one score value. The set of items is locally homogenous if there is no evidence against hypotheses of equal item parameters across different score groups *within* the r score intervals. Intervals containing more than one score value are referred to as the homogenous score intervals.

Definition 3. Consider a partition, $[1, s_1]$, $[s_1 + 1, s_2]$, $\ldots$, $[s_{r-1} + 1, k - 1]$, of the score range, $[1, k - 1]$ into r score intervals so that item responses appear to be homogeneous within score intervals. If concatenation of adjacent score intervals results in score intervals where item responses appear to be heterogeneous, we then refer to the set of score intervals as a *maximally locally homogeneous* (MLH) set of score intervals.

Note that local homogeneity is defined in terms of *empirical* findings during item analysis by RMs. These findings suggest, but do not in themselves define a stochastically ordered mixed RM. Note also that the definition permits both situations where homogeneity is found in just one extreme score interval, situations where homogeneity are found in two extreme score intervals, and situations with several homogeneous score intervals are spread across the score range.

When evidence against a conventional RM has surfaced, analysis of local homogeneity attempts to identify a set of MLH score intervals. Analysis of local homogeneity is thus supposed to be a protected procedure in the sense that it should only be performed when initial tests of the RM have rejected the model, and only if the possibility of a stochastically ordered mixed RMs makes sense. Under these conditions, the following stepwise procedure is suggested:

Initialization

Select an initial set of m_0 disjoint score intervals, $J^0 = \{J_1^0, J_2^0, \ldots, J_{m_0}^0\}$, so that $[1, k - 1] = \bigcup_i J_i^0$. Ideally, the initial score intervals should be the elementary score groups, but larger score intervals may be warranted if the number of cases in each score group is too small for estimation of item parameters to make sense.

Iterative Step

Compare item parameters in adjacent score groups using Andersen's (1973a; 1973c) conditional likelihood ratio test.

Let $L(\hat{\beta}_{[s,t]}; Y_{[s,t]})$ be the conditional likelihood function evaluated for the data, $Y_{[s,t]}$, of the $[s,t]$ where $\hat{\beta}_{[s,t]}$ are the conditional maximum estimates. The conditional likelihood ratio test comparing item parameter estimates in all score intervals is equal to

$$G^2_{1,t_1,\ldots,t_{m-1},k-1} = 2\left(\sum_{i=1}^{m} \ln\left(L\left(\hat{\beta}_{[t_{i-1},t_i]}; Y_{[t_{i-1},t_i]}\right)\right) - \ln\left(L\left(\hat{\beta}_{[1,k-1]}; Y_{[1,k-1]}\right)\right)\right) \tag{8.9}$$

where we assume that $t_0 = 1$ and $t_m = k - 1$.

We refer to (8.9) as a test of global homogeneity. It generalizes without problems to tests for local homogeneity comparing item parameters in score groups not adding up to the complete set of informative scores. We consider here a partition of a score interval $H_{[a,b]} \subset H_{[1,k-1]}$ into m disjoint score intervals by $m-1$ thresholds $t_0 = a < t_1 < t_2 < \ldots, t_{m-1} < t_m = b$ and a conditional likelihood ratio test, $G^2_{a,t_1,\ldots,t_{m-1},b}$, of homogeneity of item parameters within the $[a,b]$ score interval, where $G^2_{a,t_1,\ldots,t_{m-1},b}$ is defined as in (8.9) with $t_0 = a$ and $t_m = b$. It is shown in Andersen (1973a, Corollary 4.5, p. 127) that the arguments proving the asymptotic χ^2 distribution for the test of global homogeneity extends without problems to the test for local homogeneity. $G^2_{a,t_1,\ldots,t_{m-1},b}$ therefore is also approximately χ^2 distributed with $(m-1) \cdot (k-1)$ degrees of freedom.

If all test statistics are significant, the search for local homogeneity stops. If some test statistics are insignificant, two or more homogeneous score intervals are merged into larger score intervals followed by a new iterative step.

Several procedures for joining score intervals may be considered. Let $G^2_i(t)$ be the conditional likelihood ratio test for comparison of score intervals i and $i{+}1$ during the tth step of the procedure. One conventional procedure would be to merge score intervals i and $i{+}1$ if $G^2_i(t)$ is insignificant and smaller than all other test statistics calculated during the jth step. The score intervals for the $(t{+}1)$st step will then be

$$J^{t+1}_j = J^t_j \quad \text{for} \quad j = 1, \ldots, i-1$$
$$J^{t+1}_i = J^t_i \cup J^t_{i+1}$$
$$J^{t+1}_j = J^t_{j+1} \quad \text{for} \quad = i+1, \ldots, m_{t+1}$$

where $m_{t+1} = m_t-1$.

Another procedure, referred to as "shrinking," collapses the extreme score intervals, J_1^t and J_2^t and/or $J_{m_t-1}^t$ and $J_{m_t}^t$ before mid-range intervals are merged. Arguments supporting this strategy are discussed in the next section.

The result of a search for local homogeneity agrees with a stochastically ordered mixed RM with two latent classes if the end result is two homogeneous score intervals at extreme ends of the score range. The results of local homogeneity are particularly favorable if the end result consists of two locally homogeneous score intervals, $J_1^t \cup J_2^t = [1, k-1]$. When this happens, the upper limit of the first interval may be used as a diagnostic cut-point distinguishing persons from one latent class from persons from the other class. In most cases, things will not turn out so conveniently. One or more score intervals between the two extreme intervals comprising a mixture of persons from both classes may exist so that classification by scores in practice is doubtful or close to impossible. Even when end results appear to be unambiguous, the risk of misclassification should be acknowledged. In order to both check the adequacy of a stochastically ordered latent-class model and to evaluate the risk of misclassification, analysis of local homogeneity should be succeeded by an analysis by mixed RMs providing not only a check of the adequacy of the model but also proper estimates of class sizes and the risk of misclassification if cut-points separating homogeneous score intervals are used for classification.

8.5 Issues in Analysis by Stochastically Ordered Mixed Rasch Models

There are technical issues to be addressed before both types of analysis.

8.5.1 Analysis by Mixed Rasch Models

Analysis by mixed RMs is documented in Rost (1990) and Rost & von Davier (1995) and implemented by von Davier (1994, 2001). Results include estimates of the number of classes, estimates of class sizes, item parameters and conditional score distributions, from which it is possible to estimate sensitivity and specificity of diagnostic procedures using posterior class estimates. All is well documented and easily accessible in the references mentioned above. Two issues, however, requires deliberation.

Firstly, the estimate of the number of classes is based on Akaike information criterion (AIC) and Bayesian information criterion (BIC) that do not always provide the same answer,[2] Which is the better information criterion

---

[2] Other methods, like the parametric bootstrap (von Davier, 1997) or posterior predictive model checking (Sinharay, 2004), are available for latent-class and item response models but are computationally intensive and therefore used less frequently in practice.

therefore has to be examined. Secondly, estimates of score distribution may be either smooth, fitting a two-parameter power series distribution, or "rough," satisfying no restrictions at all except those imposed by the estimation equations. The problem is that the choice between smooth and rough distributions will have an effect, not only on the estimates of score distributions, but also on estimates of the number of classes and class sizes. Simulation results reported by Kreiner et al. (2006) unequivocally recommend the following:

1. Estimates of the number of classes should be based upon rough estimates using AIC statistics. If smooth estimates are used, the analysis will be influenced by mixtures on the latent trait scale and consequently report that more than one class is present even though item responses fit perfectly to a conventional RM. Using BIC with rough estimates of score distributions underestimate the number of classes whereas AIC always capture the correct number of classes.

2. After the number of classes has been decided upon, one should use smooth score distributions for estimation of both class sizes and score distributions.

The results of analysis by mixed RMs presented in Tables 8.4 and 8.5 below follow these recommendations.

8.5.2 Analysis of Local Homogeneity

The stepwise analysis of local homogeneity is similar to stepwise model search. The adopted strategy is a backwards model search procedure starting with the most complex situation where all score groups are assumed to have different item parameters. The search for local homogeneity then proceeds toward a simpler model where item parameters may be assumed to be the same in some score groups. Score groups will be collapsed if conditional likelihood ratio tests are insignificant. Conventional model search procedures using tests of significance to decide how to proceed would usually take the path of least resistance, by selecting the next model motivated by the test statistic with the highest p-value. It is well known, however, that such procedures lead to too complicated models because test statistics calculated at the later stages of model searching are related to test statistics calculated at the beginning of the analysis.

The situation is illustrated in Figure 8.1, describing a comparative analysis of three different groups, A, B, C. The stepwise analysis starts at the top where all groups are different and then tries to get to the bottom, where there is no dissimilarity among the groups. On the way, different likelihood ratio statistics are calculated. The test, LR_1, is thus a test of $((A = B) \neq C)$ against $(A \neq B \neq C)$. The negative association between test statistics evaluated at the beginning of the model search procedure and test statistics calculated later is due to the fact that the likelihood ratio test of $(A = B = C)$ against

$(A \neq B \neq C)$ is equal to both $LR_1 + LR_4$, $LR_2 + LR_5$, and $LR_3 + LR_6$. If the $((A = B) \neq C)$ model is selected at the first step of the procedure because LR_1 is smaller than LR_2 and LR_3, the next step will depend on a test statistic known to have a larger value than the test statistic to be considered if another path had been chosen. Consequently, the conventional p-value driven procedure has an inherent risk of stopping to soon.

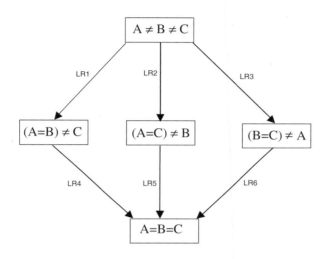

Fig. 8.1. Models and test statistics for comparison of three different score groups

We recommend using strategies that take subject matter considerations into account. Such strategies are in most cases difficult to implement and test, because subject matter considerations by nature have to be different from analysis to analysis. Analysis of stochastically ordered mixed RMs is, however, an exception to this rule. Local homogeneity is to be found at the extreme ends of the score range. It therefore makes sense to use a shrinking model search strategy, where extreme score groups collapse if test results are insignificant, even when test results relating to nonextreme score groups are more insignificant. The simulation studies referred to above suggest the conjecture that this strategy works more satisfactorily than conventional p-value driven strategies.

Another concern is the large number of significance tests calculated during analysis of local homogeneity. Some kind of p-value adjustment has to be invoked. We routinely use Benjamini & Hochberg (1995) procedures controlling the False Discovery Rate at $FDR = 0.05$ during analysis of local homogeneity and other analyses relying on large number of p-values.

8.6 The Mini-Mental State Examination

We illustrate the analyses of local homogeneity and mixed RMs with data on the Mini-Mental State Examination (MMSE) collected in connection with a survey among Danish elderly. Information on the study may be found in Schultz-Larsen et al. (2005a,b). The analysis reported in these papers suggested a two-dimensional latent structure underlying the responses to the items of which only one appeared to be related to age. In the example here, we only consider the subscale of nine items loading on the latent variable that was independent of age.

Complete responses to the MMSE items were obtained from 1148 persons. Neuropsychological assessment was completed for a total of 242 elderly, some of whom were suspected of suffering from dementia. The examination showed that 69 patients suffered from dementia to some degree. Out of these, only 25 had total MMSE scores less than 25 leading to an estimate of the sensitivity equal to 36.2%. Given this result, one is forced to conclude that MMSE would be an ineffective instrument when screening for dementia.

Table 8.2 shows the items and the frequencies of correct responses on the items in the subscale described here. The score distribution is strongly negatively skewed.

Table 8.2. The nine MMSE items included in the subscale that does not correlate with age. All items are treated as dichotomous items in this chapter.

Item/Question	Sub Item	Frequency of Correct Responses
Where are we now?	Name some nearby streets	0.97
	County	0.96
	Town/City	0.99
	Address	0.99
	Floor	0.99
Recognize and name three unrelated objects		0.99
Remember the three objects		0.33
Follow written instruction		0.99
Draw a copy of a picture		0.61

Out of the 1148 persons, 258 responded correctly to all items. Chronbach's α is equal to 0.38, which indicates very poor reliability. Loevinger's H is equal to 0.34, which also tells us that, whether or not it fits a Rasch model, MMSE is close to useless as a measure of cognitive function. Measuring cognitive function is, however, not what MMSE is meant for. Instead, the objective is to screen for cognitive impairment, and perhaps—if the cognitive function appears to be impaired—to measure the degree of impairment.

The level of cognitive function among persons without impairments is a completely different problem, and the poor performance of MMSE according to conventional psychometric requirements of good quantitative measurement of persons without impairments is less relevant here.

The RM does not fit the item responses. Table 8.3 presents Andersen's (1973c) conditional likelihood ratio test comparing parameter estimates in different groups. Differential item functioning relative to both education and gender is suggested. Departures from the RM are, however, diffuse. Tests of conditional independence of items and exogenous variables given the total score and tests of local independence as suggested by Kreiner & Christensen (2004) disclose no evidence of biased or locally dependent items. Which, by the way, is exactly what is to be expected from items fitting a mixed RM?

Table 8.3. Conditional likelihood ratio tests of homogeneity of item parameters in subpopulations. Results presented for the RM and for the graphical loglinear RM.

Variable Defining Subpopulations	CLR	df	p
Score groups (1–6,7,8)	32.6	16	0.008
Level of education—three categories	33.1	16	0.007
Gender	20.6	8	0.008
Age—five categories	28.0	32	0.669

8.6.1 Analysis of Local Homogeneity

Table 8.4 shows the analysis of local homogeneity. Prior to the analysis, score groups 1–5 were collapsed because the numbers of cases in these groups were so small that testing hypotheses concerning equivalence of item parameters was infeasible. Item responses are locally homogeneous within score groups 1–6 and 7–8, but heterogeneous across the score groups.

Next, item parameters estimated in groups defined by different levels of education, gender, and age are compared separately in each of the two score groups. The evidence of differences depending on gender disappears in both score groups as does the evidence of differences related to education among persons with scores equal to 7 or 8. There is still marginal evidence, however, that item parameters depend on the level of education for persons with scores between 1 and 5.

8.6.2 Analysis by Mixed Rasch Models

Analysis by mixed RMs suggests two latent classes as shown in Table 8.5. Figure 2 and Table 8.6 show the estimated score distribution in the two classes. Posterior class probabilities calculated conditionally given the score are included in Table 8.6. Basically, the analysis agrees with the results of the

Table 8.4. Analysis of local inhomogeneity of nine MMSE items

Comparison of	G^2	df[1]	p
Comparisons of Adjacent Score Groups			
1–5 and 6	6.6	7	0.522
6 and 7	18.1	8	0.021[+]
7 and 8	13.1	7	0.070
Tests for Combined Score Groups			
1–6 and 7–8	19.5	8	0.012[*]

[1]: Degrees of freedom have been adjusted when items have responses in both score groups.
[+]: Not significant after Benjamini–Hochberg adjustment.
[*]: Significant after Benjamini–Hochberg adjustment.

analysis of local homogeneity. Yet it raises some questions concerning what the cut-point should be. The likelihood principle selects the same cut-point as the analysis of local homogeneity, whereas the Bayesian principle prefers a cut-point one point lower.

Table 8.5. Information statistics and class size estimates of mixed RMs

Number of Classes	Class Sizes	AIC
1	1.000	4255.3
2	0.973	4125.4
	0.027	
3	0.491	4140.9
	0.483	
	0.026	

The sensitivity and specificity of diagnoses using different cut-points are easily calculated from the score distributions in Table 8.6. Table 8.7 presents the results. The results favor the 6/7 cut-point suggested by the likelihood principle and the analysis of local homogeneity because the sensitivity with this cut-point is much higher than the sensitivity obtained by the Bayesian cut-point. Table 8.7 also shows standard estimates of sensitivity and specificity in the subsample of elderly where neuropsychological examinations provided proper gold standards for the MMSE results. The similarity of estimates obtained by analysis by mixed models without gold standards and the conventional estimates is notable, but of course also to be expected, because sensitivity and specificity do not depend on the prevalence of demented per-

Table 8.6. Fitted smooth score distributions and posterior class probabilities

Score	Class 1	Class 2	P(Class2|Score)
0	0	0.15	1.00
1	0	0.50	1.00
2	0	1.32	1.00
3	0	2.75	1.00
4	0.04	4.53	0.99
5	1.89	5.91	0.76
6	44.59	6.11	0.012
7	290.26	5.00	0.017
8	521.49	3.24	0.006
9	258.62	1.67	0.006

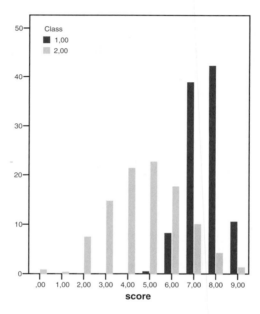

Fig. 8.2. Estimated score probabilities in two latent classes

sons. The estimates of specificity according to the mixed RM appear to be somewhat optimistic.

8.7 Discussion

Stochastically ordered mixed RMs provide a natural framework for analysis of diagnostic tests while raising a number of issues concerning conventional

Table 8.7. Comparison of estimates of sensitivity and specificity using different cut-points

Cut-point	Analysis by Mixed RMs		Elderly with Neuropsychological examination[1,2]	
	Sensitivity	Specificity	Sensitivity	Specificity
6/7	68.2 %	95.8%	71.0 % (59.4–80.6)	88.4 % (82.9–92.4)
5/6	48.6 %	99.8 %	44.9 % (33.8–56.7)	95.4 % (91.3–97.7)

[1]: The subsample consisted of 69 cases with and 173 elderly without dementia.
[2]: Parentheses contain 95% confidence intervals.

requirements of valid, well-targeted, and reliable measurements. In particular, these issues become inevitable in connection with measurements used for screening in populations containing both abnormal and normal cases. In such situations, measurements cannot be construct valid in the traditional sense because they depend on more than one quantitative latent trait variable, and sensitivity and specificity increases if items are ill-targeted for both types of cases, such that score distributions are strongly skewed in opposite directions in the two subpopulations.

Analysis of local homogeneity is a simple approach for initial analysis prior to analysis by mixed RMs aiming specifically at definition of the cut-points required for simple diagnostic procedures. One advantage of analysis of local homogeneity is that it is easily generalized to more complicated types of RMs, e.g., the family of graphical loglinear RMs (Kreiner & Christensen, 2002), which are discussed elsewhere in this volume.

Analysis by mixed RMs and analysis of local homogeneity as two different procedures validate the results of each other. Analysis by local homogeneity suggests, but does not actually fit a latent-class model. Results from analyses of local homogeneity therefore require confirmation by mixed RMs. On the other hand, results by mixed RMs resulting in score distributions that separate latent classes with scores that are higher in one class than the other should of course reappear during analysis of local homogeneity. If estimates of item parameters are not the same when calculated in score groups that, according to the analysis, are dominated by one of the latent classes, then, of course, the model cannot be a mixed RM.

The results on MMSE presented here are only a small part of the full analysis of these data. Schultz-Larsen et al. (2005a,b) tells the complete story discussing different cut-points for the complete MMSE scores, cut-points for a subscale summarizing responses to the items loading on the other MMSE dimension, and cut-points for scores using polytomous rather than dichotomous items.

A HYBRID Model for Test Speededness

Keith A. Boughton[1] and Kentaro Yamamoto[2]

[1] CTB/McGraw Hill
[2] Educational Testing Service

9.1 Introduction

Assessing speededness by simple approaches such as counting the number of missing responses near the end of a test is often inadequate because many examinees switch to a guessing or random response strategy as the testing time limit approaches. Parameter estimation within item response theory (IRT) can be greatly impacted by speededness; thus, it is crucial to assess how much speededness a test may possess (Oshima, 1994). It is also critical to correct the item-parameter estimates that may have been affected by this end-of-test speededness. Examinees who switch to random responses at the end of the test, in terms of the underlying response processes, expose a very different behavior when responding to an item when compared to examinees who try to solve the item using their cognitive skill set. In order to account for these different types of response behaviors, a HYBRID model was proposed by Yamamoto (1989) and later extended to assess test speededness more directly (Yamamoto, 1990, 1995).

It is important to note that there are many reasons why one of the key assumptions of IRT, namely that of conditional independence, may fail. Speededness is one such case, and in particular, this application of the HYBRID model addresses a specific type of speededness that will be later elaborated on. This research will show how the HYBRID model can detect examinees who have switched to a random response strategy, thereby eliminating the noise caused by end-of-test speededness, which should result in more accurate IRT parameter estimates for those end-of-test items.

9.2 Purpose and Method

This chapter will first explicate the HYBRID model, its development, and parameter estimation. The second section will demonstrate, using real data with quasi-experimental controls, the HYBRID model's accuracy and efficacy for assessing the amount of speededness and reducing its effects on item-parameter estimation. A writing assessment with 45 multiple-choice items was shortened to 38 items due to known end-of-test speededness and then readministered. The last five items of the 45-item test were placed in the middle of the shortened 38-item version, thus creating a quasi-experimental condition in which the item parameters from the middle of the 38-item test, which should not have been affected by speededness, will be used as the estimated "true" parameters. The HYBRID model item-parameter estimates for the last five items of the longer 45-item version will be compared to these "true" parameters.

9.3 The HYBRID Model

The original HYBRID model, proposed by Yamamoto (1987, 1989), was specifically developed in order to incorporate cognitive structure into the IRT methodology of that time, which up to that point, was mostly used for the scaling and reporting of scores from large-scale assessments. Yamamoto (1989) acknowledges that a multidimensional IRT (MIRT) model could be employed; however, he cautions against the use of the compensatory MIRT model, since assessments may not involve compensatory abilities. He also points out that, "the notion of single-event learning cannot be incorporated easily into a purely continuous model" (p. 4).

Yamamoto (1990) later extended the HYBRID model for diagnosing test speededness. This psychometric approach to speededness has made significant advances in this area by combining a latent-class (LC) model with an IRT model strategy. This HYBRID model has been studied through several simulations (Boughton & Yamamoto, 2004; Yamamoto, 1990, 1995; Yamamoto & Everson, 1995, 1997). As with any model, however, more research is needed in order to securely support and demonstrate its appropriateness and utility, especially with the use of real data, since simulations cannot model actual human response behavior.

Classical test theory (CTT) and item response theory (IRT) each describe the behavior of examinees based on a single model, whereas the HYBRID psychometric approach (Yamamoto, 1989) utilizes two models in the detection of speededness. That is, subsets of examinee response patterns are modeled by a discrete latent-class model (i.e., multinomial independent class), with the remaining responses modeled by an IRT model (Yamamoto & Everson, 1995, 1997). In contrast to finite-mixture-distribution IRT models that assume the same parametric model—with different parameter vectors—in each of the mixing components, HYBRID models assume different model structures in each mixture component. It is important to note that the HYBRID model does not necessarily have only two classes, but is implemented by assuming many classes with restrictions imposed across classes, each defined by a switch point in the item sequence. The HYBRID model can estimate the point in an assessment at which each examinee has switched from an ability-based response strategy to a guessing or random-response strategy. Thus, the HYBRID model provides an index to help set test lengths appropriate to the time-constraint allocations, as well as to ascertain the differential speededness for any subgroup population (Boughton et al., 2004; Yamamoto & Everson, 1995).

9.4 HYBRID Model and Parameter Estimation

The HYBRID model estimates both person and item parameters along with the parameters that define the distribution of examinees switching from an ability-based to a random-response strategy. The HYBRID model assumes that any examinee who switches to a random response strategy has conditional probabilities that are independent of their proficiency level for the remaining items. Every examinee's response can be modeled either by a continuous uni-dimensional IRT model or an LC model, and conditional independence holds, given an examinee's proficiency and strategy. The following function expresses the likelihood of a correct response on an item i given the three assumptions above:

$$p\left(x_i = 1\,|\,\theta, \beta_i, k\right) = \left(1 + \exp\left(\theta - b_i\right)\right)^{m_{ik}} c_i^{m_{ik}+1}, \tag{9.1}$$

where k indicates the last item answered under the IRT model; $M_{ik} = -1$, when $i \leq k$ and $M_{ik} = 0$, when $i > k$. x_i is a dichotomous response (i.e., 0/1) on item i; β_i represents the item difficulty parameter; θ is the examinee ability parameter; and c_i is the expected proportion correct under a patterned or random response strategy. Equation 9.1 gives the conditional probability of a response x_i, given θ, item parameters β_i, and strategy switch point k. Specifically, this function specifies that an IRT model holds until a random response occurs, with a constant conditional probability holding for the remaining random responses (Yamamoto, 1995).

The likelihood of observing a response vector x_v, given θ_v, when switching from an ability-based solution to a random-response strategy on item k_v is

$$P\left(x_v|\,\theta_v, B, k_v\right) = \prod_{i=1}^{k_v} P\left(\theta_v, \beta_i\right)^{x_{iv}} Q\left(\theta_v, \beta_i\right)^{1-x_{iv}} \prod_{i=k_v+1}^{I} c_i^{x_{iv}}\left(1 - c_i\right)^{1-x_{iv}}. \tag{9.2}$$

The marginal probability of observing x_v given model parameters B is

$$P(x_v|\,B) = \sum_{k}^{L} \int_{\theta} P(x_v\,|\theta, B, k)\, f(\theta\,|k) d\theta f(k)\,, \tag{9.3}$$

where $f(\theta\,|k)$ is the conditional probability of θ given a switch point k, and $f(k)$ is the marginal distribution of the strategy-switching population.

The joint likelihood of parameters given the observed response matrix $X = (x_1, x_2, \ldots, x_v)$ from a total of V examinees is

$$L(B \mid X) = \prod_{v=1}^{V} P(x_v \mid B).$$

The IRT item parameters can be estimated to maximize the above marginalized likelihood function using an iterative method, such as the Newton–Raphson (N-R) method. The N-R method can be described as $P^{n+1} = P^n - D_2^{-1} * D_1$, where P^{n+1} is a vector of parameters updated from P^n by a certain amount designated by the function D_2 (matrix of second derivatives) and D_1 (vector of first derivatives). However, D_2 can be quite large and the off-diagonal elements need not be zero. Consequently, a full implementation of the N-R method would be too great a computational burden. Bock & Aitkin (1981) advanced the idea of using the EM algorithm (Dempster et al., 1977) in the area of IRT parameter estimation. Within the EM algorithm, the continuous distribution of theta (i.e., the ability parameter) is approximated by a discrete distribution, in order to facilitate the numerical integration over the range of the latent-variable theta. With respect to u, a model parameter including either an item parameter or a probability of the discrete ability density, the first derivative of the log-likelihood of the above function can be expressed as

$$\frac{\partial \ln L(B \mid X)}{\partial u} = \sum_{v=1}^{V} \sum_{k=1}^{I} \int_{\theta} \frac{\partial P(x_v \mid \theta, B, k)}{\partial u} \frac{f(\theta \mid k) f(k)}{P(x_i \mid B)} d\theta.$$

Followed by the application of the empirical Bayes method and approximation of integration by summation denoted by q-quadrature points and $A(\theta_q \mid k)$ as defined as conditional weights approximating $f(\theta_q \mid k)$, the above equation for a parameter u_i can be written as

$$\frac{\partial \ln L}{\partial u_i} = \sum_{k} \sum_{q} \frac{A(\theta_q \mid k)}{P_{ik}(\theta_q) Q_{ik}(\theta_q)} \frac{\partial P_{ik}(\theta_q)}{\partial u_i} \sum_{v=1}^{V} [x_{iv} - P_{iv}(\theta_q)] f(k) P_i(\theta_q \mid x_v, k).$$

The right side of the above equation can be rewritten as follows, since x_{iv} is either 1 or 0:

$$\sum_{k} \sum_{q} \frac{1}{P_{ik}(\theta_q) Q_{ik}(\theta_q)} \frac{\partial P_{ik}(\theta_q)}{\partial u_i} f(k) (R_{iqk} - P_{ik}(\theta_q) N_{iqk}),$$

where

$$R_{iqk} = \sum_{v} x_{iv} \frac{P(x_v \mid \theta_q, B, k) A(\theta_q \mid k)}{P(x_v, B)},$$

$$N_{iqk} = \sum_{v} \frac{P(x_v \mid \theta_q, B, k) A(\theta_q \mid k)}{P(x_v, B)},$$

and

$$\frac{\partial P_{ik}(\theta_q)}{\partial a_i} = D(\theta_q - b_i) P_{ik}(\theta_q) Q_{ik}(\theta_q),$$

$$\frac{\partial P_{ik}(\theta_q)}{\partial b_i} = -Da P_{ik}(\theta_q) Q_{ik}(\theta_q).$$

The matrix of second-order derivatives can be expressed as follows:

$$\frac{\partial^2 \ln L}{\partial a_i^2} = D^2 \sum_k \sum_q f(k) (\theta_q - b_i)^2 N_{iqk} P_{ik}(\theta_q) Q_{ik}(\theta_q),$$

$$\frac{\partial^2 \ln L}{\partial b_i^2} = -b^2 \sum_k \sum_q a_i^2 N_{iqk} P_{ik}(\theta_q) Q_{ik}(\theta_q),$$

$$\frac{\partial^2 \ln L}{\partial a_i \partial b_i} = D^2 \sum_k \sum_q a_i (\theta_q - b_i)^2 N_{iqk} P_{ik}(\theta_q) Q_{ik}(\theta_q).$$

Once item parameters are estimated, estimation of an examinee's proficiency can be carried out using one of several existing methods, such as the maximum likelihood method (MLE), Bayes modal estimates (MAP), or expected a posteriori (EAP). The MLE ability estimation is described by Lord (1980), and MAP and EAP are both described by Bock & Aitkin (1981).

Prior distributions for the item parameters, proficiency, and switching population distributions can be used during the maximization phase. For example, item parameters can be assumed to be drawn from a particular distribution, and, therefore, updating parameters would be constrained to meet that particular distribution. Likewise, the proficiency distribution may be assumed as a normal distribution at each switching point, including the last item. In addition, $E(\theta|k)$ may be constrained to have a specific functional form in relation to the value of k (Yamamoto, 1995). The HYBRID model parameters for the speededness model can be estimated using the HYBILm software program (Yamamoto, 1990).

9.5 Results

The 44-item writing assessment was shortened to 38 items after the last five items were found to be greatly impacted by speededness (i.e., student reported speededness). These five items were then repositioned into the middle of the 38-item form, giving us the opportunity to demonstrate how well the HYBRID Rasch model (RM) can recover the "true" parameters (i.e., the parameter estimates obtained when calibrated in the unaffected portion of the shortened 38-item test). The parameters of the five items in the middle of the shortened 38-item test will be considered the "true" parameters, and the comparisons

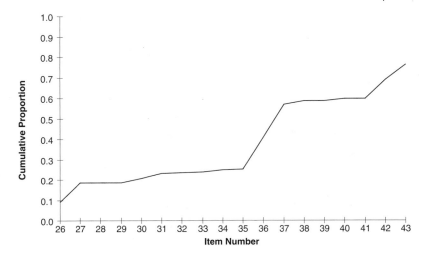

Fig. 9.1. Cumulative switching proportions across items 26–43 in the 44-item test

will be made between these five-item-parameter estimates and the estimates obtained from the end of the 44-item calibration.

Figure 9.1 displays the cumulative proportion of examinees switching from an ability-based strategy to a random-response strategy across the last 18 items. The x-axis represents the item number and the y-axis is the cumulative proportion of examinees switching strategies. As seen from the figure, this test is speeded, with over 50% switching to a random-response strategy starting at item 37. Figure 9.2 displays the cumulative proportion switching across the last 17 items of the shortened 38-item form. The proportion of switchers is considerably lower. However, there is still over 20% switching over the last four items. The HYBRID model can be used as a tool to help identify how short a test needs to be in order to give all examinees the opportunity to show their true abilities fairly. Given the switching information from Figure 9.1, it would seem reasonable to shorten the test to a length of 35 items; however, the test was only shortened to a length of 38 items, given reliability predictions and time-per-item estimations. Note that the switching proportions would suggest that the test should be shortened to 35 items, since we observe approximately 20% switching on that item. Although the 20% criterion is a somewhat arbitrary bound, given the authors' experiences with speeded assessments and their effects on item-parameter estimation, it seems a good rule of thumb. Of course, it would be more desirable to have 0%, at least for assessments in which speed of answering is not the intended construct; however, this may not be realistic. Thus, it is the impact on the item-parameter estimates that will be the defining factor in this research. It can be seen in Figure 9.2 that

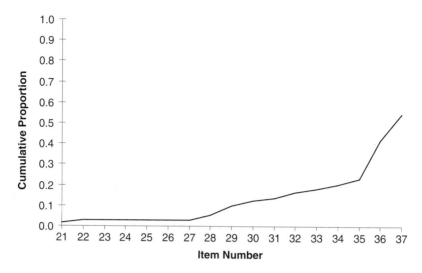

Fig. 9.2. Cumulative switching proportions across items 21–37 in the 38-item test

the shortened test was not short enough, and had it been shortened to 35 items, as the HYBRID model suggests, then the 20% criterion would most likely have been met when the test was readministered. However, it could be that, no matter how short an assessment is, there will always be examinees who cannot estimate how much time it will take to complete the test.

Figure 9.3 shows the item-characteristic curves for the five items that were removed from the end of the 44-item test and moved to the middle of the 38-item test. The actual position of item 39 in the 38-item version is (22), 40 (23), 42 (24), 43 (25), and 44 (26). Each of the five graphs has three ICCs; the "true" ICCs (i.e., recalibrated in the middle of the 38-item test), the Rasch ICCs, and the HYBRID ICCs, both calibrated in the 44-item-test version and then scaled using a Stocking & Lord (1983) transformation to the 38-item-test scale, using the first 21 nonspeeded items in both tests. All items, except for item 22, were biased when the Rasch model was used alone (i.e., items appeared more difficult). However, the HYBRID RM produced corrected item parameters that were consistent with the "true" parameters, with a slight overcorrection for items 24, 25, and 26 (i.e., the item appeared slightly easier).

Figure 9.4 displays the speeded characteristic curves. The x-axis is the ability metric, with the y-axis being the expected true score for the five items presumed speeded. The impact of the bias in the expected score would be about 0.5 for the middle of the ability range. The "Rasch-only" model is

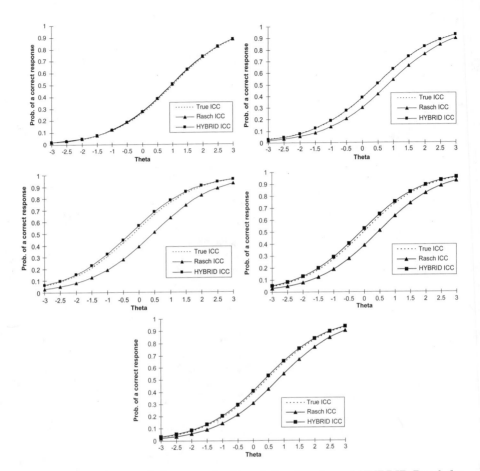

Fig. 9.3. Item characteristic curves for "true," Rasch-only, and HYBRID-Rasch for Items 22, 23, 24, 25, and 26, from left to right and down

biased and would result in a lower-ability expected score. The HYBRID model recovered the "true" five item parameters.

Figure 9.5 displays the entire 38-item-test test characteristic curve TCC, for the "true," the Rasch-only, and the HYBRID TCC. The TCC is recovered when the HYBRID model is used, while the Rasch-only is biased.

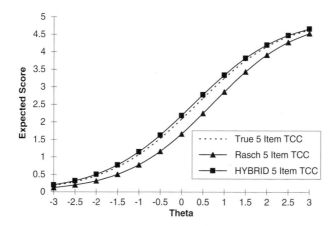

Fig. 9.4. Speeded-section characteristic curves for "true," Rasch-only, and HYBRID-Rasch

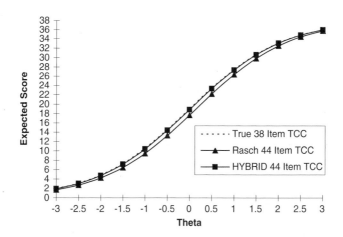

Fig. 9.5. Test characteristic curves for "true," Rasch-only, and HYBRID-Rasch

9.6 Discussion and Conclusion

The purpose of this study was to examine an estimation method that incorporates two distinct models for each examinee in the detection and then modeling of speededness. This research has demonstrated the HYBRID model's utility and appropriateness using real data with quasi-experimental controls.

The 44-item test was found to be speeded, with over 20% switching to a random response pattern on item 36. However, even the shortened 38-item version shows over 20% switching behavior before reaching the last item. These results suggest that even when examinees are given more time per item, some examinees do not pace themselves appropriately and thus fail to reach the end of the test using an ability-based response strategy. When not accounting for speededness, parameter-estimation bias was found in four of the five items studied, with the Rasch-only model overestimating the difficulty of the items. The HYBRID RM corrected all of the parameter estimates, although it slightly underestimates the item difficulty for some of the items. However, at the TCC level, the HYBRID RM matches the "true" TCC, while the Rasch-only model results in a biased TCC. These results suggest that the HYBRID model improves item-parameter estimation for speeded items located near the end of a test. These improvements coincide with the proportion of examinees switching to a random-response strategy on each form.

The HYBRID model provides a method that can reduce the effects of speededness on IRT item and ability parameters, while also mapping item/examinee switch behavior for tests with speededness. However, the HYBRID model does not work well for all testing situations. For example, if examinees responded randomly at the beginning of a test, then the current model would not be appropriate. The HYBRID model also does not work well for tests that have items ordered from easiest to most difficult, because low-ability examinees will have response patterns similar to examinees switching to a random-response strategy (Yamamoto & Everson, 1995). The tests presented in this study did not have any of these limitations. Ironically, as is the case for many studies, this research's strength is also its weakness. The application to real-world data with quasi-experimental controls is paramount in illustrating the HYBRID model's utility and appropriateness. However, the accuracy of the parameter estimates are judged in comparison with parameters that are estimates in and of themselves. In addition, position effects may hamper direct comparison between the long and shortened test length item parameters, although this was not apparent with these results. It is extremely important to ensure that test length or time is appropriate when a test's construct of interest does not include the speed with which each student answers. Searching for not-reached items at the end of a test, especially for examinees who randomly fill in unanswered responses, may not prove beneficial. In these cases, the HYBRID RM proposed here can aid test developers in setting appropriate test lengths (i.e., using the cumulative proportion switching), and/or correct any speededness-induced bias for end-of-test items.

10

Multidimensional Three-Mode Rasch Models

Claus H. Carstensen and Jürgen Rost

Leibniz Institute for Science Education, Kiel

10.1 Introduction

Rasch's measurements model has been generalized in many different ways (see Chapter 1, this volume). One direction of generalizing the Rasch model is to consider not only two factors of the response probability, i.e., persons and items, but an additional third factor. This means to extend the two-dimensional data matrix to a three-dimensional data cube and extending the RM accordingly. Those extensions have been proposed in various contexts, e.g., in the context of measuring change, where the third factor or "mode" is time (Rost & Spada, 1983, Spiel, 1994), in the context of multitrait-multimethod measurement, where the third factor or "mode" is the method (Rost & Walter, 2005), in the context of assessing inter-rater agreement, where the third factor or mode is the rater or judge (Linacre, 1989), and in the context of facet-designed tests, where the item factor is split up into two facets like content domain knowledge and cognitive processes (Rost & Carstensen, 2002).

All these examples have in common that the data structure is not a matrix, but a cube. Many analyses can be done with those data by an "intelligent application" of the ordinary RM. In contrast, the ordinary RM is not capable of explicitly modeling all ways of looking at such a three-factor data structure. For example, in the context of measuring change, the "slices" of the data cube that relate to the time points of measurement can be treated as new (virtual) persons responding to the same items or as if the same persons respond to new (virtual) items at each point of time. In either of these cases, the ordinary RM can be applied to a reorganized data matrix with tN persons or tk items, respectively, with t being the number of time points (Glück & Spiel, 1997).

In other cases it is necessary to apply a multidimensional RM in order to analyze such a data cube according to the aim and hypotheses of the investigation. The present contribution describes the family of RMs that emerges from a systematic generalization of the RM to a three-factor data structure.

We refer to this family of models as "three-mode" RMs (in analogy to three-mode factor analysis), because other terms like factor, dimension, or facet are preoccupied by other connotations. Most of the models in this family of three-mode models are multidimensional in the sense that more than one person parameter will be assigned to each person. The models of this family are special cases of the mixed-coefficients multinomial logit model presented in Chapter 4. Unidimensional three-mode models are special applications of the linear logistic test model (LLTM; Fischer, 1973). The three-mode structure of the models has its implications on the identification and estimation of its parameters (which will be discussed here). The models will be discussed and illustrated in the context of three different applications.

10.2 The Family of Three-Mode Rasch Models

Ordinary item response theory (IRT) refers to the situation where a number of persons have responded to a number of items. The resulting data can be organized in a data matrix and hence be considered as a two-dimensional data structure. However, in order to avoid confusion with the concept of multidimensionality of the trait variable to be measured, a simple data matrix is called a two-way or two-mode data structure. The generalization of two-mode IRT to a three-mode data structure emerges in many different contexts.

The most prominent context of such a generalization is measurement of change, where a test has been administered repeatedly to the same sample of persons. In this case, the data matrices obtained for each time point can be considered as slices of a three-mode data structure, where time is the third mode beside persons and items. Despite some—very common—anomalies of the data structure resulting from incomplete designs, the data structure can be represented as a cube. Rost & Spada (1983) developed the system of eight different models for measuring change by means of uni- and multidimensional RMs for this data cube (Rost, 2004; Spiel, 1994). The same system can be applied to any three-mode data structure regardless whether the third mode is to model time or any other aspect of the response process.

The present chapter focuses on facet designed tests as a special case of systematically constructed tests that produce three-mode data structures. When modeling the response process, typically the respondents and some item features will be considered to have an impact on the response process. Additional facets such as the item format, the judgments from different raters, or several measurement occasions may be taken into account, to name some examples for additional facets of the response process. An appropriate item response model parametrizes the facets that are assumed to significantly impact the response process. Mellenbergh (2001) provides a systematic approach to response process facets and appropriate response models. In this chapter, we address models with a subject facet, an item facet, and a third one that may be related to one of both, subjects or items. Considering a test with two item facets, each item represents a combination of the components of two facets like content and cognitive process or subject area and context. The set of components described by a facet may be used to construct tests where each item corresponds to exactly one component of the two facets. For each unique combination of components from these two facets, one or more items may be constructed.

One of the three examples considered in this chapter is an intelligence test, where each item refers to a *representational* mode with verbal, numeric or figural tasks and a *process* mode separating fluency, memory, analytical thinking and creativity (Jäger et al., 1997). The data structure can be organized as a cube with persons, representations and processes as the three modes. The test encloses three to five items per combination of these two modes.

Another example is a science test with each item constructed according to one content and one cognitive operation, which yields a matrix structure of i contents by j cognitive operations. In contrast to the intelligence test, only one item for each combination of these two modes is administered. We will refer to the different combinations of components as *item types* (Carstensen, 2000). Tests can be distinguished according to the number of items per item type, one or more than one.

The second and third mode from both examples above, representations and process or content and operation, respectively, will be modeled as person abilities in multidimensional models. The third example is a mathematics test again constructed according to a two-mode structure, resulting in a three-mode data cube. Unlike the other two examples, the modes will be modeled as item-difficulty modes and the response models employed will be unidimensional.

In the following, a system of generalized RMs for three-mode data structures is presented and discussed with respect to the situation of facet-designed tests. The system is shown in Fig. 10.1, where in each box a different decomposition of the exponent λ of the logistic function

$$p\left(x_{vij} = 1 \,|\lambda_{vij}\right) = \frac{\exp\left(\lambda_{vij}\right)}{1 + \exp\left(\lambda_{vij}\right)}$$

for a three-mode data structure is shown. $p\left(x_{vij} \in X\right)$ is the response probability of person v with respect to an item that is composed by component i of the second mode and component j of the third. In the notation of Fig. 10.1, θ_v is an ability parameter of person v, which may have a second index, i or j, in the case of multidimensionality. σ_i or δ_j are difficulty parameters of the components of the two facets, which may be double indexed as σ_{ij} in the case that the item difficulties are not modeled according to the facet structure of the test. Doubly indexed delta parameters, δ_{vj}, are multidimensional ability parameters.

The hierarchy of models depicted in Fig. 10.1 has four levels, the lowest and the highest represented by a single model each. Model (1) is the main effects model, i.e., a straightforward generalization of the two-mode RM. The third

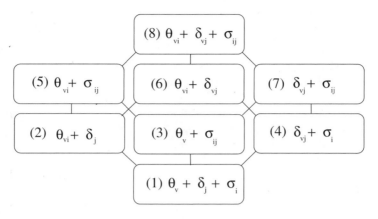

Fig. 10.1. Hierarchy of the eight three-mode RMs

mode is represented by a third parameter δ_j. Modeling the third mode like this consequently follows Rasch's idea of separating the influence of different modes on the response behavior assuming no interactions between the modes and their parameters. This assumption yields a unidimensional model.

Model (3) separates the influence of persons and items, in contrast to model (1), which does not assume the item difficulties are to be explained by the two facets. This is reflected in the doubly indexed item-parameters σ_{ij}. Models (3) and (1) are the only unidimensional model in the hierarchy, all other models are multidimensional. Both unidimensional models will be discussed and illustrated using the mathematics achievement data presented in Section 10.2.

Models (2), (4), and (6) assume the impact of the latter two modes to be either on item difficulty or on person ability. The parameters are not doubly indexed with respect to the two modes, i and j. Models (2) and (4) are multidimensional by assuming ability parameters to be specific for the components of one of the facets, whereas model (6) assumes a latent ability for each item type. These models will be discussed in context of the science test in Section 3.

The three remaining models, (5), (7), and (8), specify the same multidimensionality as models (2), (4), and (6), but do not differentiate between the modes on the level of item difficulties. Hence these models have double indexed σ_{ij} parameters and are generalizations of models (2), (4), and (6). These three models will be considered with respect to the intelligence test, the Berlin Intelligence Structure Test in Section 10.4.

10.3 Unidimensional Three-Mode RMs

In model (1), the main effects model, the probability of observing a dichotomous (correct/incorrect) response x_{vij} from person v on an item that represents component i of the first facet and component j of the second, is

Model (1) $P(X = x|\lambda_{vij}) = \frac{\exp[x(\theta_v + \delta_j + \sigma_i)]}{1 + \exp(\theta_v + \delta_j + \sigma_i)}.$

Using the notation of Fig. 10.1 for model (1), the exponent in the logistic
function is

Model (1) $\lambda_{vij} = (\theta_v + \delta_j + \sigma_i).$

In contrast, model (3) does not decompose the item parameters according
to the facet structure, the exponent in the logistic function for a correct response (in the case of 0 or 1 scored data) is given by

Model (3) $\lambda_{vij} = (\theta_v + \sigma_{ij}).$

Model (1) is a special case of model (3), because it assumes that each item
difficulty can be predicted by the specific combination of the two facets main
effects in each item, i.e., $\sigma_{ij} = \delta_j + \sigma_i$.[1] In the case of a test with one item per
item type (i.e., combination of modes i and j), each item is parametrized with
its own parameters σ_{ij} and model (3) becomes equivalent to the dichotomous
RM. In a test with more than one item for each item type, specifying only
one difficulty parameter σ_{ij} for item type obviously is a restriction, compared
to a RM.

The mathematics test of the German extension to the PISA 2003 study
(Prenzel et al., 2004) is guided by the distinction between different topics and
cognitive processes. For each of three topics (arithmetic, algebra, and geometry[2]), items were developed that require the students either to do technical
processing (of things that they should have rehearsed), to do numerical analysis (solutions with numbers), or formal modeling (solutions with abstract or
formal thinking).

The test consists of 124 items in four by three item types. For the analyses presented here, 18 items from one booklet of the data collections were
selected in order to have two items from each of three by three[2] item types.
Consequently, model (3) is a restriction of the RM specifying nine item parameters σ_{ij} for 18 items. This, however, is a typical situation, because one
observation per facet combination may not be sufficient information for estimating the trait parameters of some multidimensional models. It is important

---

[1] If two or more components are assumed for each facet

[2] A fourth topic—stochastics—was dropped from the analyses because only very
few items were administered in the booklet selected here (only 2 out of 66 items
in book 9, PISA 2003 main study 2nd day).

to note that within the family of three-mode RMs, models (1) and (3) actually constrain the parameter space and can be viewed as restricted versions of the unidimensional RM with model (1) allowing only main effects of the two item modes and model (3) allowing interactions. The other models in contrast extend the parameter space by allowing multidimensionality. It follows that models (1) and (3) will be identified whenever the RM is identified, whereas this is not necessarily the case for the other models. The notation chosen in Fig. 10.1 does not take into account more than one item in each item type. Thus, adding a third index k to the item-parameter σ_{ijk} indicates more than one item in each item type.

Table 10.1. Design matrix of model (1) for the German mathematics test PISA 2003 and parameter estimates

Parameter/ Item	Arithmetic	Algebra	Geometry	Technical processing	Numerical modeling	Formal modeling	M1 parameters	RM parameter	Difference	SE of difference
1	1			1			−1.02	−1.15	**−0.13**	0.10
2	1				1		−0.20	0.07	**0.27**	0.09
3	1					1	−0.19	−0.43	**−0.24**	0.09
4		1		1			−0.05	−0.06	**−0.01**	0.09
5		1			1		0.78	0.65	**−0.12**	0.09
6		1				1	0.78	0.69	**−0.09**	0.09
7			1	1			−0.41	−0.14	**0.26**	0.09
8			1		1		0.42	0.09	**−0.33**	0.09
9			1			1	0.43	0.58	**0.15**	0.09
10	1			1			−1.02	−1.19	**−0.17**	0.10
11	1				1		−0.20	0.41	**0.61**	0.09
12	1					1	−0.19	−0.60	**−0.41**	0.09
13		1		1			−0.05	−0.20	**−0.15**	0.09
14		1			1		0.78	0.73	**−0.05**	0.09
15		1				1	0.78	1.28	**0.50**	0.10
16			1	1			−0.41	−0.27	**0.14**	0.09
17			1		1		0.42	0.05	**−0.37**	0.09
18			1			1	0.43	0.59	**0.16**	0.09

parameter   −0.47 0.50 0.15 −0.55 0.27 0.28

Models (1) and (3) are represented by design matrices in Tables 10.1 and 10.2, respectively. In these design matrices, the rows correspond to the items and the columns to the facets components. In both tables, two items correspond to each of the nine different item types, represented by nine rows with different entries. The main effects model (1) in Table 10.1 predicts the item difficulties by six difficulty parameters[3] only, one for each component of both facets.

In order to estimate the parameters of model (1), the item or subject parameters have to be constrained; one way to do this is to constrain the mean of the latent trait distribution. Alternatively, the mean of the item difficulties, or one item parameter can be constrained (set to some constant, often zero) in order to remove the indeterminacy of the scale. In addition to the design matrix, eight model parameters are specified, six item-component parameters, a population mean and a population variance. The mean was set to zero and seven parameters were estimated using the software package ConQuest (Wu et al., 1997) assuming a Gaussian distribution for the latent trait parameters.

The estimates of the six facets parameters are given in the last column of Table 10.1. In the fourth last column the combined item parameters are printed, the parameters of a RM on these items are given in the third last row and the differences between the two with standard error are given in the second last and last column. The arithmetic and technical processing items are the easiest ones, the items combining algebra and formal modeling are the hardest. Looking at the differences between parameter estimates, that is, the RM item difficulties minus the model (1) difficulties in the last column, we find that some item difficulties are not predicted very well by model (1). Items 11 and 15 are showing the largest differences indicating the worst fit.

However, it cannot be concluded from these numbers whether these residuals are due to the facets structure being invalid for these items or to differences between the difficulties of two items within each facet. This question can be answered by applying model (3). Table 10.2 shows the design matrix of this model and provides some parameter estimates.

The differences between the parameter estimates are much smaller than for the first model, however, two items still show a poor fit, in this case item 6 and 15. Both represent formal modeling processes in algebra tasks and have the same predicted difficulty of 0.97 whereas the difference between their difficulties is about 0.6. Tasks of this type may vary in their difficulty, independently of their facets structure. The reason of the misfit of item 11 under the first model (see above) may be explained by the facets decomposition, because by model (3), the RM difficulties are predicted more accurately than by model (1).

Table 10.3 shows the fit statistics for all three models under consideration. The log-likelihood for the first model is -9461.7; six component parameters were estimated and a population variance, the population mean was set to zero. With a sample size of 882, the consistent Akaike information criterion (CAIC) value comes to 18978. In model (3), 9-item-component parameters

---

[3] We write easiness parameters in the model equations; however item-parameter estimates will reflect difficulty.

Table 10.2. Design matrix of model (3) for the German mathematics test PISA 2003 and parameters estimates

Parameter/ Items	Arithmetics tech. proc.	Arithmetics numerical m.	Arithmetics formal m.	Algebra tech. proc.	Algebra numerical m.	Algebra formal m.	Geometry tech. proc.	Geometry numerical m.	Geometry formal m.	M3 parameter	RM parameter	difference	SE of difference
1	1									-1.17	-1.15	**0.02**	0.10
2		1								0.24	0.07	**-0.17**	0.09
3			1							-0.51	-0.43	**0.08**	0.10
4				1						-0.13	-0.06	**0.07**	0.10
5					1					0.69	0.65	**-0.04**	0.10
6						1				0.97	0.69	**-0.28**	0.10
7							1			-0.20	-0.14	**0.06**	0.09
8								1		0.07	0.09	**0.02**	0.10
9									1	0.58	0.58	**-0.01**	0.10
10	1									-1.17	-1.19	**-0.02**	0.10
11		1								0.24	0.41	**0.17**	0.10
12			1							-0.51	-0.60	**-0.09**	0.10
13				1						-0.13	-0.20	**-0.07**	0.10
14					1					0.69	0.73	**0.04**	0.10
15						1				0.97	1.28	**0.31**	0.10
16							1			-0.20	-0.27	**-0.06**	0.10
17								1		0.07	0.05	**-0.02**	0.10
18									1	0.58	0.59	**0.01**	0.10

parameter -1.17 0.24 -0.51 -0.13 0.69 0.97 -0.20 0.07 0.58

Table 10.3. Fit statistics for models (1), (3), and the RM

Model	ln L	# Parameters	BIC	CAIC
Model (1) $(\theta_v + \delta_j + \sigma_i)$	-9462	7	18971	18978
Model (3) $(\theta_v + \sigma_{ij})$	-9371	10	**18810**	**18820**
RM $(\theta_v + \sigma_{ijk})$	-9350	19	18829	18848

and a population variance were estimated. For the RM, 18 item difficulties and a variance were estimated. According to these results, model (3) shows a better fit to the data than model (1). As compared with the unrestricted RM, model (3) is sufficient to describe the item difficulties (the Bayesian information criterion [BIC] and CAIC information criteria are smallest for this model). It may be concluded that the distinction of topics and modeling types does help to model the item difficulties of mathematics tasks in the sense of model (3), except for formal modeling in algebra. However, the prediction of item difficulties by simply adding facet-specific difficulties in terms of model (1) does not fit the data well.

Models (1) and (3) were estimated with ConQuest (Wu et al., 1997). Alternatively, the program LPCM-Win (Fischer, 1989) may be used for parameter estimation and model control, because both models are linear logistic test models (Fischer, 1973). For estimation with other software packages, the reader is referred to Kelderman's Chapter 5 in this volume on loglinear multivariate and mixture distribution RMs.

10.4 Multidimensional Models Separating the Two Facets

The models in this group are based on the assumption of multidimensional abilities. Either one or both of the latter two facets of the response process may be modeled as ability modes or difficulty modes. A second assumption is restricting the impact of the facets either on ability or on item difficulty. The models, according to the notation introduced in Fig. 10.1, are

Model (2) $\lambda_{vij} = (\theta_{vi} + \delta_j),$

defining I abilities and assuming J basic parameters to build up the item difficulties.

Model (4) $\lambda_{vij} = (\theta_{vj} + \sigma_i)$

defining in contrast to model (2) J abilities and I basic parameters for the item difficulties

Model (6) $\lambda_{vij} = (\theta_{vi} + \delta_{vj})$

specifies I plus J abilities and has no (explicit) difficulty parameter. However, difficulty parameters may be specified for each component within the facets if appropriate model identification constraints are chosen. In general, not defining item parameters for one or two modes is equivalent to assuming the according item difficulties to be equal and setting them to zero. With model (2), it is assumed that items do not differ in their difficulty between the components of the second facet (indicated with i's); with model (4), no differences between the components of the third facet are assumed. Model (6) defines all item difficulties to be equal and zero. These constraints will be discussed again in the context of the example presented below.

The models of this section will be illustrated by means of the German national science data of the PISA 2003 study (Rost et al., 2004). In this test, which has been constructed by a German science expert group, two facets are completely crossed, i.e., seven cognitive operations and nine content areas from the school subjects physics, chemistry, and biology. Hence, the test covers 63 items, of which only one third are used for the present example. We have chosen one content domain from each science subject, labeled "breathing and photosynthesis" from biology, "in the pool" from chemistry, and "everyday electricity" from physics.

The seven cognitive operations have been derived from an in depth analysis of the German science framework and assessment instruments used in the PISA 2000 study. A task analysis revealed five different cognitive processes necessary for solving the tasks (Prenzel et al., 2002). These cognitive operations had been extended (Rost, 2004) by the operations "divergent thinking," which is the counterpart of analytical (convergent) thinking and related to tasks that do not ask for the only correct solution but for the production of several possible solutions. The second new operation is "evaluation," where again not the single correct solution is asked for, but some good reasons have to be given for the position selected by the student.

The focus of analyzing this test was on the question, whether the cognitive operations (facet one) or the content topics (facet two) require a multidimensional test model for representing the students differences in ability. Let the cognitive operations be the second facet of the response process and the content areas the third facet. Then model (2) assumes multidimensionality for the cognitive operations only, model (4) for the contents only, and model (6) for both facets. Consequently, model (2) specifies seven abilities and three basic item-difficulty parameters, model (4) assumes seven basic parameters and three abilities, and model (6) defines ten abilities and no item-difficulty parameters.

The design matrix specifying the ability dimensions of model (6) and the parameter estimates of all three models are presented in Table 10.4. For the abilities, univariate and multivariate normal distributions were assumed. The last three rows of Table 10.4 give the parameter estimates according to the three models. For model (2), the means of seven ability distributions and two basic parameters were estimated (basic parameters are written in italics); the third basic parameter was constrained to be the negative sum of the other two as identification constraint. The ability means were not restricted, but note that for each item a basic parameter is identified and estimated in the third mode. For model (4), six basic parameters were estimated with the seventh being the negative sum of the other six, and three ability means were estimated without further restriction. For model (6), ten ability means are estimated without further restriction. As noted above, implicitly all item difficulties are assumed to be zero. Alternatively and equivalently, the ability means may be restricted to be zero, and a basic parameter may be estimated for each component of the facets, i.e., according to the design matrix in Table 10.4.

Another constraint is necessary to uniquely specify model (6). The design matrix defines ten dimensions but is only of rank nine, allowing parameter estimation for nine independent dimensions. For the estimation the last column of the design was omitted, fixing these parameters to be zero. In order to have person parameters for all ten dimensions, parameters for ten dimensions may be recomputed from the estimated parameters introducing another constraint on the ten dependent parameters for each subject (see Carstensen, 2000). The mean parameters in the last row of Table 10.4 were computed by constraining the mean of the cognitive operation parameters to be equal to the mean of the content area parameters for every subject.

The last six columns at the right-hand side of the table give the difficulties for each item composed through the design matrix and the standard errors of the difference between models (2) and (4). The item parameters of the three models are very close. This has to be expected, because both ways of modeling a facet, as item-difficulty mode or as ability mode, results in assuming all items from one component, cognitive operation or content area, to have the same difficulty. These difficulties are modeled through one parameter for each component, ability mean or a basic parameter. However, the basic parameter for number processing in model (4) does not fit into the number processing difficulty according to the other models.

From the parameter estimates, the cognitive operations "convergent thinking," "mental modeling," and "number processing" are rather difficult ones, whereas "verbalizing" and "divergent thinking" are easier to perform. The content areas do not contribute much to the variation of the task difficulties.

The question which of the facets calls for a multidimensional model can be answered by means of the fit statistics shown in Table 10.5. Comparing the models through the CAIC index, model (2) seems best in explaining the data. In particular, it is not necessary to differentiate students' science achievement with respect to the content domains as indicated by poorer fit and the lower contribution of the according parameters to the item difficulties.

The models (2), (4), and (6) seem rather restrictive in composing all item difficulties from one parameter for each component, either a mean or a basic parameter. The appropriateness of (one of) these models obviously depends on a systematic item construction with one item for each combination of the second and the third facet of the response process. More, the impact of a component of a facet has to be assumed to be the same on all items constructed. The science test presented is constructed in this way. However, how well the item construction succeeded can be evaluated in comparing models (2), (4), or (6) to a more general model defining a specific difficulty for each item. Such models are discussed in the following section.

Table 10.4. Design matrix for the German science test PISA 2003

Parameter Item	Decision making	Divergent thinking	Graphical representation	Convergent thinking	Mental modeling	Verbalizing	Number processing	Breathing & Photosynthesis	In the pool	Electricity	Model (2) parameters	Model (4) parameters	Model (6) parameters	SE of difference (M2+M4)
1	1							1			0.02	0.01	0.02	0.06
2		1						1			−0.40	−0.35	−0.38	0.04
3			1					1			0.33	0.29	0.33	0.06
4				1				1			1.30	1.26	1.30	0.06
5					1			1			0.94	0.97	0.95	0.05
6						1		1			−0.23	−0.23	−0.23	0.06
7							1	1			0.70	**0.45**	0.72	0.10
8	1								1		−0.13	−0.12	−0.12	0.06
9		1							1		−0.54	−0.48	−0.53	0.04
10			1						1		0.18	0.16	0.19	0.06
11				1					1		1.16	1.13	1.16	0.06
12					1				1		0.80	0.84	0.80	0.05
13						1			1		−0.38	−0.36	−0.37	0.06
14							1		1		0.56	**0.32**	0.57	0.10
15	1									1	0.28	0.25	0.26	0.07
16		1								1	−0.13	−0.11	−0.14	0.05
17			1							1	0.59	0.53	0.57	0.07
18				1						1	1.57	1.50	1.54	0.06
19					1					1	1.21	1.21	1.19	0.06
20						1				1	0.03	0.00	0.01	0.07
21							1			1	0.97	**0.69**	0.96	0.11
Par. M2*	0.06	-0.36	0.37	1.34	0.98	-0.19	0.74	*-0.04*	*-0.19*	*(0.23)*				
Par. M4*	*-0.33*	*-0.69*	*-0.05*	*0.92*	*0.63*	*-0.58*	*(0.11)*	0.34	0.21	0.58				
Par. M6*	-0.24	-0.64	0.07	1.04	0.68	-0.49	0.46	0.26	0.12	(0.50)				

*Note: Basic parameters (printed in italics) and negative means of latent dimensions, parameters set in brackets are constrained and not estimated; for details on the constraint in M6, see text.

10.5 Multidimensional Models with Unrestricted Item Parameters

This group of three multidimensional models shares the assumption of an ability parameter for each component of the second or the third mode or both

Table 10.5. Fit statistics for models (2), (4), and (6)

Model	ln L	Number of Parameters*	BIC	CAIC
Model (2) $(\theta_{vi} + \delta_j)$	-10045	21+7+7+2	**20340**	**20377**
Model (4) $(\theta_{vj} + \sigma_i)$	-10158	3+3+3+6	20418	20433
Model (6) $(\theta_{vi} + \delta_{vj})$	-10035	36+9+9+0	20434	20488

*Note: Printed are the numbers of covariance + variance + mean + basic.

with the previous group of models. In contrast, the item parameters of the models in this group are unrestricted with respect to the mode structure, i.e., the σ_{ij} parameters are not decomposed. The models, according to the notation introduced in Fig. 10.1, are

Model (5) $\lambda_{vij} = (\theta_{vi} + \sigma_{ij})$,

defining I abilities and different difficulties in each combination of components of the second and the third facet.

Model (7) $\lambda_{vij} = (\delta_{vj} + \sigma_{ij})$

defines J abilities in contrast and $I \times J$ difficulties, whereas

Model (8) $\lambda_{vij} = (\theta_{vi} + \delta_{vj} + \sigma_{ij})$

specifies $I + J$ abilities and I x J difficulties. In these equations, the same difficulty is assumed for any item within each item type, i.e., combination of facets I and J. If more than one item response is to be modeled within an item type, the models may be generalized further by introducing separate item parameters for each item within an item type. The item parameters shall then be indexed with k. Complete model equations are printed below for the data set analyzed.

Leaving the item parameters unrestricted implies for a given test that the difficulties of the items are not assumed to be determined by the mode structure. This situation is given in the German intelligence test developed by Jäger et al. (1997), the Berlin Intelligence Structure test BIS T4. The test is based on a structural model of human intelligence, according to which each higher cognitive process has to be performed in some representational mode, like verbal, numerical, or figural. Moreover, intelligence tasks can be classified with respect to the kind of cognitive process to be performed in a representational mode. The most central processes are creativity, memory, speed, and capacity.

The BIS model obviously is influenced by older intelligence models, like Thurstone's primary mental abilities (1941) or the structural model by Guilford (1967). In contrast to these theories, the BIS model focuses on the most

relevant processes and representational modes and explicitly states that each
intelligence task has to refer to both facets: the type of cognitive process and
the medium in which the process takes place. The theory states that any
cognitive process can only be observed when it is performed in some content
or representation. In the other direction, the ability to solve tasks in some
content area can only be assessed if a cognitive process is induced.

It is a basic assumption of the BIS-test (Jäger et al., 1997) that two intelligence traits are involved in determining the probability of each response in
the BIS, one trait related to the content and one trait related to the process
to be performed in a task. Hence, the seven dimensions, i.e., three content
related and four process related abilities, of the BIS are organized in two
modes (see Fig. 10.2). For each of the 12 cells in this model, three, four, or
five subtests have been constructed, each covering a series of items of the same
type. The BIS-test includes 45 subtests in total. According to the BIS model,
these tests contribute to a global measure of intelligence (g-factor), which is,
however, not part of the formalized model. It is just the reason for expecting
substantial correlations among the seven abilities, what is different from, e.g.,
Thurstone's theory. In the design matrix in Table 10.6, the rows correspond
to the item types (the twelve combinations of processes and representation),
the columns correspond to the abilities. The second column gives the number
of items for each item type.

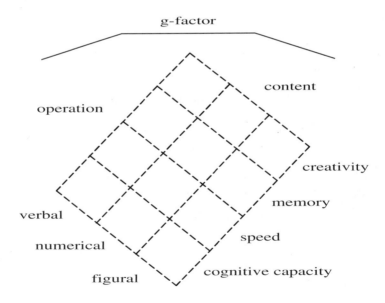

Fig. 10.2. Intelligence structure model underlying the BIS T4 intelligence test

In the following, results of a study will be presented that tries to validate the assumed psychometric structure of the BIS. Carstensen (2000) analyzed a set of data that is combined from the original data of the test authors and some data from own data collections, 650 cases in total. Multidimensional models were estimated using joint maximum likelihood (JML) procedures employing the software MULTIRA (Carstensen & Rost, 2001). In this section, however, results gained by marginal maximum likelihood (MML) procedures using the software ConQuest (Wu et al., 1997) are presented. In the MML approach, the ability distributions are assumed to be multivariate normal, so that much less parameters have to be estimated as compared to the JML method.

The tasks for the 12 types of subtests consist of more or less traditional intelligence tasks. The four cognitive processes have been assessed by means of solving analogies (cognitive capacity or reasoning), trying to find as many stimuli with a certain quality as possible in a given time (speed), reproducing stimuli after a short exposition (memory), or trying to produce as many solutions as possible according to given instruction (creativity). As the total number of item responses across subtests is quite large, the number of responses in the subtest quite different, it might be difficult to fit a response model on the item level. Because the responses within subtests are expected to be more homogeneous (locally dependent) than across subtests, the multidimensional model has not been specified on the level of single item responses but on the subtest scores. That means, the 45 subtests are treated as "items," As Andrich (1985) has proposed for locally dependent subtest responses, the equidistance RM is used on the level of subtest scores. A higher homogeneity among the items within a subtest will result in a narrower dispersion indicated by a higher dispersion parameter value.

Table 10.6. Design matrix for the BIS-T4 with 4 operations and three contents

Parameter/ Item Types*	N. of Items of This Type	Cognitive Capacity	Speed	Memory	Creativity	Verbal	Numerical	Figural
1	5	1				1		
2	3		1			1		
3	3			1		1		
4	4				1	1		
5	5	1					1	
6	3		1				1	
7	3			1			1	
8	4				1		1	
9	5	1						1
10	3		1					1
11	3			1				1
12	4				1			1

*note: (3 to 5 items from each item type in the BIS-T4).

The BIS-T4 has been analyzed with the models (5), (7), and (8) of the hierarchical system of three-mode RMs from Fig. 10.1. The assumption of model (5) is that the operations (response facet I) are related to different traits whereas the content areas (response facet J) are not. In addition to equation in Fig. 10.1, the model for the BIS data has to take into account the subtest scores for more than one subtest from each item type. The subtest scores are modeled by the equidistance model Andrich (1982), specifying a location parameter β and a dispersion parameter τ for each subtest. The subtests are indexed with k within each item type ij, and the probability of subject v getting x_{vijk} correct responses in subtest ijk then is a function of

Model (5a) $\qquad \lambda_{vijk} = \exp\left(x\theta_{vi} + x\sigma_{ijk}\right)$

with $x\sigma_{ijk} = (x\beta_{ijk} + x\left(h_{ijk} - x\right)\tau_{ijk})$, and where X_{ijk} denotes the observed count of correct solutions and h_{ijk} the maximum number of correct solutions for subtest ijk with β_{ijk} and τ_{ijk} being a difficulty and a threshold parameter for this subtest.

If in contrast the assumption of model (7) is made, i.e., the content areas correspond to latent traits and the operations do not, the probability for a BIS subtest score x_{vijk} is given by

Model (7a) $\qquad \lambda_{vijk} = \exp\left(x\delta_{vj} + x\sigma_{ijk}\right)$

with $x\sigma_{ijk}$ as above. Defining the operations as well as the contents as latent traits and allowing the item difficulties to vary without respect to the item type yields model (8), the BIS model. The probability of having x_{vijk} correct response from on subtest ijk is then a function of

Model (8a) $\qquad \lambda_{vijk} = \exp\left(x\theta_{vi} + x\delta_{vj} + x\sigma_{ijk}\right)$

with $x\sigma_{ijk}$ as above. For estimation, the means of the ability distributions were fixed to zero for all three models, whereas the item locations and dispersions were not further restricted. As a consequence, the subtest locations represent the difficulty of the subtests for each item type. The location parameters will be presented below. In analogy to the additional constraint for model (6), only six of the seven dimensions are estimated for model (8), fixing the parameters of the seventh dimension to zero. A set of seven parameters for each person may be obtained by introducing the same constraint as for model (6), i.e., fixing the sum of the operation parameters to equal the sum of the content parameters for each subject. The correlation matrix of person parameters computed according to this constraint is presented in Table 10.7.

Item dispersion certainly is also a relevant feature of subtest scores and is related to test length and subtest homogeneity. For the present data analysis, the sum scores of the subtests were grouped into six categories. These modifications of the raw data destroy the benefits of the dispersion parameters, which have no threshold interpretation with a psychological meaning any more. In the presented analysis, they are just a tool to fit the models to the data.

Table 10.8 shows the likelihoods the number of parameters and BIC and CAIC indices for model fit comparisons. The results confirm the assumptions of the BIS-T4, because model (8) with both types of traits, process and content traits, shows the closest fit to the data.

Table 10.7. Fit statistics for models (5), (7), and (8)

Model	Number of Independent Parameters*	ln L	BIC	CAIC
Model (5) operation dimensions	$6 + 4 + 0 + 45 + 45$	-40612	81872	81972
Model (7) content dimensions	$3 + 3 + 0 + 45 + 45$	-41028	82678	82774
Model (8) BIS model	$15 + 6 + 0 + 45 + 45$	-40326	**81372**	**81483**

*Note: The numbers of covariance + variance + mean + location + dispersion parameters are printed in this order.

For model fit testing reasons, model (8) should be compared to a more general model, specifying twelve dimensions, one for each item type. In the MML approach, the estimation of this 12-dimensional model did not converge properly and thus no results are available. This may be due to the small sample size of 650 subjects only, compared to the complexity of the model. However, Carstensen (2000) reports a likelihood comparison of these two models from the JML approach. He uses empirically constructed distributions of the test statistic obtained from resampling methods. According to his results, model (8) is sufficient to explain the data.

Turning to the ability distributions, Table 10.8 gives the matrix of latent correlations among the seven dimensions (see paragraph on constraints above). The general ability dimension is computed as the sum of either four operation or three content parameters for each subject. The correlations among the cognitive operations are close to zero. For example, creativity and speed show a low positive correlation, which may be due to the nature of the creativity tasks. In these tasks, respondents are asked to produce as many solutions as possible in a given time.

Note that the operation parameters for each subject add to the general ability as the content parameters do. Both sets of ability parameters, therefore, are ipsative measures and their correlations are artificially distorted in the negative direction. The content parameters show somewhat higher correlations among each other and with the general ability as the operation parameters do. Taking into account, that the artificial distortion due to ipsative measurement is higher for *three* ipsative variables (content) than for *four* (operation), the results may have a substantial interpretation: the abilities related to the four cognitive processes are easier to distinguish as the abilities related to content areas or representational modes. The correlations between operations and contents are generally positive and of medium strength, a result that may be explained by the fact that each operation can only be measured in the context of a content and vice versa.

Table 10.8. Correlation coefficients among the abilities on model (8) for the re-computed seven dimensional parameters and general ability

Correlations	Capacity	Speed	Memory	Creativity	Verbal	Numerical	Figural
Speed	0.00						
Memory	0.12	0.02					
Creativity	−0.22	0.25	−0.28				
Verbal	0.26	0.50	0.38	0.28			
Numerical	0.38	0.45	0.36	0.26	0.23		
Figural	0.38	0.37	0.22	0.39	0.21	0.43	
General	0.46	0.61	0.45	0.42	0.72	0.75	0.70

In earlier analyses, Rost & Carstensen (2002) have shown that the correlations among sum scores are quite different from, and generally higher than the correlations among the ability parameters of a multidimensional model. However, the problems of ipsative measurement are neither solved in the latter case.

10.6 Conclusion

In this chapter, a system of three-mode item response models has been introduced. A three-mode model may be applied to response data if three facets of the response process are to be modeled. The three-mode structure of the models covered in this chapter is based on extensions to the simple logistic model by Rasch (1960). The resulting system of models covers the LLTM, special cases of the RM, and multidimensional generalizations. Not in every model of the system is the separation between person abilities and item difficulties maintained. In other words, the person and item facets of the response process are not modeled independently in every model. In model (4) for example, the difficulty of items with regard to components of the third facet (indicated by j) cannot be estimated independently of the person abilities with regard to the different dimensions associated with the components of this facet.

Facet designed response data may be obtained in a variety of data collection designs and facets may be due to numerous conditions in the response process. As suggested in this chapter, the family of different three-mode models may be particularly useful for modeling different facets of the response process by assuming a multidimensional ability concept. This may include cognitive processes related to different contents. Rost & Carstensen (2002) analyzed an interest questionnaire that investigated the interest of students in different topic areas of science conditionally on different activities related to science.

A system of models like the family of three-mode models provides a framework for testing model-data fit. Different hypotheses on the mode structure, i.e., about the adequate way of relating the facets in the responses to modes in the response model, can be empirically evaluated. These questions may be addressed by likelihood comparisons as likelihood ratio tests or information indices (AIC, BIC, CAIC). Different software packages are available that produce estimates for three-mode models. In the framework of marginal maximum likelihood, the software ConQuest estimating the Mixed-Coefficients Multinomial Logit Model is capable of estimating all three-mode models. Conditional maximum likelihood estimates are available through the Software LPCM (Fischer) for LLTM models and MULTIRA (Carstensen & Rost, 2001) for multidimensional three-mode RMs.

11

(Almost) Equivalence Between Conditional and Mixture Maximum Likelihood Estimates for Some Models of the Rasch Type

Anton K. Formann

University of Vienna, Department of Psychological Basic Research

11.1 Introduction

It has been known for several years that conditional and mixture maximum likelihood estimates do agree for the dichotomous Rasch model (RM). This equivalence may be attained by a sufficient number of mixing components in a specifically restricted latent-class model. Because the principle of such a semiparametric approach is a general one (Kiefer & Wolfowitz, 1956), it also applies to some other models of the Rasch type having simple sufficient statistics. Exact equivalence regarding the parameter estimates can be shown, for example, for the linear logistic test model, a RM with linearly constrained item parameters, and for the polytomous RM; only almost equivalence is found for the mixed RM. As formal proofs of these results are difficult, the presentation focuses on numerical examples demonstrating the said (almost) equivalence.

Neyman & Scott (1948) investigated problems of consistent estimates based on partially consistent observations. The general situation can be characterized as follows. "Let x_i stand for a (possibly multivariate) random variable and assume that the variables of the sequence $x_1, x_2, \ldots, x_n, \ldots$ are mutually independent" (p. 1). "...the set of unknown parameters involved in the totality of probability laws of the random variables $\{x_i\}$ is infinite and can be split into two parts. The first part is composed of a *finite* number of parameters, say $\xi_1, \xi_2, \ldots, \xi_\nu$, each of which appears in the probability laws of an *infinity* of random variables of the sequence $\{x_i\}$. ... The second part of the set of unknown parameters is infinite and is composed of parameters θ_m each of which appears in the probability law of only a finite number of random variables considered. ... the parameters $\xi_1, \xi_2, \ldots, \xi_\nu$ will be called *structural*. All the other parameters $\theta_1, \theta_2 \ldots$ will be called incidental" (p. 2). As their main result, Neyman and Scott stated that "maximum-likelihood estimates of the structural parameters relating to a partially consistent series of observations need not be consistent" (p. 7), and that "even if the maximum-likelihood estimate of a structural parameter is consistent ... the maximum-likelihood

178 Anton K. Formann

estimate need not possess the property of asymptotic efficiency" (p. 8). The further considerations in Neyman and Scott regarding a systematic method of obtaining consistent estimates end in the statement, "... that, thus far, there does not seem to exist a systematic method of solving the ... problem" (p. 19).

Some years later, Kiefer & Wolfowitz (1956) presented such a method according to which the structural parameters have to be estimated together with the distribution of the incidental parameters. They proved for their approach "that, under usual regularity conditions, the maximum likelihood estimator of a structural parameter is strongly consistent, when the (infinitely many) incidental parameters are independently distributed chance variables with a common unknown distribution function. The latter is also consistently estimated although it is not assumed to belong to a parametric class" (p. 887).

Four years later, the book by Rasch (1960) was published, containing, among others, his famous item response model for dichotomous data. As is well-known now, the probability of answer x_{vi} ($x_{vi} = 1$ if subject S_v solved item I_i, $x_{vi} = 0$ otherwise), $v = 1, \ldots, N$, $i = 1, \ldots, k$, is governed by two parameters, the first one, θ_v, characterizing subject S_v, and the other one, σ_i, the item I_i :

$$p_{vi} = p(X_{vi} = 1|\sigma_i, \theta_v) = \frac{\exp(\theta_v + \sigma_i)}{1 + \exp(\theta_v + \sigma_i)}. \tag{11.1}$$

As the number of items, k, is fixed, but N increases with increasing sample size, the situation corresponds exactly to that of structural vs. incident parameters where the maximum likelihood (ML) estimates of the structural parameters need not be consistent. And in fact, they are not consistent when estimated together with the incidental person parameters (unconditional or joint ML method). It seems to be unknown whether Rasch was aware of the Kiefer–Wolfowitz approach or not, but it is sure that his solution to the problem of parameter estimation was another one, in some sense related to proposals derived by Neyman & Scott (1948). Rasch's favorite was the conditional ML (CML) method, which substitutes the incidental person parameters by their sufficient statistics, the raw scores, and conditions the person parameters out of the likelihood.

Another way of eliminating the subjects parameters is to integrate them out. This was done by the marginal ML (MML) method of parameter estimation in the RM. This method assumes that subjects stem from a population with continuous ability distribution $G(\theta)$, so that the marginal probability of response pattern $\mathbf{x}_v = (x_{v1}, \ldots, x_{vk})$ is given by

$$p(\mathbf{x}_v) = \int_{-\infty}^{\infty} p(\mathbf{x}_v|\theta)dG(\theta) \tag{11.2}$$

and the whole likelihood may be written as

$$L = p\{(\mathbf{X})\} = \prod_{v=1}^{N} \int_{-\infty}^{\infty} p(\mathbf{x}_v|\theta)dG(\theta). \qquad (11.3)$$

The item parameters are then estimated by applying the ML method to this marginal likelihood. Originally, the ability distribution $G(\theta)$ was assumed to be known or at least to belong to a certain family of distributions (for example, normal; cf. Bock and Lieberman, 1970). Later on, the continuous ability distribution was approximated by a discrete distribution, with an arbitrary number of support points θ_j, $j = 1, \ldots, m$, with corresponding masses w_j, $j = 1, \ldots, m$, $0 < w_j \leq 1$, $\sum_{j=1}^{m} w_j = 1$, resulting in the (nowadays called semi- or nonparametric) likelihood

$$L^* = \prod_{v=1}^{N} \sum_{j=1}^{m} w_j p(\mathbf{x}_v|\theta_j). \qquad (11.4)$$

The discrete ability distribution, that is, their support points and corresponding masses, has to be estimated along with the item parameters; see Bock & Aitkin (1981) for the normal ogive model, and Thissen (1982) and Mislevy (1984) for the RM.

For an arbitrary number of support points, this method comes close to the Kiefer–Wolfowitz (1956) approach. That it becomes the Kiefer–Wolfowitz approach and, as a consequence, that it leads to the same item-parameter estimates as obtained with the CML method, was shown independently by Leeuw & Verhelst (1986), Follmann (1988), and Lindsay et al. (1991). They derived that, apart from degenerate data, the equivalence between conditional and semiparametric ML can be attained for the dichotomous RM if the number of support points, m^*, at least is

$$m^* = \begin{cases} (k+1)/2 & \text{for } k \text{ odd,} \\ k/2 + 1 & \text{for } k \text{ even.} \end{cases} \qquad (11.5)$$

Then, the observed score distribution equals the expected one, and the item- parameter estimates agree perfectly. If k is odd, usually all parameters (support points and their masses, item parameters) are identifiable. If k is even, one parameter will be unidentifiable, and one restriction has to be imposed, see the example in Formann (1989). If m, the number of support points, is chosen to be greater than m^*, the number of unidentifiable parameters increases, and no improvement of fit is possible.

As pointed out by Formann (1989) for the dichotomous RM, the semiparametric ML approach can easily be realized by specifically restricted models within the framework of linear logistic latent-class analysis (Formann, 1982, 1985). Thereby, the individual response vectors $\mathbf{x}_v = (x_{v1}, \ldots, x_{vk})$ can be represented by the multinominal distribution of the 2^k response patterns $\mathbf{x}_s$ and their observed frequencies n_s. Because of the assumption of local independence, the likelihood results in

$$L^* = \prod_{s=1}^{2^k} \left[\sum_{j=1}^{m} w_j \prod_{i=1}^{k} p_{i|j}^{x_{si}} (1 - p_{i|j})^{1-x_{si}} \right]^{n_s}, \qquad (11.6)$$

with $p_{i|j}$ denoting the probability of a positive response, given membership to class C_j. Linear logistic latent-class analysis constrains the $p_{i|j}$ according to

$$\ln[p_{i|j}/(1 - p_{i|j})] = \sum_{t=1}^{u} q_{ijt}\eta_t, \qquad (11.7)$$

so that for models analogous to the dichotomous RM,

$$\ln[p_{i|j}/(1 - p_{i|j})] = \theta_j + \sigma_i \qquad (11.8)$$

has to be chosen.

In the following, three numerical examples are given. The first one demonstrates that the CML and the semiparametric ML methods with a certain number of latent classes are equivalent for the linear logistic test model (LLTM). Unsurprisingly, this is the case for the same saturation point as found for the RM: both the RM and the LLTM have in common the sufficient statistic for the person parameters; they differ only regarding their structural parameters. The second example demonstrates the equivalence of the CML and semiparametric ML approaches for the polytomous RM. This example differs from the first one regarding the dimensionality of parameters. In the polytomous RM, the parameters are vectorial, but the principle of the Kiefer–Wolfowitz approach remains applicable. The third example, in contrast, referring to the mixture RM for dichotomous data, shows that an approximate solution, lying near to the CML solution, can be found even in cases where the Kiefer–Wolfowitz method does not apply: in the mixture RM, the parameters do not stem from a common distribution, but are recruited from a mixture distribution.

11.2 Example 1: The Linear Logistic Test Model

The linear logistic test model (LLTM) is a RM with linearly restricted item parameters σ_i,

$$p_{vi} = \frac{\exp(\theta_v + \sum_{r=1}^{t} q_{ir}\eta_r)}{1 + \exp(\theta_v + \sum_{r=1}^{t} q_{ir}\eta_r)}, \qquad (11.9)$$

with the weights q_{ir}, $i = 1, \ldots, k$, $r = 1, \ldots, t$, being known constants. The q_{ir} state a specific structural hypothesis regarding the item parameters σ_i of the RM. Such structural hypotheses may be derived from the experimental setting under which the data have been collected (e.g., in the measurement of change when the same items were presented repeatedly to the same subjects), or they may be inferred from the items themselves (e.g., when different types of cognitive operations are involved in solving the items of an intelligence test).

When the N person parameters θ_v, $v = 1, \ldots, N$, of the LLTM are replaced by only m parameters θ_j, $j = 1, \ldots, m$, describing the ability of the classes $C_1, \ldots, C_m$, then one gets the latent-class/linear logistic test model (LC/LLTM) with its specification equation

$$
p_{i|j} = \frac{\exp(\theta_j + \sum_{r=1}^{t} q_{ir}\lambda_r)}{1 + \exp(\theta_j + \sum_{r=1}^{t} q_{ir}\lambda_r)}. \tag{11.10}
$$

To estimate its parameters, linear logistic LCA for dichotomous data (Formann, 1982, 1985, 1989) is appropriate. Increasing the number of classes has the same effect as it has in the case of the LC/RM: the larger the number of classes, the better the fit of the expected raw score distribution to the observed raw score distribution, but only up to a certain saturation point; this saturation point is the same as it is in the LC/RM. When it is reached, the CML estimates of the parameters η_r of the LLTM and those of the parameters λ_r of the LC/LLTM agree perfectly. Knowing the analogue result for the RM, these findings are not surprising because both the RM and the LLTM have the raw score as the sufficient statistic for the person parameter.

As an example, consider six items of a nonverbal intelligence test similar to Raven's progressive matrices. Each item consists of a 3-by-3 scheme in which eight figures are arranged following certain rules. The ninth, missing figure has to be found out from a given set of alternatives by the examinee. The matrices possess varying difficulty due to different types and, within each type, different numbers of cognitive operations required for their solution. The six items chosen for our example contain two cognitive operations each, whereby three different types of them were distinguished (A, B, C).

To illustrate the specification of the LC/RM and the LC/LLTM in the sense of linear logistic LCA for dichotomous data, the weights corresponding to these models with two classes each can be seen in Table 11.1. In the parametrization of the LC/LLTM, the cognitive operation of type A is used as the reference operation with difficulty equal to 0, and the weights for parameters λ_1 and λ_2 describe the increase in the item difficulty in the presence of one additional cognitive operation of type B or C.

Table 11.2 shows the behavior of the expected raw score distribution for increasing number of latent classes under the LC/LLTM. As under the LC/RM, for four classes the raw score distribution is fitted perfectly and the estimates of the structural parameters λ coincide with those under the CML approach for the LLTM. The corresponding goodness-of-fit statistics, see Table 11.3, indicate bad fit. As increasing the number of classes does not lead to better fit, it is to be concluded that the hypothesized structure of items cannot explain their difficulty to a statistically sufficient amount.

Table 11.1. Matrices items—Weights for the LC/RM and the LC/LLTM assuming two classes

		LC/RM					LC/LLTM				
			σ				θ	λ			θ
Class	Item	1	2	3	4	5	1 2	B	C	1	2
1	1	1					1	1	1	1	
	2		1				1	0	0	1	
	3			1			1	2	0	1	
	4				1		1	1	0	1	
	5					1	1	0	2	1	
	6	−1	−1	−1	−1	−1	1	0	1	1	
2	1	1					1	1	1		1
	2		1				1	0	0		1
	3			1			1	2	0		1
	4				1		1	1	0		1
	5					1	1	0	2		1
	6	−1	−1	−1	−1	−1	1	0	1		1

Table 11.2. Matrices items—Observed frequencies of the raw scores and their expectations for increasing number of classes $(m = 1, \ldots, 4)$ under the LC/LLTM

Score	Observed	Expected Frequencies			
r	Frequency	$m = 1$	$m = 2$	$m = 3$	$m = 4$
0	37	7.1	23.8	36.2	37.0
1	118	72.0	132.2	121.0	118.0
2	238	251.1	252.9	231.6	238.0
3	300	398.2	276.5	308.3	300.0
4	259	308.5	256.1	253.3	259.0
5	148	111.4	172.9	150.3	148.0
6	63	14.7	48.6	62.4	63.0

Table 11.3. Matrices items—Goodness-of-fit statistics for the LC/LLTM with increasing number of classes (X^2 = Pearson's chi-squared statistic, G^2 = likelihood ratio statistic)

Classes	X^2	G^2	df	χ^2_{95}
1	453.8	342.0	60	79.1
2	118.7	118.7	58	76.8
3	101.6	100.7	56	74.5
4	101.2	100.0	54	72.2

11.3 Example 2: The Polytomous Rasch Model

The sufficient statistic for the person parameter is scalar in both in the dichotomous RM and the LLTM. It is shown in the following for the polytomous RM that the semiparametric ML method may also become equivalent to the CML method in the case of vectorial incidental parameters. In this model, each subject S_v is characterized by its vectorial person parameter $\theta_v = (\theta_{v1}, \ldots, \theta_{vg})$, expressing the tendency for showing reactions in each one of the categories $K_1, \ldots, K_g$, and each item I_i is represented by its vectorial parameter $\sigma_i = (\sigma_{i1}, \ldots, \sigma_{ig})$, reflecting the amount to which it provokes answers in each one of the categories. The probability for observing an answer of subject S_v at item I_i in category K_h, derived by Rasch (1961) from the principle of specific objectivity, is

$$p_{vih} = \frac{\exp(\theta_{vh} + \sigma_{ih})}{\sum_{l=1}^{g} \exp(\theta_{vl} + \sigma_{il})}, \tag{11.11}$$

with the normalization conditions $\sum_h \sigma_{ih} = 0$ for $i = 1, \ldots, k$ (items), $\sum_i \sigma_{ih} = 0$ for $h = 1, \ldots, g$ (categories), $\sum_h \theta_{vh} = 0$ for $v = 1, \ldots, n$ (subjects).

The semiparametric or latent-class equivalent of this model, call it the polytomous latent-class/RM (P-LC/RM), assumes the subject parameters to be concentrated on a few location parameters θ_j, $j = 1, \ldots, m$, referring to the response behavior of latent classes $C_1, \ldots, C_m$. Hence, θ_j together with their prevalence rates π_j, $j = 1, \ldots, m$, replace the subjects parameters θ_v, $v = 1, \ldots, n$, of the polytomous RM, while the item parameters σ_i, $i = 1, \ldots, k$, have the same meaning as they have in the polytomous RM. In this sense, the class specific probability $p_{ih|j}$ for observing an answer at item I_i in category K_h is given by

$$p_{ih|j} = \frac{\exp(\theta_{jh} + \sigma_{ih})}{\sum_{l=1}^{g} \exp(\theta_{jl} + \sigma_{il})}, \tag{11.12}$$

with normalization conditions analogous to those above.

As will be shown by example of the life-satisfaction data, given in Table 11.4 and previously analyzed by Clogg (1979), among others, the P-LC/RM becomes equivalent to the polytomous RM, in that for more than a certain number of classes, the P-LC/RM estimates of the item parameters equal the CML estimates in the polytomous RM.

Considering all side conditions, for k items each having g categories, there are $(k-1)(g-1)$ item parameters σ to be estimated by the CML method in the polytomous RM. Assuming m classes, under the P-LC/RM the same number of item parameters plus $m(g-1)$ class parameters θ plus $(m-1)$ class sizes, in total $(k-1)(g-1) + mg - 1$ parameters, are to be estimated. Conditioning on the persons' raw scores (which are the sufficient statistics for the persons' parameters) in the CML method for the polytomous RM is tantamount to fitting perfectly the raw score distribution by the P-LC/RM. Because the item parameters are common under both approaches, the location parameters and class sizes of the P-LC/RM are free to fit the raw score distribution. In order to be able to do that, the number of the location parameters plus the number of class sizes, $mg - 1$, must at least be equal to the number, say o,

Table 11.4. Life-satisfaction—Response patterns and their observed frequencies; $N = 1472$. Satisfaction with hobbies (item 1), residence (item 2), and family (item 3); categories: positive (1), neutral (2), and negative (3)

Response Pattern	Observed Frequency	Response Pattern	Observed Frequency	Response Pattern	Observed Frequency
111	466	211	126	311	54
112	27	212	31	312	12
113	16	213	5	313	7
121	191	221	117	321	49
122	38	222	58	322	26
123	14	223	12	323	11
131	64	231	45	331	23
132	18	232	23	332	16
133	5	233	3	333	15

of (independent) elements of the (vectorial) raw score distribution. From this inequality, $m \geq (o + 1)/g$, the minimal number of classes for the P-LC/RM necessary to fit the raw score distribution can be derived (cf. Table 11.5). While for dichotomous data o is simply equal to the number of items, for polytomous data it depends in a more complicated way upon the number of items and the number of categories.

Table 11.5. Number of parameters in the polytomous RM (CML) and in the P-LC/RM

Model	Number of	m Classes k Items g Categories	m Classes $k = 3$ $g = 3$
RM, P-LC/RM	Item Parameters	$(k-1)(g-1)$	4
P-LC/RM	Location parameters	$m(g-1)$	$2m$
	Class sizes	$m-1$	$m-1$
	Loc. par. + Class sizes	$mg - 1$	$3m - 1$
RM, P-LC/RM indep. elements of the	Raw score distribution	o	9
Raw score distribution can be fitted	by the P-LC/RM if	$mg - 1 \geq o$ $m \geq (o+1)/g$	$3m - 1 \geq 9$ $m \geq 4$

For $k = g = 3$, which is the case for the life-satisfaction data, the following raw scores (r_1, r_2, r_3) are observable, whereby r_1 denotes the number of answers in category K_1 given by a single subject, summed over the items, and so on: $(3, 0, 0)$, $(0, 3, 0)$, $(0, 0, 3)$, $(2, 1, 0)$, $(2, 0, 1)$, $(1, 2, 0)$, $(1, 0, 2)$, $(0, 2, 1)$, $(0, 1, 2)$, and $(1, 1, 1)$. Therefore, the raw score distribution consists of 9 independent elements, from which it follows that m, the number of classes, at least must be four. Because for $m = 4$ the number of location parameters θ plus the number of class sizes equals 11, the model will be overparameterized by two parameters; in other words, two parameters will be unidentifiable, so that the number of degrees of freedom for the goodness-of-fit tests will be 13 instead of $11 = (g^k - 1) - \{(k-1)(g-1) + mg - 1\} = 3^3 - 2 \cdot 2 - 4 \cdot 3$. If m is chosen to be greater than four, the number of unidentifiable parameters increases such that the number of degrees of freedom remains 13, and no improvement of fit can be reached.

Table 11.6. Life-satisfaction—Goodness-of-fit tests for some P-LC/RMs (X^2 = Pearson's chi-squared statistic, G^2 = likelihood ratio statistic)

Model	Classes	Number of Parameters			X^2	G^2	df	χ^2_{95}
		For classes	For items	Total				
P-LC/RM(2)	2	1	8	9	40.72	36.91	17	27.59
P-LC/RM(3)	3	2	10	12	18.00	18.99	14	23.68
P-LC/RM(4)	4	3	10	13^a	17.96	18.96	13	22.36
P-LC/RM(5)	5	4	9	13^b	17.96	18.96	13	22.36

Notes:
[a] Two parameters not identifiable.
[b] Five parameters not identifiable.

Numerical results are given for the data on life-satisfaction, with respect to the goodness-of-fit statistics in Table 11.6, and with respect to the raw score distributions in Table 11.7. The latter ones illustrate that for an increasing number of classes, the expected raw score distribution comes closer to the observed one. For four classes, both are identical, while this is not true with respect to the expected and the observed distribution of the response patterns. Estimating the item parameters according to the CML method, and estimating them by linear logistic LCA for polytomous data Formann (1992), assuming P-LC/RM with four or more classes, leads to the same numerical results for the item parameters: $\sigma_1 = (-.23, .00, .23)$, $\sigma_2 = (-.43, .21, .22)$, $\sigma_3 = (-.66, -.21, -.45)$.

11.4 Example 3: The Mixed Rasch Model

The models in the two previous examples are based on the assumption that the sample has been drawn from a population that is heterogeneous with respect to the subjects' abilities but is homogeneous with respect to the scaling model and its parameters. In contrast, the mixed RM (MRM; Rost, 1990), in the following considered for dichotomous data only, assumes that the population

Table 11.7. Life-satisfaction—Observed and expected frequencies of the scores for increasing number of classes ($m = 1, \ldots, 4$) under the P-LC/RM

Score	Observed Frequency	Expected Frequencies $m = 1$	$m = 2$	$m = 3$	$m = 4$
300	466	327.0	464.5	466.0	466.0
030	58	24.9	51.9	57.4	58.0
003	15	1.8	5.2	15.0	15.0
210	344	462.2	351.2	343.8	344.0
201	134	201.5	130.1	134.2	134.0
120	186	199.2	171.5	186.9	186.0
102	35	37.3	35.6	35.1	35.0
021	61	31.7	73.2	61.7	61.0
012	30	13.3	34.1	29.9	30.0
111	143	173.1	154.7	142.0	143.0

under investigation comprises two or more subpopulations in each of which the RM holds for a given set of items. Across subpopulations, the items are allowed to have different parameters.

Comparable models can be formulated within the latent-class framework. Such latent-class/mixed RMs (LC/MRM) can be stated by assuming that subjects are located at a few discrete points on the latent continuum. However, instead of postulating the same item parameters for all classes as was in the LC/RM and LC/LLTM, two or more sets of item parameters are provided corresponding to the Rasch homogeneous subpopulations of the MRM (in the following called item difficulty types). For each item difficulty type, two or more ability parameters are allowed (in the following called ability levels). In contrast to the LC/RM and the LC/LLTM, where the possible heterogeneity of the persons is caught by ability levels only (for all persons, the same set of item parameters is assumed to be valid), the LC/RM considers the possible heterogeneity in two ways: by allowing more than one item difficulty type and by allowing more than one ability level within each item difficulty type. In this sense, the specification equation of the LC/MRM can be stated as follows:

$$p_{i|j(L)} = \frac{\exp\{\theta_{j(L)} + \sigma_{i(L)}\}}{1 + \exp\{\theta_{j(L)} + \sigma_{i(L)}\}}, \tag{11.13}$$

where $\sigma_{i(L)}$ is the parameter of item I_i for the L-th item difficulty type, and $\theta_{j(L)}$ is the ability parameter of the j-th ability level within the L-th item difficulty type. As an example, Table 11.8 gives the weights of linear logistic LCA for the LC/MRM assuming six items, two item difficulty types, and two ability levels within each item difficulty type, resulting in altogether four classes.

As for the six matrices items in this analysis, the observed and expected score distributions shown in Table 11.9 for increasing number of classes illus-

Table 11.8. Matrices items—Weights for the LC/MRM (two item difficulty types, two ability levels) in linear logistic LCA

Diff. Type	Class	Item	σ_1					θ_1		σ_2					θ_2	
			1	2	3	4	5	1	2	1	2	3	4	5	1	2
I	1	1	1					1								
		2		1				1								
		3			1			1								
		4				1		1								
		5					1	1								
		6	−1	−1	−1	−1	−1	1								
	2	1	1						1							
		2		1					1							
		3			1				1							
		4				1			1							
		5					1		1							
		6	−1	−1	−1	−1	−1		1							
II	3	1								1					1	
		2									1				1	
		3										1			1	
		4											1		1	
		5												1	1	
		6								−1	−1	−1	−1	−1	1	
	4	1								1						1
		2									1					1
		3										1				1
		4											1			1
		5												1		1
		6								−1	−1	−1	−1	−1		1

trate that the LC/MRMs does not allow fixing the score distribution as is the case under the LC/RM and the LC/LLTM. As a result, the LC/MRM can only approximate the observed score distribution, and with it, the estimates of the item parameters for the two difficulty types. Under the LC/MRM, they come close to their CML estimates obtained for the MRM. Note that this almost equivalence regarding the item-parameter estimates is already met when assuming two ability levels for each one of the two difficulty types; see Table 11.10.

The five-classes LC/MRM (one item difficulty type with two ability levels, another item difficulty type with three ability levels) is nearly equivalent to the two-classes MRM with respect to fit. More than five classes of the LC/MRM are not identifiable. This can be concluded from the result that increasing the number of classes up to eight does not improve the fit statistics and from analyzing the matrix of second-order partial derivatives of the log-likelihood function; regarding identifiability in latent-class models, see Goodman (1974), Formann (1985, 1992, 2003), and G.-H. Huang & Bandeen-Roche (2004). Fi-

188   Anton K. Formann

Table 11.9. Matrices items—Observed score frequencies as well as expected score frequencies under the LC/MRM and the MRM assuming two item difficulty types

		Expected Frequencies			
		LC/MRM		MRM	
Score	Observed	Ability Levels per Item Difficulty Type			
r	frequency	$1+1$	$2+2$	$2+3$	
0	37	26.0	34.7	37.0	37.0
1	118	131.6	120.8	118.0	118.0
2	238	247.9	238.4	238.2	238.0
3	300	276.3	300.2	300.1	300.0
4	259	260.8	257.2	258.2	259.0
5	148	174.1	148.9	148.5	148.0
6	63	46.3	62.8	63.0	63.0

Table 11.10. Matrices items—Item-parameter estimates under the LC/MRM and the MRM assuming two item difficulty types

			LC/MRM			
			Ability Levels per Item Difficulty Type			
	Type	Item	$1+1$	$2+2$	$2+3^*$	MRM
Item-parameter	I	1	-1.15	-1.24	-1.26	-1.22
estimates		2	3.26	4.12	11.37	3.92
		3	$-.38$	3.96	20.49	4.87
		4	1.50	2.85	10.02	2.66
		5	-1.79	-2.09	-2.12	-2.07
		$6^\#$	0	0	0	0
	II	1	$-.94$	-1.05	-1.05	-1.05
		2	1.05	1.06	1.14	1.10
		3	$-.61$	-1.22	-1.14	-1.25
		4	.12	.12	.16	.14
		5	-1.81	-1.87	-1.85	-1.86
		$6^\#$	0	0	0	0
Prevalence type	I		.420	.238	.181	.239

Notes: * More parameters not identifiable.
       # Normalized to 0.

nally, Table 11.11 displays the statistics of the goodness-of-fit tests for the LC/MRM and the MRM. In contrast to the LC/LLTM, the four- and five-classes LC/MRMs fit the data on the six matrices items well.

Table 11.11. Matrices items—Goodness-of-fit statistics for the LC/MRM for increasing number of ability levels and for the MRM, in both cases assuming two item difficulty types

Ability Levels per Item Difficulty Type	Number of Classes	X^2	G^2	df	χ^2_{95}
$1+1$	2	79.9	81.4	50	67.5
$2+2$	4	48.2	54.5	46	62.8
$2+3$	5	45.8	51.5	44	60.5
MRM	2	46.4	51.8	42	58.1

11.5 Final Remarks

Linear logistic latent-class analysis for dichotomous (Formann, 1982, 1985) as well as for polytomous data (Formann, 1992) provides a very general framework for modeling item latent probabilities and class sizes. In addition to the models explicitly mentioned above, most of the classic latent-class models and most of item response models that have been formulated previously for dichotomous and polytomous data, e.g., threshold models, but also more general models, such as hybrid models, can be restated in terms of linear logistic latent-class analysis; see Formann & Kohlmann (1998). Therefore, it would be rather easily possible to search for further types of models for which (almost) equivalence of CML and semiparametric ML is attainable, and to investigate empirically under which conditions this equivalence is attained. But doing this will be of theoretical importance only. From the practical point of view of parameter estimation, the semiparametric ML method must be rated inferior as compared to the CML method. Estimating the item parameters according to the CML method involves computing the symmetric functions, a task that in the early days of the RM (and similar models) was demanding: The "difference algorithm" (Fischer & Allerup, 1968) proved very prone to numerical errors and, thus, usually worked well for rather small numbers of items only. However, the more recent "summation method" (Andersen, 1972; Gustafsson, 1980) is numerically stable and remains applicable even in the presence of large numbers of items. So, getting the CML parameter estimates has become routine, whereas parameter estimation according to the mixture ML method, e.g., via restricted latent-class models, is more involved. In contrast, employing the mixture approach seems to be more promising when thinking of multivariate extensions of the Rasch model. Especially, when there do not exist simple sufficient statistics—as they do, for example, in the polytomous RM-, the CML approach may prove difficult or even impossible to be made applicable. In such situations, the semiparametric ML-method promises to be quite useful having in mind the possible disadvantages of existing alternatives, particularly of the unconditional ML method and the marginal ML method with prespecified latent-ability distribution.

12

Rasch Models for Longitudinal Data

Thorsten Meiser

Friedrich-Schiller-Universität Jena

12.1 Introduction

The chapter gives an overview of Rasch models for the measurement of change across repeated observations of the same individuals and items. The models described herein include extensions of the original Rasch model that allow one to analyze multidimensional latent constructs and to incorporate heterogeneity of change across individuals. In particular, the use of mixture-distribution Rasch models in longitudinal research allows one to model quantitative interindividual differences in a latent trait at each occasion, together with qualitative interindividual differences in the course of development. A mover–stayer mixed-Rasch model can be specified as a special case that reflects the assumption that change over time occurs for some latent subpopulation but not for another. An empirical example illustrates that the mover–stayer mixed-Rasch model can provide a parsimonious and viable account of observed heterogeneity of change.

12.2 Rasch Models for Repeated Observations

The Rasch model (RM, Rasch, 1968, 1980) is usually applied to the responses of individuals to items observed at one point in time. However, the RM can also be used in situations in which a set of items is repeatedly administered to the same sample of individuals. In those longitudinal designs, the RM specifies the probability that item i, $i = 1, \ldots, I$, is solved by person v, $v = 1, \ldots, N$, at occasion t, $t = 1, \ldots, T$:

$$P(X_{vit} = 1 | \theta_{vt}, \beta_{it}) = \frac{\exp(\theta_{vt} - \beta_{it})}{1 + \exp(\theta_{vt} - \beta_{it})}. \tag{12.1}$$

The parameter θ_{vt} denotes person v's latent ability at occasion t, and β_{it} denotes item i's difficulty at occasion t.

Modeling changes in ability or item difficulty over time is the aim of extensions of the RM and other IRT models, such as those by Fischer (1983, 1995d), Wilson (1989), and Embretson (1991). This chapter gives an overview of RMs for modeling change and presents an application of some of the presented models to a longitudinal data set. Additional applications of this class of models can be found in the chapters by Draney and Wilson, and Glück and Spiel in this volume.

12.2.1 Modeling Homogeneous and Person-Specific Change

Aside from specifying the probability of solving an item at a particular measurement occasion t in terms of Equation 12.1, the RM and its extensions allow one to measure change from one occasion to another and to test hypotheses about the latent course of development. In the simplest case, one may assume that the person and item parameters are invariant over time, that is, $\theta_{vt} = \theta_v$ and $\beta_{it} = \beta_i$ for all occasions t, which means that no change occurs at all. Alternatively, one can specify the hypothesis that all individuals exhibit the same amount of change on the latent continuum by introducing a change parameter λ_t that is constant across individuals and items:

$$P(X_{vit} = 1|\theta_v, \beta_i, \lambda_t) = \frac{\exp(\theta_v + \lambda_t - \beta_i)}{1 + \exp(\theta_v + \lambda_t - \beta_i)}. \tag{12.2}$$

The model in Equation 12.2 represents a linear logistic test model (LLTM; Fischer, 1983, 1995d,b; Spada & McGaw, 1985) that decomposes the item parameter β_{it} into basic parameters that capture the item's initial difficulty β_i and the change λ_t that has occurred until occasion t, $\beta_{it} = \beta_i - \lambda_t$ with $\lambda_1 = 0$. Technically, the person parameter θ_v is considered constant over time in the linear logistic model, so that the relative position of person v is preserved across the measurement occasions. Because change in overall item difficulty is equivalent to global change in latent-person ability, however, the model reflects the assumptions that change may occur and that change is homogeneous across persons. Accordingly, λ_t can be interpreted as the average increase (or decrease) in ability from the first measurement occasion until occasion t for all individuals. Due to the additive decomposition of β_{it} into item difficulty β_i and the change effect λ_t, the relative positions of the items are also maintained over time. The latter assumption can be dropped by allowing for time-specific item parameters.

The linear logistic RM in Equation 12.2 is based on a unidimensional latent space. That is, the position of person v on the one latent trait θ underlies her or his responses to all items i at all occasions t, although the person's absolute position on the latent continuum may shift from one occasion to another.

In many applications, however, it may be plausible to assume that different items measure different latent constructs, such as distinct aspects of a syndrome in clinical research or specific cognitive abilities in educational assessment. To measure time or treatment effects across repeated observations in such cases, the linear logistic test model with relaxed assumptions (LLRA; Fischer, 1983, 1995c) accommodates multidimensionality of items. This model allows for item-specific latent traits by specifying interactions between persons and items, θ_{iv}. To measure time or treatment effects, the model contains change parameters that are considered constant across the items and their latent dimensions. Although such generalizations of the RM to incorporate multidimensionality in an item set are suitable specifications in many instances, the remainder of this chapter will largely focus on the issue of homogeneity versus heterogeneity of change across individuals, which can also be addressed by modeling and testing for particular types of multidimensionality in longitudinal RMs.

The RM in Equation 12.2 contains the rather restrictive assumption that change is homogeneous across persons, that is, that the amount of change λ_t is supposed to be the same for all persons v. This restrictive assumption can be dropped by specifying a multidimensional latent space that contains one latent-trait continuum for each measurement occasion (e.g., Andersen, 1985). The resulting model reflects the concept of person-specific change that can be written as

$$P(X_{vit} = 1|\theta_{vt}, \beta_i) = \frac{\exp(\theta_{vt} - \beta_i)}{1 + \exp(\theta_{vt} - \beta_i)}. \qquad (12.3)$$

Formally, the parameter θ_{vt} represents an interaction between person v and measurement occasion t, which implies that change in the latent ability θ may be person-specific rather than homogeneous, whereas item difficulty β_i is assumed to remain constant over time. In contrast to the linear logistic RM (12.2), the relative position of person v may therefore change from one occasion to another in Equation 12.3, so that the amount of change cannot be measured by means of a global change parameter λ_t. The model of person-specific change in Equation 12.3 is appropriate in longitudinal research designs in which the items form a unidimensional scale at each occasion with stationary item parameters, and in which the speed or direction of development may vary between persons, for example because individuals profit to different degrees from training or intervention programs.

The models of homogeneous change in Equation 12.2 and of person-specific change in Equation 12.3 result from particular restrictions of the person parameters θ_{vt} and the item parameters β_{it} in the general RM for repeated observations as defined in Equation 12.1. Alternative restrictions are also possible, including the decomposition of the item parameters β_{it} into linear combinations of specific treatment effects and general trends (e.g., Fischer, 1995c).

12.2.2 Loglinear Rasch Models for Measuring Change

The loglinear representation of RMs (Cressie & Holland, 1983; Kelderman, 1984; see also the chapter by Kelderman in this volume) forms a suitable framework for the specification and test of hypotheses about change in longitudinal data. In the loglinear notation of the conditional RM, the expected probabilities of response vectors are reparameterized as linear combinations of item parameters and of parameters representing the total scores of the response vectors. This notation facilitates the specification of theoretical assumptions concerning latent change and affords straightforward statistical tests especially for small item sets (Meiser, 1996; Meiser et al., 1998).

To illustrate, let a set of I items be administered to a sample of individuals at $T = 2$ measurement occasions. Because the total score $R_v = \sum_t \sum_i x_{vit}$ forms the sufficient statistic for person parameter θ_v under the unidimensional RM of homogeneous change in Equation 12.2, the probability of a given response vector $x = (x_{11}, \ldots, x_{I1}, x_{12}, \ldots, x_{I2})$ with total score R can be expressed without latent-person parameter θ_v. In the loglinear reparameterization of the RM of homogeneous change, the logarithm of the expected probability of response vector x can therefore be written as

$$\ln P(x = (x_{11}, \ldots, x_{I1}, x_{12}, \ldots, x_{I2})) = u - \sum_{t=1}^{2} \sum_{i=1}^{I} x_{it}\beta_i + \sum_{i=1}^{I} x_{i2}\lambda_2 + u_R.$$
(12.4)

Likewise, the sufficient statistic of the two-dimensional latent-ability vector $(\theta_{v1}, \theta_{v2})$ in the model of person-specific change (12.3), for two occasions is given by the pair of total scores (R_{v1}, R_{v2}), with $R_{v1} = \sum_i x_{i1}$ being the total score at the first occasion and $R_{v2} = \sum_i x_{i2}$ being the total score at the second occasion. The conditional RM of person-specific change can therefore be specified by the following loglinear model for the expected probability of response vector x with the two total scores R_1 and R_2:

$$\ln P(x = (x_{11}, \ldots, x_{I1}, x_{12}, \ldots, x_{I2})) = u - \sum_{t=1}^{2} \sum_{i=1}^{I} x_{it}\beta_i + u_{(R_1, R_2)} \quad (12.5)$$

To achieve identifiability of the loglinear RMs in (12.4) and (12.5), some parameter restrictions need to be imposed. The usual restrictions include the constraints that the set of item parameters and the set of total score parameters sum to zero, that is, $\sum_i \beta_i = 0$, $\sum_R u_R = 0$, and $\sum_{R_1} \sum_{R_2} u_{(R_1, R_2)} = 0$.

The loglinear framework facilitates straightforward specifications and tests of hypotheses about change, such as stationarity of the change parameters or invariance of item parameters across measurement occasions. Stationarity of latent change is reflected by the constraints $\lambda_t = \lambda$ for all $t > 1$ in Equation 12.4. Invariance of the item parameters can be tested by introducing time-specific difficulty parameters β_{it} in Equations 12.4 and 12.5 and by comparing the resulting more-general model variants with the models assuming constant item parameters.

For model-testing purposes, it is of particular importance to note that the loglinear model of homogeneous change in (12.4) can be derived as a special case from the loglinear model of person-specific change in Equation 12.5. That is, imposing the restrictions $u_{(R_1,R_2)} = u_{(R_1+R_2)} + R_2\lambda_2$ in Equation 12.5 yields Equation 12.4. This hierarchical relation between the loglinear models (12.4) and (12.5) allows one to test for homogeneity of change across persons by means of a statistical model comparison.

12.2.3 Extensions to Multiple Response Categories and Multidimensional Latent Traits

Linear logistic RMs for the measurement of change have been extended from the analysis of dichotomous items to the analysis of items with several response categories (Fischer & Parzer, 1991; Fischer & Ponocny, 1994, 1995). For that purpose, the item and category parameters in the rating-scale model (Andrich, 1978) or the partial-credit model (Masters, 1982) for polytomous items are specified with regard to different points in time, analogous to the item parameter in Equation 12.1. The item and category parameters are then decomposed into basic parameters that reflect item and category difficulty on the one hand and change or treatment effects over time on the other hand.

Moreover, longitudinal RMs can be extended to include more than one latent trait at each occasion, as in the linear logistic model with relaxed assumptions. Generalizing the concepts of homogeneous and person-specific change from unidimensional RMs, change can be specified to be homogeneous across persons or person-specific within each of the latent traits of a multidimensional latent-trait model.

In very general terms, the probability to observe response category x in item i with $m + 1$ response categories $0, \ldots, m$ at occasion t can be specified by a longitudinal RM with D latent traits at each measurement occasion:

$$P(X_{vit} = x|\theta_{\mathbf{vt}}, \tau_{\mathbf{ist}}) =$$
$$\frac{\exp(\sum_{d=1}^{D}\sum_{s=1}^{x} w_{isd}\theta_{vtd} - \sum_{d=1}^{D}\sum_{s=1}^{x} w_{isd}\tau_{istd})}{\sum_{y=0}^{m}\exp(\sum_{d=1}^{D}\sum_{s=1}^{y} w_{isd}\theta_{vtd} - \sum_{d=1}^{D}\sum_{s=1}^{y} w_{isd}\tau_{istd})}. \quad (12.6)$$

In Equation 12.6, θ_{vtd} denotes the latent-ability parameter of person v at occasion t on the latent dimension d, and τ_{istd} represents the difficulty of the threshold between categories $s-1$ and s for item i at occasion t on dimension d. The values w_{isd} are weights that reflect the degree to which the latent-ability dimensions are involved in reaching the various response categories.

These weights are determined a priori by the researcher and are thus part of the model specification. Usually, the weights are restricted to the binary values of zero and one, indicating whether a particular trait is involved in reaching a category or not (see Meiser, 1996; Meiser et al., 1998).

The polytomous multidimensional latent-trait model for longitudinal data in Equation 12.6 serves as a superordinate framework, or metastructure, to derive more specific models by sets of parameter constraints. For example, a multidimensional model of homogeneous change within each latent trait can be specified by setting $\theta_{vtd} = \theta_{vd}$ and by decomposing the threshold parameters into their initial difficulty and change parameters, $\tau_{istd} = \tau_{isd} - \lambda_{td}$. The resulting model reflects global change with persisting relative positions of the persons and items on each of the D latent traits (Meiser, 1996; Meiser & Rudinger, 1997). Together with a theory-based and parsimonious selection of the weights w_{isd}, such parameter constraints are often necessary to yield identifiable submodels of the superordinate framework in Equation 12.6 for a given data set.

12.3 Mixture-Distribution Rasch Models for the Analysis of Change

The aforementioned distinction between change that is completely homogeneous across persons versus change that is purely person-specific marks two extremes of homogeneity and heterogeneity, respectively. In a given population, a limited number of latent-developmental trajectories may coexist, so that change is neither completely homogeneous nor completely person-specific. Instead, the direction and the amount of change may be rather homogeneous within each of several subpopulations, whereas the course of change may differ between the subpopulations.

In some cases, relevant subpopulations can be defined by manifest extraneous grouping variables, such as gender, socioeconomic status, or treatment group, so that differences in the developmental trajectories can be analyzed by parameter comparisons between groups (e.g., Fischer, 1983, 1995d). In other cases, either extraneous grouping variables may either not be available, or they may not account for observed heterogeneity of change in the population (e.g., Wilson, 1989). Then, the subpopulations are latent and have to be identified by statistical modeling techniques in order to separate the developmental patterns that are mixed in the total population.

The goal to identify latent subpopulations and to measure change within each subpopulation can be pursued by means of finite mixture-distribution models (McLachlan & Peel, 2000; Titterington et al., 1985). Finite mixture-distribution models characterize the probabilities of events in terms of a weighted sum of component distributions. Each component distribution is specified to hold within a subpopulation c, $c = 1, \ldots, C$, and the weights correspond to the proportions of the subpopulations in the entire population, π_c.

12.3.1 Class-Specific Homogeneous Change

Applying the notion of finite mixture-distribution models to longitudinal RMs, one may assume that a population consists of C latent subpopulations and that change is homogeneous within each subpopulation. This assumption can be specified by a mixed RM (Rost, 1990, 1991; von Davier & Rost, 1995; see also the chapter by von Davier & Yamamoto in this volume) of the form

$$P(X_{vit} = 1) = \sum_{c=1}^{C} \pi_c P(X_{vit} = 1 \mid c)$$

with component probabilities

$$P(X_{vit} = 1|c, \theta_{v|c}, \beta_{i|c}) = \frac{\exp(\theta_{v|c} + \lambda_{t|c} - \beta_{i|c})}{1 + \exp(\theta_{v|c} + \lambda_{t|c} - \beta_{i|c})}. \tag{12.7}$$

The mixed RM for longitudinal data in Equation 12.7 combines the unidimensional RM, which allows for quantitative differences among persons while implying homogeneity of change, and the latent-class approach, which allows for qualitatively distinct patterns of change (see Meiser et al., 1995, for a discussion of Rasch and latent-class models in longitudinal research).

More specifically, in contrast to the model of homogeneous change in Equation 12.2, the parameters of the mixed RM in Equation 12.7 are specified conditional on latent class c that contains a proportion π_c of the entire population. By introducing class-specific change parameters $\lambda_{t|c}$, the model accounts for qualitative differences in change. In contrast to usual latent-class models, however, the mixed RM also allows for quantitative differences between individuals of the same subpopulation in terms of the person parameter $\theta_{v|c}$. Together, the mixed longitudinal RM (12.7) integrates interindividual differences and homogeneous change within each latent subpopulation with qualitative differences in change between subpopulations.

12.3.2 A Mover–Stayer Mixed-Rasch Model

With appropriate parameter restrictions, mixed RMs can be used to disentangle latent subpopulations of "movers" and "stayers" within a latent-trait framework that incorporates quantitative interindividual differences as well as differences in change over time.

The distinction between a latent subpopulation that exhibits change over time, the "movers," and a latent subpopulation that shows invariant response behavior over time, the "stayers," has been incorporated into mixed Markov chain models (e.g., Langeheine & van de Pol, 1994; van de Pol & Langeheine, 1990) to express the idea that observed heterogeneity of change may reflect the coexistence of two simple mechanisms in a given population: change and no change. The distinction between a latent class of movers and a latent class of stayers can easily be transferred to the mixed longitudinal RM in Equation 12.7 by setting $C = 2$ and imposing the restriction $\lambda_{t|2} = 0$ for all t. Thereby, the change parameters for the first subpopulation $\lambda_{t|1}$ are free to differ from zero, which means that the latent class $c = 1$ may exhibit global change in the latent ability across the measurement occasions. Thus, class 1 represents a subpopulation of movers. By restricting $\lambda_{t|2}$ to zero, the latent ability is constrained to be invariant over time in class $c = 2$. Thereby, class 2 forms a subpopulation of stayers. Extending mover–stayer models in the framework of mixed Markov models, the mover–stayer mixed RM admits persisting interindividual differences in latent ability within both subpopulations of movers and stayers.

Mover–stayer mixed RMs were successfully applied to longitudinal data concerning the development of observed activity in childhood (Meiser & Rudinger, 1997) and concerning the development of mathematical problem-solving skills in primary school (Meiser et al., 1998). The latter analysis is briefly summarized in the following section in order to illustrate the various RMs for the measurement of change that were discussed throughout this chapter. For further applications of RMs to longitudinal data, see the chapters by Draney and Wilson and by Glück and Spiel in this volume.

12.4 An Empirical Illustration

In an analysis of mathematical problem-solving skills in primary-school children, Meiser et al. (1998) applied a series of longitudinal RMs to investigate the course of latent development. The empirical data were taken from a large-scale longitudinal study on the cognitive abilities and achievements of school children in Germany (Weinert & Helmke, 1997). The selected items encompassed three arithmetic word problems that were administered to a sample of 1030 children in the second and third grades. The series of models was specified as conditional RMs in their loglinear representation, and the analyses were run with the software LEM (Vermunt, 1997a). This software facilitates loglinear model specification in terms of design matrices (see Meiser, 2005; Rindskopf, 1990) and allows the inclusion of latent-class variables in the loglinear modeling framework.

In a first step, we applied the conditional RM of homogeneous change in its loglinear representation (see Equation 12.4) to the three items at the two occasions. This model was rejected on grounds of a poor overall goodness of fit, as revealed by the likelihood ratio statistic of $G^2(54) = 72.53$, $p = .047$. The loglinear RM of person-specific change (see Equation 12.5), in contrast, showed a satisfactory goodness of fit with $G^2(46) = 54.84$, $p = .175$. As delineated above, the two loglinear models are hierarchically related. A model comparison by means of the conditional likelihood ratio statistic therefore yields a focused test of homogeneity of change across persons. The model comparison showed a significant difference in model fit, $\Delta G^2(8) = 17.69$, $p = .024$, which indicated that the homogeneity assumption was violated for the given data set.

To analyze the structure of developmental heterogeneity further, we specified a mover–stayer mixed RM that follows from Equation 12.7 with the specification of two latent subpopulations and with the restriction $\lambda_{t|2} = 0$ for the stayer class $c = 2$. In addition, we imposed equality restrictions on the item parameters across the latent classes $c = 1$ and $c = 2$, $\beta_{i|1} = \beta_{i|2}$, which reflect the assumption that the items form an invariant scale not only across time but also across the different latent subpopulations. The resulting model provided an acceptable overall goodness of fit to the data, $G^2(49) = 64.79$, $p = .065$. The latent subpopulation of movers comprised an estimated proportion of $\hat{\pi}_1 = .43$ of the children, and the latent subpopulation of stayers comprised the complementary estimated proportion of $\hat{\pi}_2 = .57$.

The mover–stayer mixed RM cannot be compared with the models of global change and person-specific change by means of a conditional likelihood ratio test using the chi-square distribution. This is due to the fact that the mover–stayer mixed RM is not hierarchically related to the other models, so that the regularity conditions for a statistical model comparison are not met. Therefore, a descriptive comparison between the model of person-specific change and the mover–stayer mixed RM was conducted with the information criterion CAIC (Burnham & Anderson, 2002). This model comparison demonstrated that the mover–stayer mixed RM provided a better balance between model fit and model parsimony, CAIC=7740.27, than did the model of person-specific change, CAIC=7442.36.

Together, the empirical results of the Rasch analysis of the given data set on arithmetic problem-solving highlight that the mover–stayer mixed RM may offer a parsimonious account of observed heterogeneity in change by specifying the two simple underlying mechanisms of change and no change in a given population. In fact, the subpopulation of movers, $c = 1$, showed an estimated change parameter of $\hat{\lambda}_{2|1} = 1.19$ that was significantly larger than zero, as indicated by a z-value of 4.01. In terms of the expected probabilities to solve the arithmetic problems, the movers improved their chances to provide the correct responses to the three items from an average of .47, .35, and .43 at second grade to an average of .72, .61, and .69 at third grade. Because the change parameter was fixed to zero for the subpopulation of stayers, $c = 2$ with $\lambda_{2|2} = 0$, the expected probabilities of successful item solution did not differ between the two assessment occasions for stayers. Children in this latent subpopulation had average chances of .41, .34, and .38 to solve the three items at both second grade and third grade.

The mover–stayer mixed RM allows for differences in item difficulty and person ability at each measurement occasion, and it separates qualitatively different patterns of development. In the school data analyzed by Meiser et al. (1998), a latent subpopulation of children who improved performance from one grade to the next could be distinguished from another latent subpopulation of children whose performance remained unchanged. The separation of latent subpopulations with different developmental trajectories by mixed RMs can also be used to investigate possible associations between qualitative patterns of development and external variables such as gender and socioeconomic indices (e.g., Meiser et al., 1995). The combination of RMs for measuring change in a (sub)population and finite-mixture models for analyzing heterogeneity between latent subpopulations thus provides a flexible framework for specifying and testing hypotheses about change in longitudinal data.

13

The Interaction Model

Shelby J. Haberman

Educational Testing Service

13.1 Introduction

The interaction model, a generalization of the Rasch model (RM) for binary responses, retains many of the attractive features of the RM but does not assume local independence. Like the RM, the interaction model has simple sufficient statistics and a relatively straightforward interpretation. Computation of conditional maximum-likelihood estimates is a task of comparable difficulty to the corresponding computation for the Rasch model.

The interaction model can be used to test the validity of the RM (Rasch, 1960) by use of conventional conditional likelihood-ratio tests, and the interaction model can also be used to examine the size of the error of the RM in an information-theoretic sense (Gilula & Haberman, 1994, 1995). The interaction model has interest in its own right as an alternative to the 2PL model, which requires much less computation in large samples.

In Section 13.2, the interaction model is defined, and its relationship to the RM and to common loglinear models is discussed. In Section 13.3, computational methods are considered for the interaction model. Section 13.4 examines use of the interaction model to test the RM. Section 13.5 illustrates results by use of a multiple-choice examination with 45 items and 8,686 examinees. The examination is from the Praxis series of examinations for teacher training and certification.

13.2 Basic Properties of the Interaction Model

To define the interaction model, consider a test with $I \geq 3$ items and $N \geq I$ examinees. For examinee v, $1 \leq v \leq N$, and item i, $1 \leq i \leq I$, let x_{vi} be 1 if the response to item i is correct, and let x_{vi} be 0 otherwise. Let $\mathbf{x}_v$ be the I-dimensional response vector with coordinates x_{vi}, $1 \leq i \leq I$. Let θ_v be a one-dimensional measure of the ability of examinee v, and assume that the θ_v are random variables and the $\mathbf{x}_v$ are random vectors. Let the pairs $(\mathbf{x}_v, \theta_v)$,

$1 \leq v \leq N$, be independent and identically distributed. Let the common distribution function of θ_v be F, let $p(\mathbf{x})$ be the probability that $\mathbf{x}_v = \mathbf{x}$ for $\mathbf{x}$ in the set Γ of I-dimensional vectors with coordinates 0 or 1, and let $p(\mathbf{x}|\theta)$ be the conditional probability that $\mathbf{x}_v = \mathbf{x}$ given that $\theta_v = \theta$. Let $x_v. = \sum_{i=1}^{I} x_{vi}$ be the number of items correctly answered by examinee v, and for $0 \leq r \leq I$, let $\Gamma(r)$ be the set of $\mathbf{x}$ in Γ such that $x. = \sum_{i=1}^{I} x_i = r$, so that $\mathbf{x}_v$ is in $\Gamma(r)$ if $r_v = x_v. = r$. For $0 \leq r \leq I$, let $p^R(r)$ be the probability that $r_v = r$, and let p_j be the probability that $x_{vi} = 1$ for $1 \leq i \leq I$. For I-dimensional vectors $\mathbf{a}$ and $\mathbf{b}$ with respective coordinates a_i and b_i, $1 \leq i \leq I$, let

$$\mathbf{a}'\mathbf{b} = \sum_{i=1}^{I} a_i b_i.$$

In the RM, for unknown real β_i, $1 \leq i \leq I$, it is assumed that the conditional probability that $x_{vi} = 1$ given that $\theta_v = u$ is $[1 + \exp(-u + \beta_i)]^{-1}$, and it is assumed that the x_{vi}, $1 \leq i \leq I$, are conditionally independent given θ_v. It follows that

$$\log p_\theta(\mathbf{x}) = \alpha(\boldsymbol{\beta}, \theta) + \sum_{i=1}^{I} x_i(\theta - \beta_i) = \alpha(\boldsymbol{\beta}, \theta) + x.\theta - (\boldsymbol{\beta}'\mathbf{x}), \quad (13.1)$$

where $\boldsymbol{\beta}$ is the I-dimensional vector with coordinates β_i, $1 \leq i \leq I$, and

$$\alpha(\boldsymbol{\beta}, \theta) = -\sum_{i=1}^{I} \log[1 + \exp(\theta - \beta_i)]. \quad (13.2)$$

To identify parameters, the convention may be adopted that $\beta_1 = 0$. As is well known, if, for any I-dimensional vector $\mathbf{a}$,

$$s_r(\mathbf{a}) = \sum_{\mathbf{x} \in \Gamma(r)} \exp(-\mathbf{a}'\mathbf{x}),$$

then the conditional probability that $\mathbf{x}_v = \mathbf{x}$ in $\Gamma(r)$ given that $r_v = r$ and $\theta_v = \theta$ is

$$p(\mathbf{x}|r) = p(\mathbf{x})/p^R(r) = \frac{\exp(-\boldsymbol{\beta}'\mathbf{x})}{s_r(\boldsymbol{\beta})},$$

so that $\mathbf{x}_v$ and θ_v are conditionally independent given r_v (Andersen, 1972).

In the interaction model, an additive interaction term is added for each pair of items, so that for unknown β_i and γ_i, $1 \leq i \leq I$,

$$\log p_\theta(\mathbf{x}) = \alpha(\boldsymbol{\beta}, \boldsymbol{\gamma}, \theta) + \sum_{i=1}^{I} x_i(\theta - \beta_i) + \sum_{i=2}^{I} \sum_{j=1}^{i-1} (\gamma_i + \gamma_j) x_i x_j$$
$$= \alpha(\boldsymbol{\beta}, \boldsymbol{\gamma}, \theta) + x.\theta - \boldsymbol{\beta}'\mathbf{x} + (x. - 1)\boldsymbol{\gamma}'\mathbf{x}, \quad (13.3)$$

where $\boldsymbol{\gamma}$ is the I-dimensional vector of γ_i, $1 \leq i \leq I$, and

$$\alpha(\boldsymbol{\beta}, \boldsymbol{\gamma}, \theta) = -\log \left[\sum_{r=0}^{I} \exp(r\theta) s_r(-\boldsymbol{\beta} + (r-1)\boldsymbol{\gamma}) \right]. \qquad (13.4)$$

To identify parameters, the convention is adopted that β_1 and γ_1 are 0. Thus the RM holds if the interaction model holds and $\boldsymbol{\gamma}$ is the zero vector $\mathbf{0}$.

The interaction model is not a conventional item response model, for the local independence assumption does not hold; that is, the x_{vi}, $1 \le i \le I$, are not assumed conditionally independent given the latent variable θ_v. Nonetheless, the interaction model retains the conditioning properties of the RM. The conditional probability that $\mathbf{x}_i = \mathbf{x}$ in $\Gamma(r)$ given that $r_v = r$ and $\theta_v = \theta$ is

$$p(\mathbf{x}|r) = \frac{\exp[-\boldsymbol{\beta}'\mathbf{x} + (r-1)\boldsymbol{\gamma}'\mathbf{x}]}{s_r(\boldsymbol{\beta} - (r-1)\boldsymbol{\gamma})}, \qquad (13.5)$$

so that $\mathbf{x}_v$ and θ_v are conditionally independent given r_v.

The interaction model implies that the loglinear-interaction model

$$\log p(\mathbf{x}) = \tau_r - \boldsymbol{\beta}'\mathbf{x} + (r-1)\boldsymbol{\gamma}'\mathbf{x} \qquad (13.6)$$

holds for $\mathbf{x}$ in $\Gamma(r)$ and $0 \le r \le I$ for some $(I+1)$-dimensional vector $\boldsymbol{\tau}$ with coordinates τ_r, $0 \le r \le I$, and some I-dimensional vectors $\boldsymbol{\beta}$ and $\boldsymbol{\gamma}$ with $\beta_1 = \gamma_1 = 0$. It is readily seen that under (13.3) and (13.4),

$$\tau_r = \log \int \exp(r\theta) \exp[\alpha(\boldsymbol{\beta}, \boldsymbol{\gamma}, \theta)] dF(\theta).$$

The interaction model is equivalent to the model that (13.6) holds and the vector $\boldsymbol{\tau}$ satisfies the condition that $\exp(\tau_r - \tau_0)$ is $E(Z^r)$, $0 \le r \le I$, for some positive random variable Z (Cressie & Holland, 1983).

13.2.1 The Interaction Model as an Approximation

Even if the loglinear-interaction model does not hold, this model can be used to approximate the common distribution of the $\mathbf{x}_v$ (Gilula & Haberman, 2000). Let S be the population of probability arrays $\mathbf{p}$ with elements $p(\mathbf{x}) > 0$, $\mathbf{x}$ in Γ, such that $\sum_{\mathbf{x} \in \Gamma} p(\mathbf{x}) = 1$ and (13.6) holds for some τ_r, $\boldsymbol{\beta}$, and $\boldsymbol{\gamma}$ with $\beta_1 = \gamma_1 = 0$. Consider the actual probability vector $\mathbf{p}$ such that $p(\mathbf{x})$ is the probability that $\mathbf{x}_v = \mathbf{x}$ for $\mathbf{x}$ in Γ. For a probability array $\mathbf{q}$ with nonnegative coordinates $q(\mathbf{x})$, $\mathbf{x}$ in Γ, with sum 1, let

$$H(\mathbf{q}) = -I^{-1} E(\log q(\mathbf{x}_v))$$

be the expected penalty per item if a probability prediction $\mathbf{q}$ is employed and a penalty of $-\log q(\mathbf{x})$ is incurred whenever $\mathbf{x}_v = \mathbf{x}$. The minimum achievable value H_* of $H(\mathbf{q})$ for a probability prediction $\mathbf{q}$ in the set S is attained by the unique $\mathbf{p}_*$ in S such that

$$p_{*j} = \sum_{\mathbf{x} \in \Gamma} x_i p_*(\mathbf{x}) = p_j,$$

$$p_*^R(r) = \sum_{\mathbf{x} \in \Gamma} p_*(\mathbf{x}) = p^R(r),$$

and

$$\sum_{r=0}^{I} \sum_{\mathbf{x} \in \Gamma(r)} r x_i p_*(\mathbf{x}) = \sum_{r=0}^{I} \sum_{\mathbf{x} \in \Gamma(r)} r x_i p(\mathbf{x}).$$

If $\mathbf{x}_*$ is a random vector with values in Γ such that $\mathbf{x}_* = \mathbf{x}$ in Γ with probability $p_*(\mathbf{x})$, if coordinate i of $\mathbf{x}_*$ is x_{j*}, and if $r_* = \sum_{i=1}^{I} x_{i*}$, then x_{i*} and x_{vi} have the same distribution for each integer i from 1 to I, r_* and r_v have the same distribution, and the point-biserial correlation of x_{i*} and r_* is the same as the point-biserial correlation of x_{vi} and r_v for each integer i from 1 to I. Unique τ_r, $0 \leq r \leq I$, β_i, $1 \leq i \leq I$, and γ_i, $1 \leq i \leq I$, exist such that $\beta_1 = \gamma_1 = 0$ and

$$\log p_*(\mathbf{x}) = \tau_r - \boldsymbol{\beta}'\mathbf{x} + (r-1)\boldsymbol{\gamma}'\mathbf{x} \tag{13.7}$$

holds for $\mathbf{x}$ in $\Gamma(r)$ and $0 \leq r \leq I$.

By the information inequality, it is always true that

$$H_* \geq H_M = I^{-1} E(-\log p(\mathbf{x}_v)),$$

where H_M is the Shannon entropy per item associated with $\mathbf{x}_v$ (Shannon, 1948), and $H_* = H_M$ if and only if $\mathbf{p}$ is in S, so that the loglinear-interaction model holds. Thus $\Delta = H_* - H_M$ is a measure of model error per item.

This information-theoretic argument can also be applied to the RM. The RM can hold only if the loglinear model holds in which (13.6) holds and $\boldsymbol{\gamma}$ is the zero vector. Let S_R be the population of probability arrays $\mathbf{p}$ with elements $p(\mathbf{x}) > 0$, $\mathbf{x}$ in Γ, such that $\sum_{\mathbf{x} \in \Gamma} p(\mathbf{x}) = 1$ and (13.6) holds for some τ_r, $\boldsymbol{\beta}$, and $\boldsymbol{\gamma}$ with $\beta_1 = 0$ and $\boldsymbol{\gamma}$ the zero vector. Let H_R be the minimum of $H(\mathbf{q})$ for $\mathbf{q}$ in S_R. Because S_R is obviously a subset of S, $H_R \geq H_*$, and $\Delta_R = H_R - H_*$ provides a measure of the improvement of the loglinear-interaction model over the loglinear RM.

It is of particular note that the loglinear-interaction model provides an approximation to a 2PL model (Holland, 1990a). Consider the case of x_{vi} conditionally independent given θ_v for $1 \leq i \leq k$. For each item i, $1 \leq i \leq i$, let real β_{i+} and positive real a_i be defined such that

$$P_i(\theta) = [1 + \exp(-a_i\theta + \beta_{i+})]^{-1}$$

is the conditional probability that $x_{vi} = 1$ given that $\theta_v = \theta$, and let $\mathbf{P}(\theta)$ be the vector with coordinates $P_i(\theta)$ for $1 \leq i \leq I$. Let $\mathbf{a}$ be the I-dimensional vector of a_i, $1 \leq i \leq I$, and let $A_v = \mathbf{a}'\mathbf{x}_v$ be the weighted sum of the x_{vi} that corresponds to the a_i. Let ρ_R be the correlation of A_v and r_v, let μ_A and σ_A be the respective mean and standard deviation of the A_v, and let μ_R and σ_R

be the respective mean and standard deviation of the r_v. Let $\alpha = \sigma_A \rho_R / \sigma_R$ be the slope of the linear regression of A_v on r_v, let $\zeta = \mu_A - \alpha \mu_R$, let σ_d be the standard deviation of the residual

$$d_v = A_v - \zeta - \alpha r_v$$

that results from regression of the weighted sum A_v on the unweighted sum r_v, let $\delta_i = a_i - \alpha$, and let $\boldsymbol{\delta}$ be the I-dimensional vector with coordinates δ_i for $1 \leq i \leq I$. Note that each δ_i is 0 and $\sigma_d = 0$ if the item discriminations a_i are all equal, as is the case for an RM. The quality of the approximation of the 2PL model by the interaction model may be measured by Δ. Results depend on the distribution of the ability parameter θ_v.

The initial case to consider is one in which the Dutch identity is very easily applied (Holland, 1990a). For some real μ, some real $\sigma^2 > 0$, and some $\mathbf{y}$ in Γ, let the conditional distribution of θ_v given $\mathbf{x}_v = \mathbf{y}$ be normal with mean μ and variance σ^2. By Bayes's theorem, for $\mathbf{x}$ in Γ, the conditional distribution of θ_v given $\mathbf{x}_v$ is normal with mean $\mu + \sigma^2 \mathbf{a}'(\mathbf{x} - \mathbf{y})$ and variance σ^2 (Cornfield et al., 1967). In the desired approximation, let $\boldsymbol{\gamma}$ be the vector with coordinates $\gamma_i = \alpha \sigma^2 \delta_i$ for $1 \leq i \leq I$. Then real τ_r, $0 \leq r \leq I$, and β_i, $1 \leq i \leq I$, can be defined such that

$$\log p(\mathbf{x}) = \tau_r - \boldsymbol{\beta}'\mathbf{x} + (r-1)\boldsymbol{\gamma}'\mathbf{x} + \sigma^2[\boldsymbol{\delta}'\mathbf{x} - \zeta]^2/2$$

for $\mathbf{x}$ in $\Gamma(r)$ and $0 \leq r \leq I$. It is readily verified that

$$\Delta \leq \sigma^2 \sigma_d^2/(2I). \tag{13.8}$$

Thus the 2PL model in this case is increasingly well approximated by the loglinear model as the variability of the item discriminations a_i decreases or as the variance σ^2 of the conditional distribution of θ_v given $\mathbf{x}_v = \mathbf{y}$ decreases.

The pattern for the conditional normal case is also observed if the number of items is large (Holland, 1990a). Assume that θ has a mean μ_θ, a variance σ_θ^2, and a continuous distribution with a density that is positive and continuous at μ. Let positive real constants c_1, c_2, and c_3 exist such that $c_1 < a_i < c_3$ and $|\beta_{i+}| < c_3$ for all i. Let

$$J = \sum_{i=1}^{I} a_i^2 P_i(\mu)[1 - P_i(\mu)],$$

and let $\mathbf{y}$ be selected such that $\mathbf{a}'\mathbf{y}$ is as close as possible to $\mathbf{a}'\mathbf{P}(\mu)$. Then the distribution of $J^{1/2}(\theta - \mu)$ given $\mathbf{y}$ is readily shown to converge in distribution to a standard normal random variable. It can also be shown that (13.8) remains approximately true in the sense that the conditional variance σ^2 is approximately J^{-1} and, for any real $c > 1$, $\Delta \leq c\sigma_d^2/(2IJ)$ for I sufficiently large.

A variety of bounds on σ_d^2 may be established. For example, let

$$\alpha_0 = \frac{\sum_{i=1}^{I} a_i P_i(\mu)}{\sum_{i=1}^{I} P_i(\mu)}.$$

Then Taylor's theorem and standard arguments from probability theory may be used to show that

$$\sigma_d^2 \leq (16)^{-1} \sigma_\theta^2 \left(\sum_{i=1}^{I} |a_i - \alpha_0| a_i \right)^2 + 4^{-1} \sum_{i=1}^{I} a_i^2.$$

Thus Δ can be forced to be arbitrarily small for sufficiently large I if the variance of the ability parameter θ is sufficiently small, if all item discriminations a_i are sufficiently small, or if the variability of the a_i is sufficiently small.

13.2.2 Maximum Likelihood

Under the loglinear model (13.6), the log-likelihood

$$\ell = \sum_{v=1}^{N} \log p(\mathbf{x}_v)$$

is readily decomposed into a conditional log-likelihood

$$\ell_C = \sum_{v=1}^{N} \log p(\mathbf{x}|x_v.)$$

and a marginal log-likelihood

$$\ell_U = \sum_{v=1}^{N} \log p^R(r_v),$$

for

$$\ell = \ell_C + \ell_U.$$

Let f_{ri} be the number of examinees v for whom $r_v = r$ and $x_{vi} = 1$, let n_r be the number of examinees v with $r_v = r$, let $f_{\cdot i}$ be the number of v with $x_{vi} = 1$, and let

$$g_i = \sum_{r=0}^{I} r f_{ri}$$

be the total number of correct responses provided on all items by examinees who answered item i correctly. Then

$$\ell_C = \sum_{i=1}^{I} [-(\beta_i - \gamma_i) f_{\cdot i} + \gamma_i g_i] - \sum_{r=0}^{I} n_r \log s_r (\boldsymbol{\beta} - (r-1)\boldsymbol{\gamma})$$

and

$$\ell_U = \sum_{r=0}^{I} n_r \log p^R(r).$$

Thus the conditional log-likelihood ℓ_C, the marginal log likelihood ℓ_U, and the log-likelihood ℓ are determined by the sufficient statistics n_r, $0 \leq r \leq I$, $f_{\cdot i}$, $1 \leq i \leq I$, and g_i, $1 \leq i \leq I$. Under the loglinear model, maximization of ℓ is achieved by independent maximization of ℓ_C and ℓ_U (Haberman, 1973). Thus if $\hat{\ell}$, $\hat{\ell}_U$, and $\hat{\ell}_C$ denote the respective maxima of ℓ, ℓ_C, and ℓ_U under the loglinear-interaction model, then $\hat{\ell}$ is $\hat{\ell}_C + \hat{\ell}_U$. It is easily verified that

$$\hat{\ell}_U = \sum_{r=0}^{I} n_r \log \hat{p}^R(r),$$

where $\hat{p}^R(r) = n_r/N$. If a maximum-likelihood estimate $\hat{\mathbf{p}}$ of $\mathbf{p}$ exists, then

$$\hat{p}(\mathbf{x}) = \hat{p}^R(r)\hat{p}(\mathbf{x}|r)$$

for $\mathbf{x}$ in $\Gamma(r)$ and $0 \leq r \leq I$, where $\hat{p}(\mathbf{x}|r)$ is the conditional maximum-likelihood estimate of $p(\mathbf{x}|r)$ under (13.5) and $n_r > 0$ for $0 \leq r \leq I$.

To determine $\hat{p}(\mathbf{x}|r)$, some preliminary definitions are helpful. For any I-dimensional vector $\mathbf{a}$, let

$$s_{ri}(\mathbf{a}) = \sum_{\mathbf{x} \in \Gamma(r)} a_i \exp(-\mathbf{a}'\mathbf{x})$$

and

$$m_{ri}(\mathbf{a}) = s_{ri}(\mathbf{a})/s_r(\mathbf{a})$$

for $1 \leq i \leq I$, and let

$$s_{rij}(\mathbf{a}) = \sum_{\mathbf{x} \in \Gamma(r)} a_i a_j \exp(-\mathbf{a}'\mathbf{x})$$

and

$$c_{rij}(\mathbf{a}) = s_{rij}(\mathbf{a})/s_r(\mathbf{a}) - m_{ri}(\mathbf{a})m_{rj}(\mathbf{a})$$

for $1 \leq i \leq I$ and $1 \leq j \leq I$. Then $m_{ri}(\boldsymbol{\beta} - (r-1)\boldsymbol{\gamma})$ is the conditional expectation of x_{vi} given $r_v = r$, and $c_{rij}(\boldsymbol{\beta} - (r-1)\boldsymbol{\gamma})$ is the conditional covariance of x_{vi} and x_{vj} given $r_v = r$. Let R_+ be the set of integers r, $0 \leq r \leq I$, such that $n_r > 0$. Standard arguments for loglinear models may be employed to show that if the conditional maximum-likelihood estimates $\hat{p}(\mathbf{x}|r)$ exist for $\mathbf{x}$ in $\Gamma(r)$ and $0 \leq r \leq I$, then, for some I-dimensional vectors $\hat{\boldsymbol{\beta}}$ and $\hat{\boldsymbol{\gamma}}$ such that $\hat{\beta}_1 = \hat{\gamma}_1 = 0$,

$$\sum_{r=0}^{I} n_r m_{ri}(\hat{\boldsymbol{\beta}} - (r-1))\hat{\boldsymbol{\gamma}}) = f_{\cdot i} \qquad (13.9)$$

for $1 \leq i \leq I$,

$$\sum_{r=0}^{I} r n_r m_{ri}(\hat{\boldsymbol{\beta}} - (r-1))\hat{\boldsymbol{\gamma}}) = g_i \qquad (13.10)$$

for $1 \leq i \leq I$, and

$$\hat{p}(\mathbf{x}|r) = \frac{\exp\{[-\hat{\boldsymbol{\beta}} + (r-1)\hat{\boldsymbol{\gamma}}]'\mathbf{x}\}}{s_r(\hat{\boldsymbol{\beta}} - (r-1)\hat{\boldsymbol{\gamma}})} \qquad (13.11)$$

for $\mathbf{x}$ in $\Gamma(r)$ and $0 \leq r \leq I$ (Haberman, 1973). The estimates $\hat{p}(\mathbf{x}|r)$ are uniquely determined by (13.9) to (13.11). If $n_0 + n_I < N$, then (13.9) to (13.11) also uniquely determine $\hat{\boldsymbol{\beta}}$ and $\hat{\boldsymbol{\gamma}}$.

It is possible but not necessarily true that $\hat{\mathbf{p}}$, if it exists, is also the maximum-likelihood estimate of $\mathbf{p}$ under the interaction model as well as under the loglinear model. Consider

$$\hat{\tau}_r = \log(n_r/N) - \log[s_r(\hat{\boldsymbol{\beta}} - (r-1)\hat{\boldsymbol{\gamma}})].$$

Then

$$\log \hat{p}(\mathbf{x}) = \hat{\tau}_r - \hat{\boldsymbol{\beta}}'\mathbf{x} + (r-1)\hat{\boldsymbol{\gamma}}'\mathbf{x}$$

for $\mathbf{x}$ in $\Gamma(r)$ and $0 \leq r \leq I$. If a positive random variable Z exists such that $\exp(\hat{\tau}_r - \hat{\tau}_0)$ is $E(Z^r)$ for each integer r from 0 to I, then $\hat{\mathbf{p}}$ is also the maximum-likelihood estimate of $\mathbf{p}$ under the interaction model. In practice, it is convenient to employ $\hat{\mathbf{p}}$ even if it is not the maximum-likelihood estimate of $\mathbf{p}$ under the interaction model, for computations are simplified, and asymptotic results for $\hat{\mathbf{p}}$ are rather satisfactory.

Interpretation of the equations for the maximum-likelihood estimates is straightforward. Equation 13.9 implies that the estimated expected number of examinees who correctly answer item i is equal to the observed number $f_{.i}$ of examinees who correctly answer item i. Given (13.9), (13.10) implies that the estimated point-biserial correlation of x_{vi} and $x_{v.}$ is equal to the sample point-biserial correlation of x_{vi} and $x_{v.}$. Under the loglinear model, the estimated marginal distribution of $x_{v.}$ is the sample marginal distribution of the $x_{v.}$. In contrast, in the case of the RM, the corresponding loglinear model requires that (13.6) hold for $\boldsymbol{\gamma} = \mathbf{0}$. Under this loglinear model, the maximum-likelihood estimate $\hat{\mathbf{p}}_R$ of $\mathbf{p}$, if it exists, satisfies

$$\sum_{r=0}^{I} n_r m_{ri}(\hat{\boldsymbol{\beta}}_R) = f_{.i} \qquad (13.12)$$

for $1 \leq i \leq I$, $\hat{\beta}_{R1} = 0$, and

$$\hat{p}_R(\mathbf{x}|r) = \frac{\exp(-\hat{\boldsymbol{\beta}}_R'\mathbf{x})}{s_r(\hat{\boldsymbol{\beta}}_R)} \qquad (13.13)$$

and

$$\hat{p}_R(\mathbf{x}) = (n_r/N)\hat{p}_R(\mathbf{x}|r) \tag{13.14}$$

for $\mathbf{x}$ in $\Gamma(r)$ and $0 \le r \le I$. The estimates $\hat{p}_R(\mathbf{x}|r)$ and $\hat{p}_R(\mathbf{x})$ are uniquely determined by (13.12) to (13.14). If $n_0 + n_I < N$, then (13.12) to (13.13) also uniquely determine $\hat{\boldsymbol{\beta}}_R$. Thus the loglinear model corresponding to the interaction model involves a fit of the point-biserial correlation that is not found in the loglinear model corresponding to the RM.

Given results for maximum-likelihood estimation, the minimum expected log penalty H_* for the loglinear interaction model may be estimated by $\hat{H}_* = -\hat{\ell}/(NI)$. If $\hat{\ell}_R$ denotes the maximum of ℓ under the loglinear RM, then H_R may be estimated by $\hat{H}_R = -(NI)^{-1}\hat{\ell}_R$, so that the difference Δ_R in expected penalty per item may be estimated by $\hat{\Delta}_R = \hat{H}_R - \hat{H}_*$. No fully satisfactory estimate of Δ or H_M exists unless I is quite small.

For a given examinee v, θ_v may be estimated by $\hat{\theta}_v$, where $\hat{\theta}_v$ maximizes

$$\log \hat{p}_\theta(\mathbf{x}) = \alpha(\hat{\boldsymbol{\beta}}, \hat{\boldsymbol{\gamma}}, \theta) + x.\theta - \hat{\boldsymbol{\beta}}'\mathbf{x} + (x.)\hat{\boldsymbol{\gamma}}'\mathbf{x}$$

over θ for $\mathbf{x} = \mathbf{x}_v$. Provided that $0 < r_v < I$ and $n_0 + n_I < N$, $\hat{\theta}_v$ is the unique solution of

$$\sum_{\mathbf{x} \in \Gamma} x.\hat{p}_{\hat{\theta}_v}(\mathbf{x}) = r_v.$$

13.2.3 Large-Sample Approximations

For fixed I and large N, large-sample properties of maximum-likelihood estimates can be derived quite readily from standard results for loglinear models. Results are straightforward whether or not the model holds. Results are somewhat more challenging to derive if both I and N are large (Haberman, 1977b).

To begin, consider the case of I fixed, (13.6) true, and N large. To simplify numerical and asymptotic work, let $\boldsymbol{\eta}$ be the $2(I-1)$-dimensional vector with coordinates $\eta_i = \beta_{i+1} - (I/2-1)\gamma_{i+1}$ and $\eta_{I+i-1} = -I\gamma_{i+1}$ for $1 \le i \le I-1$. Let $\hat{\boldsymbol{\eta}}$ be the maximum-likelihood estimate of $\boldsymbol{\eta}$, so that $\hat{\eta}_i = \hat{\beta}_{i+1} - (I/2-1)\hat{\gamma}_i$ and $\hat{\eta}_{I+i-1} = -I\hat{\gamma}_{i+1}$ for $1 \le i \le I-1$. Let $\boldsymbol{\nu}_r$ be the I-dimensional vector with elements $\nu_{ir} = 0$ for $i = 1$ and $\nu_{ir} = \eta_{i-1} + (r/I - 1/2)\eta_{i+I-2}$ for $i > 1$. Thus, conditional on $r_v = r$, the probability is $m_{ri}(\boldsymbol{\mu}_r)$ that $x_{vi} = 1$. Thus ν_{ir} can be regarded as the relative difficulty of item $i + 1$ compared to item 1 given that the total score r_v equals r. Let $\hat{\boldsymbol{\nu}}_r$ be the I-dimensional vector with elements $\hat{\nu}_{ir} = 0$ for $i = 1$ and $\hat{\nu}_{ir} = \hat{\eta}_{i-1} + (r/I - 1/2)\hat{\eta}_{i+I-2}$ for $i > 1$. Let $\mathbf{C}$ be the $2(I-1) \times 2(I-1)$ matrix with elements

$$C_{ij} = E(c_{r_v ij}(\boldsymbol{\nu}_{r_v})),$$

$$C_{(I-1+i)j} = C_{j(I-1+i)} = E(I^{-1}(r_v - I/2)c_{r_v ij}(\boldsymbol{\nu}_{r_v})),$$

and

$$C_{(I-1+i)(I-1+j)} = E(I^{-2}(r_v - I/2)^2 c_{r_v ij}(\boldsymbol{\nu}_{r_v})).$$

Then the probability that $\hat{\boldsymbol{\eta}}$ is defined approaches 1, and $N^{1/2}(\hat{\boldsymbol{\eta}}-\boldsymbol{\eta})$ converges in distribution to a normal random vector with zero mean and with covariance matrix $\mathbf{C}^{-1}$ (Haberman, 1977b). For a nonzero vector $\mathbf{w}$ of dimension $2(I-1)$, let

$$\sigma(\mathbf{w}'\hat{\boldsymbol{\eta}}) = [\mathbf{w}'\mathbf{C}^{-1}\mathbf{w}]^{1/2}.$$

Then

$$z(\mathbf{w}'\hat{\boldsymbol{\eta}}) = \frac{N^{1/2}(\mathbf{w}'\hat{\boldsymbol{\eta}} - \mathbf{w}'\boldsymbol{\eta})}{\sigma(\mathbf{w}'\hat{\boldsymbol{\eta}})}$$

converges in distribution to a standard normal random variable.

Let $\hat{\mathbf{C}}$ be the $2(I-1) \times 2(I-1)$ matrix with elements

$$\hat{C}_{ij} = N^{-1} \sum_{r=0}^{I} n_r c_{rij}(\hat{\boldsymbol{\nu}}_r)),$$

$$\hat{C}_{(I-1+i)j} = \hat{C}_{j(I-1+i)} = N^{-1} \sum_{r=0}^{I} n_r I^{-1}(r - I/2)c_{rij}(\hat{\boldsymbol{\nu}}_r)),$$

and

$$\hat{C}_{(I-1+i)(I-1+j)} = N^{-1} \sum_{r=0}^{I} n_r (I^{-2}(r - I/2)^2 c_{rij}(\hat{\boldsymbol{\nu}}_r)).$$

Then $\hat{\mathbf{C}}^{-1}$ converges in probability to $\mathbf{C}^{-1}$. If

$$\hat{\sigma}(\mathbf{w}'\hat{\boldsymbol{\eta}}) = [\mathbf{w}'\hat{\mathbf{C}}^{-1}\mathbf{w}]^{1/2},$$

then $\hat{\sigma}(\mathbf{w}'\hat{\boldsymbol{\eta}})$ converges in probability to $\sigma(\mathbf{w}'\hat{\boldsymbol{\eta}})$ and

$$\hat{z}\mathbf{w}'\hat{\boldsymbol{\eta}} = \frac{N^{1/2}(\mathbf{w}'\hat{\boldsymbol{\eta}} - \mathbf{w}'\boldsymbol{\eta})}{\hat{\sigma}(\mathbf{w}'\hat{\boldsymbol{\eta}})}$$

converges in distribution to a standard normal random variable. Thus approximate confidence intervals for $\mathbf{w}'\boldsymbol{\eta}$ are readily obtained. The term $\hat{\sigma}(\mathbf{w}'\hat{\boldsymbol{\eta}})/N^{1/2}$ may be termed the estimated asymptotic standard deviation of $\mathbf{w}'\hat{\boldsymbol{\eta}}$ (Haberman, 1978b).

If I is increasing, (13.6) is true, and N is large, then arguments for the RM can be used to show that $\hat{\boldsymbol{\eta}}$ continues to behave well, although results must be changed to treat the variable dimension of $\hat{\boldsymbol{\eta}}$ (Haberman, 1977b, 2004). It is simplest to assume that, for a fixed positive constant c, $|\beta_i|$ and $I|\gamma_i|$, $2 \leq i \leq k$, never exceed c. This assumption on γ_i is reasonable if one notes results for the 2PL approximation. The probability approaches 1 that $\hat{\boldsymbol{\eta}}$ is defined. If t_i and u_i are fixed real constants for $1 \leq i \leq s$ for an integer $s \geq 1$, if some t_i or u_i is not zero, and if $\mathbf{w}$ is the $2(I-1)$-dimensional vector such that $w_i = 0$ if $s + 1 \leq i \leq I - 1$ or $I + s \leq i \leq 2(I-1)$, $w_i = t_i$ for

$1 \leq i \leq s$, and $w_{I+i-1} = u_i$ for $1 \leq i \leq s$, then $z(\mathbf{w}'\hat{\boldsymbol{\eta}})$ and $\hat{z}(\mathbf{w}'\hat{\boldsymbol{\eta}})$ converge in distribution to a standard normal random variable, and $\hat{\sigma}(\mathbf{w}'\hat{\boldsymbol{\eta}})$ converges in probability to $\sigma(\mathbf{w}'\hat{\boldsymbol{\eta}})$. Again confidence intervals for parameters may be obtained.

Asymptotic results remain available even if the model does not hold. The simplest case is for I fixed. Let $\mathbf{C}_+$ be the covariance matrix of the $2(I-1)$-dimensional vector $\mathbf{d}_v$ with coordinates $d_{vi} = x_{v(i+1)}$ and $d_{v(I-1+i)} = (r_v - I/2)x_{vi}$ for $1 \leq i \leq I-1$. Then $N^{1/2}(\hat{\boldsymbol{\eta}} - \boldsymbol{\eta})$ converges in distribution to a normal random variable with zero mean and covariance matrix $\mathbf{C}^{-1}\mathbf{C}_+\mathbf{C}^{-1}$. A similar result can be obtained for I large under quite mild conditions.

In all cases under study, $\hat{\Delta}_R - \Delta_R$ converges in probability to 0. Normal approximations and asymptotic confidence intervals for $\hat{H}_*$, $\hat{H}_R$, and $\hat{\Delta}_R$ are available (Gilula & Haberman, 1994, 1995).

Normal approximations for $\hat{\theta}_v$ are available only if I increases. Let

$$\hat{\sigma}(\hat{\theta}_v) = \left[\sum_{\mathbf{x} \in \Gamma}(x. - r_v)^2 \hat{p}_{\hat{\theta}_v}(\mathbf{x})\right]^{1/2}.$$

If the interaction model holds and N and I are large, then

$$\hat{z}(\hat{\theta}_v) = \frac{I^{1/2}(\hat{\theta}_v - \theta_v)}{\hat{\sigma}(\hat{\theta}_v)}$$

has an approximate standard normal distribution. This result is easily applied to asymptotic confidence intervals.

13.3 Computation of Conditional Maximum-Likelihood Estimates

The Newton–Raphson algorithm is readily applied to computation of $\hat{\boldsymbol{\eta}}$. Given an initial starting value $\boldsymbol{\eta}_0$, a sequence of $\boldsymbol{\eta}_t$, $t \geq 1$, is generated from the equations

$$\nu_{irt} = \begin{cases} 0, & i = 1, \\ \eta_{(i-1)t} + (r - I/2)\eta_{(i+I-2)t}, & : 2 \leq i \leq I, \end{cases}$$

$$nd_{it} = \begin{cases} f_{i\cdot} - \sum_{r=0}^{I} n_r m_{r(i+1)}(\boldsymbol{\nu}_{rt}), & 1 \leq i \leq I-1, \\ g_{i-I+1}/I - f_{(i-I+1)\cdot}/2- & \\ \sum_{r=0}^{I}(r/I - 1/2)n_r m_{r(i-I+2)}(\boldsymbol{\nu}_{rt}), & I \leq i \leq 2(I-1), \end{cases}$$

$$nC_{ijt} = \begin{cases} \sum_{r=0}^{I} n_r c_{r(i+1)(j+1)}(\boldsymbol{\nu}_{rt}), & 1 \leq i \leq I-1, 1 \leq j \leq I-1, \\ \sum_{r=0}^{I} n_r I^{-1}(r - I/2) & \\ \quad \cdot c_{r(i-I+2)j}(\boldsymbol{\nu}_{rt})), & I \leq i \leq 2(I-1), 1 \leq j \leq I-1, \\ nC_{jit}, & 1 \leq i \leq I-1, I \leq j \leq 2(I-1), \\ \sum_{r=0}^{I} n_r(I^{-2}(r - I/2)^2 & \\ \quad \cdot c_{r(i-I+2)(j-I+2)}(\boldsymbol{\nu}_{rt})), & \end{cases}$$

and

$$\sum_{j=1}^{2(I-1)} C_{ijt}(\eta_{j(t+1)} - \eta_{jt}) = d_{it}, : 1 \leq i \leq 2(I-1).$$

Computation of the $c_{rij}(\boldsymbol{\nu}_{rt})$ is performed as in the RM (Liou, 1994).

In cases in which the loglinear interaction model is examined after the RM is examined, it is reasonable to let η_{i0} be the maximum-likelihood estimate of β_{i+1} under the RM for $i < I$ and to let other η_{i0} be 0. An alternative approach is to consider the number h_{rij}, $1 \leq i \leq I$, $1 \leq j \leq I$, $1 \leq r \leq I - 1$, of observations with $x_{vi} = 1$, $x_{vj} = 0$, and $r_v = r$. Then it is readily verified that $\log[(h_{rij}+0.5)/(h_{rji}+0.5)]$ provides an estimate of $\nu_{rj} - \nu_{ri}$. Use of these estimates for all $j > 1$, for $i = 1$, and for at least two values of r suffices to construct starting values.

The Newton–Raphson algorithm may also be employed to obtain $\hat{\theta}_v$ for each examinee v. In practice, no more than $I - 1$ distinct finite values of $\hat{\theta}_v$ exist, for $\hat{\theta}_v$ depends on r_v, and $\hat{\theta}_v$ is defined only for $1 \leq r_v \leq I - 1$. One may let $\hat{\theta}_v$ be $-\infty$ for $r_v = 0$ and ∞ for $r_v = \infty$.

13.4 Tests of Fit

The likelihood-ratio chi-square statistic

$$L^2 = 2NI\hat{\Delta}_R$$

provides a formal test of the RM. If the RM holds and I is fixed, then a straightforward application of general results for loglinear models permits a demonstration that L^2 converges in distribution to a chi-square random variable with $I-1$ degrees of freedom (Haberman, 1974, Chapter 4). A more complicated case has I increasing but I^2/N approaching 0. In this case, one may show that $(L^2 - I + 1)/[2(I - 1)]^{1/2}$ converges in distribution to a standard normal random variable (Haberman, 1977a,b; Portney, 1988). The normal approximation supports use of the chi-square approximation, for a chi-square random variable χ_ν^2 with ν degrees of freedom satisfies the condition that $(\chi_\nu^2 - \nu)/(2\nu)^{1/2}$ converges in distribution to a standard normal variable as ν approaches ∞.

The proposed likelihood-ratio chi-square is similar in spirit to the likelihood-ratio chi-square statistic for the RM in which the alternative hypothesis is that

$$p(\mathbf{x}|r) = p(\mathbf{x})/p^R(r) = \frac{\exp(-\boldsymbol{\beta}_r'\mathbf{x})}{s_r(\boldsymbol{\beta}_r)}$$

for $\mathbf{x}$ in $\Gamma(r)$ and $0 \leq r \leq I$ for some I-dimensional $\boldsymbol{\beta}_r$, $0 \leq r \leq I$, with initial coordinates 0 (Andersen, 1973c); however, the proposed test has the potential advantage, especially for large I, that far fewer degrees of freedom are involved.

Tests of the interaction model may be based on a model that includes both two-factor and three-factor interactions. Analysis may also employ generalized residuals based on comparison of the counts f_{ri} and fitted expected counts $n_r m_{ri}(\hat{\nu}_r)$, $1 \leq r \leq I - 1$, $1 \leq i \leq I$ (Haberman, 1978a, 2004). In this comparison, for $d_{ri} = f_{ri} - n_r m_{ri}(\hat{\nu}_r)$, the estimated standard deviation $\hat{\sigma}(d_{ri})$ of d_{ri} is computed and the generalized residual $\hat{z}_{ri} = d_{ri}/\hat{\sigma}(d_{ri})$ is examined. In large samples, if the loglinear-interaction model holds, then each $\hat{z}_{ri}$ has an approximate standard normal distribution.

13.5 An Application to a Writing Test

For the example under study, results for item parameters are summarized in Tables 13.1. The location value is $\hat{\eta}_{i-1}$, and the slope value is $\hat{\eta}_{I+i-2}$ for item $i > 0$. The RM comparison uses $\hat{\beta}_i$. Estimated asymptotic standard deviations are in parentheses. Corresponding values of $\hat{\eta}_{i-1}$ and $\hat{\beta}_i$ are reasonably close; however, the values of $\hat{\eta}_{I+i-2}$ are rather large, rather variable, and relatively well determined. Conditional on the total score r_v, the relative difficulty of items varies considerably.

Results for ability parameters are summarized in Table 13.2 for the total scores observed in the sample. The results are rather strikingly different in terms of range of parameters and in terms of the estimated asymptotic standard deviations shown in parentheses. A significant issue appears to be that the behavior of $\hat{\theta}_v$ is somewhat sensitive to which item is designated the first item. For example, an interchange of the first and third items leads to values of $\hat{\theta}_v$ much more similar to those found with the RM. The general issue involved is a difference between the effects of changes in parameters in the interaction and RMs. In the Rasch model, if the restraint that $\beta_1 = 0$ is replaced by a constraint that $\beta_i = 0$ for some $i > 1$, then each $\hat{\theta}_v$ is changed by a constant amount. In the interaction model, if the restraints that $\beta_1 = \gamma_1 = 0$ are replaced by restraints that $\beta_i = \gamma_i = 0$ for some $i > 1$, then the change in $\hat{\theta}_v$ is a function of the score total r_v rather than a constant. In general, estimates of θ_v more similar to those in the RM are likely if the constraint $\gamma_1 = 0$ is replaced by the constraint that $\sum_{i=1}^{I} \gamma_i = 0$.

To study predictive power, observe that the interaction model yields an estimated expected log penalty per item of $\hat{H}_* = 0.591$, while the loglinear RM yields 0.596. The normal 2PL model yields 0.592, so that the the loglinear interaction model is quite competitive with the standard 2PL model. The value of $\hat{\Delta}_R$ is 0.005, so that the difference between the Rasch and interaction models appears fairly small. Nonetheless, $L^2 = 3,905$ on 44 degrees of freedom, so that overwhelming evidence exists that the RM does not hold.

Some perspective on model comparisons may be obtained by examination of the trivial model that all responses x_{vi} are independent, $1 \leq i \leq I$, for each examinee v. In this case, the estimated expected log penalty per item is

Table 13.1. Item-parameter estimates for a writing test

Item	Rasch location difficulty	Interaction location	Interaction slope
2	−0.374 (0.033)	−0.359 (0.033)	0.484 (0.208)
3	−0.755 (0.033)	−0.609 (0.033)	−3.304 (0.151)
4	−1.326 (0.033)	−1.206 (0.034)	−4.091 (0.151)
5	−0.395 (0.033)	−0.233 (0.034)	−3.316 (0.151)
6	−2.352 (0.037)	−2.316 (0.040)	−4.522 (0.151)
7	−0.055 (0.034)	−0.071 (0.033)	0.478 (0.151)
8	0.800 (0.037)	0.818 (0.039)	−1.109 (0.151)
9	−0.297 (0.033)	−0.130 (0.035)	−3.332 (0.151)
10	−1.778 (0.035)	−1.687 (0.036)	−4.079 (0.151)
11	−1.686 (0.034)	−1.549 (0.034)	−1.837 (0.151)
12	−0.083 (0.034)	0.119 (0.036)	−3.755 (0.151)
13	−1.299 (0.033)	−1.171 (0.033)	−2.747 (0.151)
14	0.566 (0.036)	0.682 (0.039)	−2.241 (0.151)
15	−1.897 (0.035)	−1.744 (0.035)	−0.988 (0.151)
16	−3.190 (0.045)	−3.461 (0.060)	−7.379 (0.151)
17	−0.886 (0.033)	−0.800 (0.032)	−0.337 (0.151)
18	−0.438 (0.033)	−0.352 (0.033)	−1.323 (0.151)
19	−1.251 (0.033)	−1.138 (0.035)	−5.934 (0.151)
20	−1.151 (0.033)	−1.036 (0.033)	−0.944 (0.151)
21	−1.249 (0.033)	−1.123 (0.033)	−1.707 (0.151)
22	−0.009 (0.034)	0.135 (0.035)	−2.711 (0.151)
23	−2.597 (0.039)	−2.571 (0.043)	−4.465 (0.151)
24	−1.525 (0.034)	−1.390 (0.033)	−1.224 (0.151)
25	−1.553 (0.034)	−1.430 (0.034)	−2.918 (0.151)
26	0.168 (0.034)	0.395 (0.037)	−3.856 (0.151)
27	−0.989 (0.033)	−0.883 (0.033)	−1.001 (0.151)
28	−1.003 (0.033)	−0.855 (0.034)	−4.650 (0.151)
29	0.040 (0.034)	0.029 (0.034)	0.154 (0.151)
30	−0.753 (0.033)	−0.662 (0.033)	−0.946 (0.151)
31	−2.064 (0.036)	−2.003 (0.038)	−4.384 (0.151)
32	−2.191 (0.036)	−2.068 (0.037)	−2.666 (0.151)
33	−1.857 (0.035)	−1.761 (0.036)	−3.727 (0.151)
34	−0.844 (0.033)	−0.697 (0.033)	−3.522 (0.151)
35	0.413 (0.035)	0.550 (0.038)	−2.518 (0.151)
36	−0.553 (0.033)	−0.361 (0.034)	−4.456 (0.151)
37	−0.222 (0.033)	−0.127 (0.034)	−1.736 (0.151)
38	−2.028 (0.036)	−2.018 (0.038)	−5.610 (0.151)
39	−0.434 (0.033)	−0.218 (0.035)	−4.735 (0.151)
40	−1.206 (0.033)	−1.077 (0.034)	−3.869 (0.151)
41	0.329 (0.035)	0.375 (0.036)	−1.218 (0.151)
42	−0.843 (0.033)	−0.717 (0.033)	−2.378 (0.151)
43	−0.273 (0.033)	−0.182 (0.034)	−1.622 (0.151)
44	−0.358 (0.033)	−0.209 (0.034)	−2.937 (0.151)
45	−0.567 (0.033)	−0.423 (0.034)	−2.968 (0.151)

Table 13.2. Ability-parameter estimates for a writing test

Total score	Rasch ability	Interaction ability
4	−3.538 (0.545)	−2.571 (0.400)
5	−3.268 (0.497)	−2.447 (0.302)
6	−3.038 (0.462)	−2.380 (0.216)
7	−2.837 (0.436)	−2.380 (0.216)
8	−2.656 (0.415)	−2.322 (0.137)
9	−2.491 (0.398)	−2.306 (0.119)
10	−2.339 (0.384)	−2.293 (0.107)
11	−2.195 (0.373)	−2.283 (0.098)
12	−2.060 (0.363)	−2.273 (0.092)
13	−1.931 (0.355)	−2.265 (0.087)
14	−1.808 (0.348)	−2.258 (0.084)
15	−1.689 (0.342)	−2.251 (0.081)
16	−1.573 (0.338)	−2.245 (0.078)
17	−1.460 (0.334)	−2.239 (0.077)
18	−1.350 (0.330)	−2.233 (0.075)
19	−1.242 (0.328)	−2.228 (0.075)
20	−1.135 (0.326)	−2.222 (0.074)
21	−1.030 (0.324)	−2.217 (0.074)
22	−0.925 (0.323)	−2.211 (0.074)
23	−0.821 (0.323)	−2.206 (0.074)
24	−0.716 (0.323)	−2.200 (0.075)
25	−0.611 (0.324)	−2.194 (0.076)
26	−0.506 (0.326)	−2.188 (0.078)
27	−0.399 (0.328)	−2.182 (0.080)
28	−0.290 (0.331)	−2.176 (0.083)
29	−0.180 (0.334)	−2.168 (0.087)
30	−0.067 (0.339)	−2.160 (0.091)
31	0.050 (0.344)	−2.152 (0.097)
32	0.170 (0.350)	−2.141 (0.105)
33	0.295 (0.358)	−2.129 (0.116)
34	0.426 (0.367)	−2.114 (0.131)
35	0.565 (0.378)	−2.094 (0.155)
36	0.713 (0.391)	−2.064 (0.191)
37	0.872 (0.408)	−2.017 (0.245)
38	1.047 (0.428)	−1.942 (0.303)
39	1.241 (0.455)	−1.833 (0.355)
40	1.463 (0.489)	−1.833 (0.355)
41	1.725 (0.537)	−1.495 (0.472)
42	2.052 (0.610)	−1.232 (0.559)
43	2.495 (0.733)	−0.844 (0.697)
44	3.226 (1.018)	−0.162 (0.996)

$$\hat{H}_I = -(NI)^{-1} \sum_{i=1}^{I} f_{\cdot i} \log(f_{\cdot i}) = 0.625,$$

and the estimated difference in expected log penalty per item between the Rasch and independence models is 0.028, so that the RM accounts for about 85% of the change in estimated log penalty from use of the interaction model rather than the independence model.

The interaction model does not appear to be true, although it is not clear that major improvement is readily achieved. The generalization of the loglinear-interaction model to include additive three-factor interactions results in only a very small improvement in estimated expected log penalty, but the likelihood-ratio chi-square that compares the two models is 263 on 44 degrees of freedom, so that clear evidence against the interaction model does exist.

Multilevel Rasch Models

Akihito Kamata[1] and Yuk Fai Cheong[2]

[1] Florida State University
[2] Emory University

14.1 Introduction

Over the past few years, several studies have investigated and demonstrated the relationships between generalized linear mixed models (GLIMM) and item response modeling. Some benefits associated with this GLIMM-based modeling framework include the modeling of nested structure of data, such as examinees nested within schools (Kamata, 2001), of multidimensional measures (Cheong & Raudenbush, 2000), and of wider class of item response models, such as 2PL item response model (Rijmen et al., 2003). Applications of this modeling approach include the detection and investigation of differential item functioning (e.g., Cheong, 2006), item-parameter drift (Pastor & Beretvas, 2006), and test equating (Chu & Kamata, 2005). In this chapter, we describe how researchers can use GLIMM to estimate multilevel, multidimensional RMs. We first provide a modeling framework for the Rasch based on the general GLIMM framework. We then discuss how the GLIMM based RM can be applied to study multidimensional constructs in multilevel settings. To illustrate the modeling approach, we analyze data collected by a statewide testing program on mathematics and reading proficiencies. Implications of the approach are discussed.

14.2 Background

Multilevel RMs can be considered as a special case of generalized RMs. However, it is distinct from other generalizations of the RM to the extent that the multilevel RM allows researchers to treat person abilities as randomly varying parameters and accommodate the nested structure often found in data in the social sciences. One typical example is data from educational surveys where primary sampling units are schools, and students are sampled from within these units.

Also, the multilevel formulation of item response models, here the Rasch model, can be viewed from several different perspectives. The first perspective is characterized by the treatment of person abilities as random effects (e.g., Adams, Wilson, & Wu, 1997; Hedeker & Gibbons, 1993; Spiegelhalter et al., 1996). One view of the original intention of this treatment was to facilitate maximum marginal likelihood estimation (MMLE) of item parameters (Bock & Lieberman, 1981; Bock & Aitkin, 1981). This approach avoids the so-called "Neyman-Scott problem" (Neyman & Scott, 1948); namely, the inconsistency of estimators that occurs when item and person parameters are estimated simultaneously. However, this treatment also gives rise to an interpretation of the item response model as a mixed-effects model formulation because, in this framework, item parameters are fixed effects and person abilities are random effects.

When person parameters are considered to randomly vary, they may be decomposed into a linear combination of fixed and random effects, in the same framework as is seen with mixed-effects and multilevel generalized linear models. This approach, which enables one to perform a one-step analysis of person characteristic variables on test data, can be considered as the second perspective on multilevel IRT formulation. For example, Zwinderman (1991) and Hoijtink & Boomsma (1996) demonstrated a decomposition of a random person ability into a linear combination of fixed person-characteristic variables and a random effect.

More recently, Adams & Wilson (1996) proposed a more general model, the random coefficient multinomial logit model (RCMLM), which subsequently was further generalized to its multidimensional form (MRCMLM) (Adams, Wilson, & Wang, 1997). Similar to Zwinderman's approach, both the RCMLM and the MRCMLM are formulated so that person parameters are random variables. They also allow person-characteristic variables to be included in the model as predictors. These models are general enough to include different classes of RMs, including those with dichotomous and polytomous outcomes, and have been implemented in ConQuest software (Wu et al., 1997). The models, however, are applicable only to a hierarchical data structure with two levels of random variation (items nested within persons) and could include only random effects at the person level.

The third perspective on multilevel formulation of IRT models is represented by the multiple-group IRT model (Bock & Zimowski, 1997). A multiple-group IRT model assumes that individuals are grouped by a common characteristic, such as ethnic group or school attended. Operationally, the model assumes separate latent distributions for groups in estimating item parameters. One special case of the model is the group-level IRT model (Mislevy, 1983; Mislevy & Bock, 1989), used in instances when the primary purpose is to estimate group-level abilities rather than individual-level abilities. Duplex design (Bock & Mislevy, 1989) can similarly be considered a special case of the multiple-group IRT in which individual- and school-level abilities are estimated simultaneously using multiple-matrix sampling. Yet another variation on the multiple-group IRT model is the item-parameter drift model (Bock, Muraki, & Pfeiffenberger, 1988), which models changes of item-parameter values over time. In this model, people that were given a test at the same time are considered to be in the same group. Differential item functioning (DIF) analysis can be thought of as a special case of multiple-group IRT (Thissen et al., 1993) in which individuals are grouped by gender and race/ethnicity. The mixed RMs (Rost, 1990; von Davier & Rost, 1995) and mixture IRT models (Mislevy & Verhelst, 1990) are also multiple-group models in which the outcomes of the grouping variable are unknown. Models following this approach can be viewed as examples of hierarchical IRT models with missing values on higher-level variables (see von Davier & Yamamoto, 2004b).

The decomposition of item parameters into more than one component parameter in IRT modeling represents the fourth perspective on multilevel formulation of IRT models. Fischer's (1973; 1983; 1995d) linear logistic test model (LLTM) can be classified under this perspective. Fischer generalized the standard binary RM by decomposing an item-difficulty parameter into linear combinations of more than one item-component parameter. This modeling approach allows the inclusion of multiple item-characteristic variables; as such, models of this type are multilevel in items rather than in persons. Accordingly, it is possible to estimate the effect of item characteristics on the probability of correct responses. Swanson et al. (2002) used a similar idea in their development of a two-level hierarchical framework to study differential item functioning.

Adopting one or several of these perspectives, researchers have demonstrated the relationships between generalized linear mixed models (GLIMM) and item response modeling. Kamata (2001), for example, formulated the RM as a two-level hierarchical generalized linear model (HGLM) and extended it to a three-level model by incorporating between and within cluster variations at the student and school level, thus a multilevel RM. This three-level extension has been demonstrated to include person- and group- characteristic variables embedded into a RM. Also, Raudenbush & Sampson (1999) and Cheong & Raudenbush (2000) described and illustrated how a multidimensional RM can be embedded in a hierarchical model, such that more than one latent trait can be modeled. Raudenbush and Sampson incorporated item response models in measuring and modeling two social organization aspects of neighborhoods: physical and social disorder. In their study, an item response model that constituted the level-1 model was used to describe the log-odds of finding disorder on individual items measuring the organizational aspects. This item response model was cast as a within-face-block model, where a face-block was defined as the block segment on one side of the street. The item response/within-face-block model was then combined with a between-face-block (level-2) model and a between neighborhood cluster (level-3) model that investigated the variability among face-blocks and among neighborhood clusters, and the correlates of the level of physical and social order.

Multilevel RMs offer several advantages over models that do not account for clustered data when analyzing complex samples. First, multilevel RMing has the ability to incorporate hierarchically structured (clustered) data, such as students nested within schools. Similar to the models developed and discussed in Zwinderman (1991) and Hoijtink & Boomsma (1996), a multilevel RM allows modeling latent variable(s) as dependent variable(s). Second, this approach potentially improves estimates of the relationships between latent traits and predictors, by considering both between and within cluster variations. Technically, observations from clustered samples may show smaller within cluster variance than between cluster variance. Third, multilevel RMs have the flexibility to include covariates, as well as random effects at the measurement units (for example, students), and social units/cluster (for example, schools) levels.

14.3 Model

14.3.1 The Rasch Model as an HGLM

Let

$$\tau_{iv} = \theta_v - \delta_i, \tag{14.1}$$

where $\tau_{iv} = \text{logit}(\mu_{iv})$ with $\mu_{iv} = P(Y_{iv} = 1|\theta_v, \delta_i)$, θ_v is the ability of person v, δ_i is the difficulty of item i, and Y_{iv} is a dichotomous response of person v on item i. It is the RM and can be expressed as a special case of HGLM with different formulations. Kamata (2001), for instance, has postulated the following formulation of a two-level RM. The level-1 model is an item-level model

$$\tau_{iv} = \pi_{0v} + \sum_{q=1}^{I-1} \pi_{qv} X_{qv}, \tag{14.2}$$

and the level-2 models are person-level models

$$\begin{cases} \pi_{0v} = \beta_{00} + u_{0v} \\ \pi_{qv} = \beta_{q0}, \end{cases} \tag{14.3}$$

where X_{qv} is the qth item-indicator dummy variable for person v, with values of 1 when $i = q$, and 0 otherwise. The coefficient π_{0v} is an intercept term, and π_{qv} is a coefficient associated with X_{qv}, where $q = 1, \ldots, I-1$. Here, there are I items in the test, but a dummy variable is not assigned for the Ith item in order to achieve a "full rank" of the design matrix, because of the presence of the intercept term. It is possible to parameterize by not including the intercept term, but with all item-dummy variables (e.g., Rijmen et al., 2003). Also, u_{0v} is a random component of π_{0v} and distributed as $N(0, \sigma^2)$, that is, u_{0v} is normally distributed with zero mean and the variance of σ^2. Here, the random effect u_{0v} is a latent variable. When the level-1 and level-2 models are combined for a specific person v and a specific item i (where $i = q$), the model becomes

$$\tau_{iv} = \beta_{00} + \beta_{q0} + u_{0v}. \tag{14.4}$$

This is equivalent to the RM, where $u_{0v} = \theta_v$, and $\delta_i = -(\beta_{00} + \beta_{q0})$ for $i = q$.

One can further include person characteristic variables in the level-2 model, similar to the two-level IRT model with covariates suggested by Adams, Wilson, & Wu (1997). Whereas main effects of person characteristic variables could be investigated with the level-2 model for π_{0v}, as given in Equation 14.3, item-by-person interaction effects could be studied using the model for the appropriate π_{qv}, as specified in the same equation.

14.3.2 Extension to a Three-Level Model

The above framework can be extended to a three-level model by adding an additional level in the data structure. The level-1 and level-2 models are identical to the two-level model, except additional subscripts are needed to represent the level-3 unit. Here, we use s for the level-3 unit $(s = 1, \dots, S)$. Then, the level-1 and level-2 models are written as

$$\tau_{ivs} = \pi_{0vs} + \sum_{q=1}^{I-1} \pi_{qvs} X_{qvs}, \tag{14.5}$$

and

$$\begin{cases} \pi_{0vs} = \beta_{00s} + u_{0vs} \\ \pi_{qvs} = \beta_{q0s} , \end{cases} \tag{14.6}$$

where $u_{vs} \sim N(0, \ \omega)$. The level-3 model is

$$\begin{cases} \beta_{00s} = \gamma_{000} + \upsilon_{00s} \\ \beta_{q0s} = \gamma_{q00} , \end{cases} \tag{14.7}$$

where $\upsilon_{00s} \sim N(0, \ \xi)$. For a specific person v in a specific level-3 unit s, for a specific item i (where $i = q$), the combined model can be written as

$$\tau_{ivs} = \gamma_{000} + \gamma_{q00} + u_{0vs} + \upsilon_{00s}. \tag{14.8}$$

Again, this is equivalent to the RM, where $\upsilon_{00s} + u_{0vs} = \theta_v$, and $\delta_i = -(\gamma_{000} + \gamma_{q00})$ for $i = q$. Group-characteristic variables, as well as person characteristic variables, can be included in the models as expressed in Equations 14.6 and 14.7. To ensure identifiability, the mean of the ability parameter is constrained to be zero with this formulation.

Alternatively, researchers can formulate the three-level RM with each X_{qvs} centered around the grand mean of the indicators, or equivalently, the reciprocal of the number of items or $1/I$ (e.g., Cheong & Raudenbush, 2000). For example, if there are 10 items in the test or $I = 10$, X_{qvs} will be centered around $1/10 = 0.2$; consequently, $X_{qvs} = 0 - .2 = -.2$ when $i \neq q$ and

$X_{qvs} = 1 - .2 = .8$ when $i = q$. If this centering is employed, the intercept γ_{000} is interpreted as the overall mean ability, and u_{0vs} and v_{00s} as the deviations in ability for person v in level-3 unit s, and for level-3 unit s, from the overall mean, respectively. In this formulation, with reference to Equation 14.1, the ability of person v in level-3 unit s is $\gamma_{000} + u_{0vs}$, and the difficulty of item i, δ_i is a function of γ_{q00}.[3] To ensure identifiability, the mean of the item difficulties is constrained to be zero with this parametrization. This formulation allows researchers to estimate and directly model the mean latent ability.

14.3.3 Multidimensional Model

The two models introduced above assume that test items measure only one latent trait. However, it is possible that a test consists of items that measure more than one latent trait. To illustrate, we assume a case where one group of items is measuring a particular trait, and another is measuring a different one. An example is subscales in an academic test, such as in a mathematics test and a science test. This type of multidimensional structure, where each item is associated with only one dimension, is known as a form of between-item multidimensionality (Adams, Wilson, & Wang, 1997).

For K dimensions,

$$\tau_{iv} = \sum_{k=1}^{K} \pi_{0_k v} + \sum_{k=1}^{K} \sum_{q_k=1}^{I_k-1} \pi_{q_k v} X_{q_k v}, \qquad (14.9)$$

and

$$\begin{cases} \pi_{0_k v} = \beta_{0_k 0} + u_{0_k v} \\ \quad \pi_{q_k v} = \beta_{q_k 0} . \end{cases} \qquad (14.10)$$

This multidimensional version can be also extended to a three-level model in a similar manner that is described above. Also, person-characteristic and group-characteristic variables can be included in the level-2 and level-3 models.

14.4 Data Analysis

The data in our example are from reading and mathematics assessments in one grade level of a state-wide testing program, and we will use the Reference/Research and Measurement subscales of the assessments. We first set up

---

[3] Specifically, the item difficulty for item i, δ_i can be shown to be equal to, for $i = q$,

$$\delta_i = -\frac{I-1}{I}\gamma_{q00} - \frac{1}{I}\sum_{of\ all\ q'} \gamma_{q'00},$$

where I is equal to the number of test items and $q' \neq q$. For more details, see Cheong (2006).

a psychometric model to simultaneously study the two proficiencies. Then, with a structural model, we investigate whether there is a contextual effect of school poverty on both skills and whether the two effects, if any, are similar.

14.4.1 Data

Data used in the following illustrative analyses were sampled from the 2003 administration of reading and mathematics assessment for 4th graders in a statewide testing program in a southeastern state in the United States. The reading test consisted of 45 items based on 4 subscales of skills, including Reading Content Words/Phrases, Main Idea/Purpose, Comparisons, and Reference/Research. The mathematics test consisted of 40 items based on 5 subscales of skills, including Number Sense, Measurement, Geometry, Algebraic Thinking, and Data Analysis. A majority of the items in the tests were in multiple-choice format and scored dichotomously. All nonresponded items were scored as incorrect answers. Here, only two subscales, Reference/Research and Measurement, were used for data analysis. With the Reference/Research subscale, skills and knowledge in organization and interpretation of presented information were measured. With the Measurement subscale, skills to recognize measurements and units of measure, as well as skills to compare, contrast, and convert measurements were measured. All items in these two subscales were scored dichotomously. There were a total of 3,166 examinees from 30 schools. Table 14.1 summarizes the descriptive statistics for the sample. Fifty-seven percent of the sampled students were enrolled in free or subsidized lunch programs. The sampled schools had an average of 59% of theirs students enrolled in free or reduced-lunch programs.

Table 14.1. Descriptive statistics for student- and school-level variables

Variable	Range	M	SD
Student-Level Measure ($N = 3,166$)			
Student Disadvantage*	$0 = $ no, $1 = $ yes	.57	.49
School-Level Measure (No. of Schools $= 30$)			
School Disadvantage**	(.20, 1.00)	.59	.29

*Enrolled in a free or subsidized lunch program.
**Proportion of students enrolled in free or subsidized lunch programs.

14.4.2 Modeling Procedure

In our illustrative analysis, we adopt a three-level extension of the multidimensional model as specified in Equations 14.9 and 14.10 with the number of dimensions $K = 2$. The baseline model constitutes an unconditional three-level hierarchical logistic regression. The level-1 units are item responses within students, the level-2 units are students, and the level-3 units are schools. The model is unconditional as it does not include any student or school-level explanatory variables. To investigate the relationships of the factors to various individual and contextual factors and covariates, we then add the relevant explanatory variables to the unconditional model and evaluate their associations with the two measures.

14.4.3 Unconditional Model

Level-1 Model

The level-1 model represents predictable and random variation among item responses within each child. This is a one-parameter item response model and might be termed a RM (Rasch, 1960) with random effects.

Let $Y_{ivs} = 1$ if the ith response is correct for student v of school s, otherwise let $Y_{ivs} = 0$. Let μ_{ivs} denote the probability of $Y_{ivs} = 1$. This probability varies randomly over students. However, conditioning on this probability, we have

$$Y_{ivs}|\mu_{ivs} \sim Bernoulli,$$

$$E\left(Y_{ivs}|\mu_{ivs}\right) = \mu_{ivs}, \quad \text{and}$$

$$Var\left(Y_{ivs}|\mu_{ivs}\right) = \mu_{ivs}\left(1 - \mu_{ivs}\right). \tag{14.11}$$

As is standard in logistic regression, we define τ_{ivs} as the log-odds of the probability of the ith response being correct for student v in school s. Thus, we have $\tau_{ivs} = \log\left(\frac{\mu_{ivs}}{1-\mu_{ivs}}\right)$. The structural model at level 1 accounts for predictable variation within student across responses. It views the log-odds of correct response i as depending on which subscale is of interest (Reference/Research or Measurement) and which specific item is involved. Let D_{RRivs} take on a value of 1 if the ith response is to an item-measuring reference and research skills and 0 otherwise and let $D_{MEASivs} = 1 - D_{RRivs}$ similarly indicate whether that response is to an item-measuring measurement skills. The D matrices may be viewed as dummy coded design matrices that define which item was responded to and to which scale this item belongs. Then we have

$$\tau_{ivs} = D_{RRivs}\left(\pi_{RRvs} + \sum_{q=1}^{3} \pi_{RRqvs}X_{ivs}\right)$$

$$+ D_{MEASivs}\left(\pi_{MEASvs} + \sum_{q=1}^{5} \pi_{MEASqvs}Z_{ivs}\right),$$

where X_{ivs} and Z_{ivs} are indicator variables representing the items in the scales. As we are interested in estimating the mean latent scores and how they are related to covariates at the student- and school-level, we center X_{ivs}

and Z_{ivs} around the mean of these indicator variables or equivalently, the reciprocal of the number of the items of each corresponding scale, i.e., $1/I$ (1/4 or 0.25 for the Reference/Research subscale and 1/6 or 0.17 for the Measurement subscale).[4] Consequently, π_{RRvs} and π_{MEASvs} are *"Reference/ Research"* and *"Measurement"* proficiencies defined as the adjusted log-odds of the correct response to a "typical item" for respective skills for student v of school s. The "difficulty" of item i is a function of π_{RRqvs} and $\pi_{MEASqvs}$ within each subscale. Given the constraint of the mean of the item difficulties to be zero, the "typical item" will have an item difficulty of 0. Note that 3 item indicators represent the 4 items in the Reference/Research subscale and 5 item indicators represent 6 items in the Measurement subscale.

Level-2 Model

The level-2 model accounts for variation between students within schools on the latent reference/research and measurement skills. The level-2 model is

$$\pi_{RRvs} = \beta_{RRs} + u_{RRvs}, \quad \text{and}$$

$$\pi_{MEASvs} = \beta_{MEASs} + u_{MEASvs}, \quad (14.12)$$

where β_{RRs} and β_{MEASs} are the intercepts for school s on the two latent skills, respectively. The random effects u_{RRvs} and u_{MEASvs} are assumed bivariate normally distributed with zero means, with student-level variances ω_{RR} and ω_{MEAS}, and covariance $\omega_{RR\bullet MEAS}$. We constrain the item effects, the values π_{RRqvs} and $\pi_{MEASqvs}$ to be invariant across the students and across schools, $\pi_{RRqvs} = \pi_{RRq}$ and $\pi_{MEASqvs} = \pi_{MEASq}$ for all v and s. As Raudenbush and Bryk (2002) indicate, this constraint reflects the belief that for a "good" test, an item should have the same difficulty for different groups of examinees that have the same ability. With these constraints in place, the model is similar to a multigroup Rasch model in the sense that item difficulties are the same across groups. By lifting this constraint, researchers can investigate whether

---

[4] We implemented the following procedure to assess the fit of the RM to the data for each subscale. We began by fitting two full-information one-factor factor analytic models with factor loadings allowed to vary across items in the first but not the second one. We then used Akaike's information criteria (AIC) and Bayesian information criteria (BIC) to compare the fit of the two models. The results showed that both AIC and BIC were smaller for the model with varying factor loadings, indicating the RM did not fit well. We then proceeded to identify which items displayed different magnitudes of factor loadings. We re-ran and compared the fit of another two full-information factor-analytic models with the flagged items removed, one with varying factor loadings and one without. One item from the Reference/Research subscale and two items from Measurement subscale were flagged. After excluding the flagged items, AIC and BIC became smaller for the model with uniform factor loadings, indicating a good fit of the RM. Consequently, those three items were excluded from our illustrative analyses.

individual item difficulty varies at the child and/or school-level and can study its correlates. Similarly, the items should function the same for all schools after holding constant the performance level. By lifting the constraint and modeling it as a function of school factor allows one to investigate the effects of school-level factors on item effects. Such variation is known as differential item functioning (DIF) in the literature of educational testing (e.g., Cheong, 2006; van der Linden & Hambleton, 1997).

Level-3 Model

The level-3 model accounts for variation between schools on the latent measures of the two abilities:

$$\beta_{RRs} = \gamma_{RR} + \upsilon_{RRs}, \quad \text{and}$$

$$\beta_{MEASs} = \gamma_{MEAS} + \upsilon_{MEASs}, \tag{14.13}$$

where γ_{RR} and γ_{MEAS} are the grand mean levels of the two latent scores on reference/research and measurement skills in schools. The random effects υ_{RRs} and υ_{MEASs} are assumed bivariate normally distributed with zero means, school-level variances ξ_{RR} and ξ_{MEAS} and covariance $\xi_{RR \bullet MEAS}$.

Combined Model

The above models can be combined through substitutions of terms and expressed as

$$\tau_{ivs} = D_{RRivs} \left(\gamma_{RR} + \sum_{q=1}^{3} \gamma_{RRq} X_{ivs} + u_{RRvs} + \upsilon_{RRs} \right)$$
$$+ D_{MEASivs} \left(\gamma_{MEAS} + \sum_{q=1}^{5} \gamma_{MEASq} Z_{ivs} + u_{MEASvs} + \upsilon_{MEASs} \right). \tag{14.14}$$

This equation shows that the log-odds of a correct response to an item for a particular subscale depends on item effects plus individual student and school contributions to the reference/research and measurement skills.

14.4.4 Estimation Approach and Algorithm

The analysis uses a sixth order approximation to the likelihood for the model based on a Laplace transform (Raudenbush et al., 2000). Simulations by Raudenbush et al. show that this approach, when compared with approximations based on penalized quasi-likelihood, Gauss-Hermite quadrature, and adaptive Gauss-Hermite quadrature, produced remarkably accurate approximation to maximum likelihood, and therefore provides efficient (or nearly efficient) estimates in terms of mean squared errors of all parameters (see also Breslow, 2003).

Table 14.2. Results for the unconditional model

a. Fixed effect estimates—Reference/Research

	Coefficient	se	t	Approx. df
Intercept	0.08	0.11	0.78	29

b. Fixed effect estimates—Measurement

	Coefficient	se	t	Approx. df
Intercept	0.27	0.14	1.94	29

c. Variance estimates of random effects

	Reference/Research	Measurement
Within School	0.87 ($se = 0.13$)	0.77 ($se = 0.06$)
Between School	0.12 ($se = 0.06$)	0.19 ($se = 0.08$)

d. Correlation estimates

	Coefficient
Between student (within schools)	0.83
Inter-scale at School level	0.98

e. Reliability estimates

	Reference/Research	Measurement
Between student (average)	0.42	0.43
Between school (average)	0.83	0.90

14.4.5 Results for the Unconditional Model

Results for the unconditional model are summarized in Table 14.2. The results show that the expected logit of a correct response to a typical reference and research item for a typical student is 0.08, which is not statistically significant from 0. The logit of a correct response to a typical measurement skill item is 0.27, which is also not statistically significant. A log odds of 0 could be translated to an odds of answering a typical item in both scales of $\exp(0) = 1$.

The results of two multivariate tests comparing model deviances (-2 log likelihood at convergence) indicate that the models with the random effects v_{RRs} and v_{MEASs} provided a better fit than the ones without either of them. The results for the multivariate test associated with the Reference/Research subscale were $\chi^2_{(2,N=3,166)} = 123.81$, $p < 0.001$ (with v_{RRs} deleted). The results for the Measurement subscale $\chi^2_{(2,N=3,166)} = 242.90$, $p < 0.001$ (with v_{MEASs} deleted). Note that each test simultaneously assessed whether there was significant variation in each skill and whether the two latent skills covaried at the school level. The estimates of the variation as well as covariation (expressed as correlations) are given in Table 14.2. The two skills manifest high intercorrelation at the between-student and between-school level, .83, and .98. These correlations capture the associations between the latent scores at the student (between π_{RRvs} and π_{MEASvs}) and school level (between β_{RRs} and β_{MEASs}) and thus are adjusted for measurement errors specified in the level-1 sampling model. Furthermore, between student (within schools), the average reliabilities for the Reference/Research and Measurement subscales are .42 and .48 respectively.[5] These indicate the reliability with which we can discriminate between students within a school. Between schools, the corresponding average reliabilities are .83 and .90. The results suggest that one can distinguish among schools in the general level of reference and research and measurement skills with high reliability.[6]

14.4.6 Conditional Model

To study the relationship between the scales and student- and school-level factors, we add relevant explanatory variables to the unconditional model and evaluate their association with the scales. In the illustrative analysis, we study whether there are compositional effects due to the socioeconomic composition of the body of the student. Such effects exist when there is a significant relationship between the aggregate of a student-level characteristic with the outcome, controlling for the effect of the characteristics at the student level (Raudenbush & Bryk, 2002). As Harker & Tymms (2003) summarized from a review of literature, such effects may arise through differences in peer-peer

---

[5] An approximate formula for computing the reliabilities for the reference/research skill measure at the student level is

$$\lambda_{RRvs} = \frac{\xi_{RR} + \omega_{RR}}{\xi_{RR} + \omega_{RR} + (n_{vs} w_{vs})^{-1}},$$

where λ_{RRvs} is the internal consistency of the reference/research measure for student v in school s, n_{vs} is the number of items on reference/research skill attempted by student v in school s, and w_{vs} is the average within student v in school s of $\mu_{ivs}(1 - \mu_{ivs})$ on reference/research items. Thus, the reliability depends on the proportion of intra-school correlation but also on the number of items per scale, and the item effects. Our summary measure of reliability is the average of the student-level reliabilities.

[6] An approximate formula for computing the reliabilities for the reference/research skill measure at the student level is

$$\lambda_{RRs} = \frac{\omega_{RR}}{\xi_{RR} + \omega_{RR} J_s^{-1} + (n_s J_s w_s)^{-1}},$$

where λ_{RRs} is the internal consistency of the reference/research measure for student v in school s, n_s is the average number of items on reference/ research skills per student in school s, J_s is the number of student sampled within school s, and w_s is the average within school s of $p_{ivs}(1 - p_{ivs})$ on reference/research items. Thus, the reliability depends on the intra-school correlation but also on the number of students sampled, the number of items per scale, and the item effects. The summary measure of reliability is the average of the school-specific reliabilities.

and student-teacher interactions and resources among schools with different compositions. The effects could be phantom ones or are merely results of misleading statistical procedures. The characteristic considered in this analysis is student disadvantage, as defined by enrollment in free or subsidized school lunch programs.

Level-1 Model

The level-1 model remains the same as given in Equation 14.12. It models the log-odds of a correct response to item i as a function of the type of skill, reference and research and measurement, and the specific item involved.

Level-2 Model

At the student level, student disadvantage is entered as a dichotomous covariate, centered around its sample mean or the overall proportion of students enrolled in a free-lunch program. The level-2 model for latent reference/research skill,π_{RRvs}, and latent measurement skill, π_{MEASvs}, are:

$$\pi_{RRvs} = \beta_{RRs} + \theta_{RR1s}(Student\ Disadvantage)_{vs} + u_{RRvs},\ \text{and}$$

$$\pi_{MEASvs} = \beta_{MEASs} + \theta_{MEAS1s}(Student\ Disadvantage)_{vs} + u_{MEASvs},$$
$$\tag{14.15}$$

where β_{RRs} and β_{MEASs} are the intercepts for school s on the two latent abilities, respectively, adjusted for student disadvantage, and θ_{RR1s} and θ_{MEAS1s} capture the relationship between student disadvantage and the latent reference/research and measurement abilities of student v within school s. Following the model specifications of Raudenbush and Bryk (2002) for compositional effects, we constrain these regression coefficients to be invariant across the schools, $\theta_{RR1s} = \theta_{RR1}$ and $\theta_{MEAS1s} = \theta_{MEAS1}$ for all s to investigate school compositional effects in this illustrative analysis.[7] The random effects u_{RRvs} and u_{MEASvs} are assumed bivariate normally distributed with zero means, and residual student-level variances ω_{RR} and ω_{MEAS}, and covariance $\omega_{RR \bullet MEAS}$.

Level-3 Model

To assess school compositional effect, we enter school poverty as a continuous variable, again centered around the overall sample mean, into the model to study if and how the school characteristic relates to the subscales. For the intercepts, β_{RRs} and β_{MEASs},

$$\beta_{RRs} = \gamma_{RR} + \gamma_{RR1}(School\ Disadvantage)_s + \upsilon_{RRs},\ \text{and}$$

---

[7] Results of exploratory analyses suggested that the two coefficients for student disadvantage as well as the variance for the measurement scale did not randomly vary over schools.

$$\beta_{MEASs} = \gamma_{MEAS} + \gamma_{MEAS1}(School\ Disadvantage)_s + v_{MEASs}. \quad (14.16)$$

Here, γ_{RR} and γ_{MEAS} are the grand mean levels of the two latent scores on reference/research and measurement skills in school. γ_{RR1} and γ_{MEAS1} capture the compositional effects associated with the socioeconomic composition of the student body in schools. The random effects v_{RRs} and v_{MEASs} are assumed bivariate normally distributed with zero means, and school-level variances ξ_{RR} and ξ_{MEAS} and covariance $\xi_{RR \bullet MEAS}$.

Combined Model

The combined model now becomes

$$\tau_{ivs} = D_{RRivs}[\gamma_{RR} + \theta_{RR1}(Student\ Disadvantage)_{vs}$$
$$+\gamma_{RR1}(School\ Disadvantage)_s + \sum_{q=1}^{3} \pi_{RRq}X_{ivs} + u_{RRvs} + v_{RRs}]$$
$$+D_{MEASivs}[\gamma_{MEAS} + \theta_{MEAS1}(Student\ Disadvantage)_{vs}$$
$$+\gamma_{MEAS1}(School\ Disadvantage)_s + \sum_{q=1}^{5} \pi_{MEASq}Z_{ivs} + u_{MEASvs} + v_{MEASs}].$$
$$(14.17)$$

The above equation shows that the log odds of a correct response to an item for a particular subscale depends on item difficulties and student and school disadvantage plus individual student and school contributions to the reference/research and measurement skills.

Table 14.3. Results for the conditional model

a. Fixed effect estimates—Reference/Research

	Coefficient	se	t	Approx. df
Predictor of Level-1 Intercept				
Intercept	0.10*	0.03	3.05	28
School disadvantage	−0.57*	0.24	−2.44	28
Predictor of student disadvantage slope				
Intercept	−0.46*	0.15	−4.97	3164

*$p < 0.05$

b. Fixed effect estimates—Measurement

	Coefficient	se	t	Approx. df
Predictor of Level-1 Intercept				
Intercept	0.29*	0.08	3.48	28
School disadvantage	−0.63	0.34	−1.85	28
Predictor of student disadvantage slope				
Intercept	−0.58*	0.10	−5.55	3164

*$p < 0.05$

14.4.7 Results for the Conditional Model

Results for the fixed effects that allow us to assess the associations between student and school disadvantage and the two proficiency scales are summarized in Table 14.3. The results suggests that there is a compositional effect for reference/research ($\hat{\gamma}_{RR1} = -.57, se = .24$), but not measurement skills ($\hat{\gamma}_{MEAS1} = -.63, se = .34$). After controlling for the effects of student disadvantage, a one standard deviation increase in school disadvantage, which is reported to be equal to .29 in Table 14.1, reduces the odds of a correct response to a typical reference/research item by $\exp(-.57 \times .29) = .85$ times. There is evidence that the magnitude of the school-level disadvantage-achievement relationship, as captured by γ_{RR1}, differs significantly from the student-level disadvantage-achievement effect, as captured by θ_{RR1} (Raudenbush & Bryk, 2002). Being enrolled in a free-lunch program reduces the odds of correctly answering a typical measurement item by $exp(-0.46) = 0.63$ times.

The fact that school disadvantage is related significantly to reference/research skill but not measurement skill does not imply that the estimates of the corresponding coefficients for each subscale (γ_{RR1} and γ_{MEAS1}) in Equation 14.17 are significantly different from each other. We therefore tested the null hypothesis that there was no difference in the school disadvantage effects for reference/research and measurement skills. Specifically, $H_0 : \gamma_{RR1} - \gamma_{MEAS1} = 0$. The result indicated that one failed to reject the null hypothesis that there was no difference in the effects of school disadvantage for the two subscales; $\chi^2_{(1,N=3,166)} = .16, p > 0.05$.

14.5 Summary

In this chapter, we provided a brief discussion on how the HGLM framework of the RM is related to the development of other item response models. We outlined and illustrated with a statewide assessment data set on reading and mathematics a general approach to study testing in multilevel settings and with multidimensional latent traits. To begin, the item response model is recast as a three-level logistic regression model that embeds its item response portion within a hierarchical structure in which the secondary units of measurement, the student, are nested within the schools. The combined model extends the usual item response model in allowing for multiple abilities to be measured. In our illustrative example case, we studied reference/research and measurement skills simultaneously, rather than investigating either of them as a single, unidimensional proficiency. The model also allows researchers to gauge the variability of the latent traits at the student and school level. It provides information on how those abilities correlate with one another and estimates of useful psychometric properties such as reliabilities for the subscales as well.

The framework accommodates the nested data structure present in most large-scale data and thus the design effects in the estimation of the standard errors of the fixed effects. It also allows the use of an integrated approach for studying measurement properties as well as structural relationships. In our illustrative example, we showed how researchers can build on the psychometric model to study how covariates at different levels are related to the constructs of interests. Specifically, we investigated whether there was a compositional effect due to school disadvantage. We found a significant contextual effect for the reference and research but not the measurement skills, even though there did not seem to be a difference in the effects. The approach could be useful to studies of school effects and evaluations of systemic reform efforts or social programs, in which there are multiple components as well as multiple outcomes.

Part III

Applications of Multivariate and Mixed Rasch Models

15

Mixed Rasch Models for Measurement in Cognitive Psychology

Susan E. Embretson

Georgia Institute of Technology

To apply standard unidimensional IRT models to ability measurement, it must be assumed that individuals at the same level of performance are in fact comparable. That is, individuals with the same estimate on the latent trait are interchangeable and thus can have identical interpretations given to their scores. Such interpretations, of course, depend on the construct validity of the trait measure, which includes both the construct representation and nomothetic span aspects (Embretson, 1983). The construct representation aspect of validity involves the meaning of the construct, in terms of the processes, strategies, and knowledge that are directly involved in performance. Construct representation is an aspect of internal validity. The nomothetic span aspect concerns the significance of the trait, which includes the relationship of trait scores to other measures, demographics and criteria. Nomothetic span is primarily the external validity of the measure.

It is well known in cognitive psychology that individuals at the same level of performance may differ qualitatively in the mechanisms underlying their performance. In the 1980s, Sternberg (1985), for example, elaborated several sources of individual differences that lead to incomparable performances, including different strategies for solving the problems and different patterns of component strengths. As applied to intelligence and ability measures, qualitative differences between examinees implies that construct representation differs. Further, since nomothetic span depends on construct representation, differences in the external relationships for test scores may be expected as well.

Differing patterns of item difficulty can be indicative of differences in the underlying mechanisms of performance. For example, items that are relatively hard under one strategy may be much easier under another strategy. Mixture-distribution-measurement models, such as the mixed Rasch model (Rost, 1990, 1991), can identify latent classes in which item difficulties have different orders. The individuals within a class have response patterns that are consistent with the same ordering of item difficulty, while individuals in other classes have response patterns that are consistent with different orders of item difficulty.

Mixed RMs have been developed for both binary (see Rost & von Davier, 1995) and polytomous (see von Davier & Rost, 1995) data.

Both aspects of construct validity, construct representation, and nomothetic span (Embretson, 1983), are relevant to the latent-class structure of item responses. First, if only one class exists, then a single meaning is supported for construct representation. The uniform order of item difficulty across persons supports performance as involving the same strategies, components, or knowledge structures. However, if more than one latent class exists, the underlying basis of performance may no longer be uniform. That is, the different orders of item difficulties may result from different strategies, components, and knowledge structures being involved in performance. In this case, the nature of the construct depends on the class to which the person belongs. Second, when two or more latent classes exist, nomothetic span may differ by class. That is, the test may be differentially correlated with other measures and hence constitute a moderator variable.

As yet, little research has concerned the impact of multiple latent classes on the construct validity of an ability test. In this chapter, two illustrative applications of mixture RMs for ability measurement will be presented. An application to spatial ability and to abstract reasoning will be presented. The implications of latent classes for both construct representation and nomothetic span will be explored.

In the studies described below, the mixed RM for binary data was used to examine the latent class structure of the ability measurements (see Rost & von Davier, 1995). The mixed RM is given as follows:

$$P_i\left(x = 1 | \theta_s\right) = \sum_g B_g \frac{\exp\left(\theta_s - \beta_{ig}\right)}{1 + \exp\left(\theta_s - \beta_{ig}\right)}, \tag{15.1}$$

where θ_s is the trait level for person s, β_{ig} is the difficulty for item i in group g, and B_g is the class size parameter or mixing proportion. Thus, the primary estimates from the model are the class proportions and the item difficulties within each class. Class membership for individual response patterns are estimated post hoc from their relative likelihood in the different classes.

15.1 Spatial Ability

Spatial ability often is assumed to be an analogue process. That is, the mental activities mirror the physical activities in manipulating the objects. Typical spatial tasks include figure manipulations, such as figure rotation, cube-folding, and comparisons. As stated by McGee (1979), spatial visualization encompasses "the ability to mentally manipulate, rotate, twist, or invert a pictorially presented stimulus object." However, for some individuals, spatial ability tasks are not solved by spatial methods. These individuals employ problem-solving methods that have been described as verbal-analytic processes (Barratt, 1953; Just & Carpenter, 1985). That is, the individual develops an orientation-free verbal description of the figures and then verbalizes their altered appearance under varying degrees of rotation. Even the spatial strategy is not necessarily homogeneous. According to Just and Carpenter's theory (1985), the folding and rotation process may follow traditional trajectories, folded first in the plane represented in the two-dimensional view, followed by folding in a perpendicular plane. Some individuals, however, appear to employ unique trajectories that lessen the burden of the folding process.

Despite the long-standing interest in strategies as applied to spatial tasks, little research has concerned the systematic impact on construct validity. The purpose of the study reported below (see also Embretson, 2004) is to explicate the role of strategies on the construct validity of a spatial ability test by examining the latent class structure of item responses. Impact of the latent classes on both the construct representation and the nomothetic span aspects of validity will be assessed.

15.1.1 Methods

Instrument

The Spatial Learning Ability Test (SLAT; Embretson, 1994) was developed to measure spatial ability. SLAT consists of a large item bank that was scaled with the RM. The form of SLAT that was used in this study consists of 28 cube-folding items (see Figure 15.1).

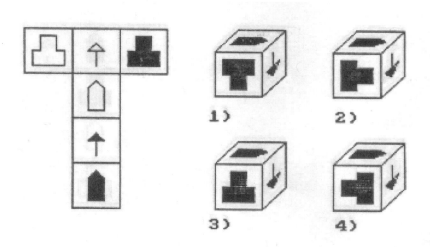

Fig. 15.1.

The examinee is instructed to fold the stem down and then find the three-dimensional view of the cube that is obtained. A cognitive model of spatial processing, the attached folding model, was developed for the SLAT items (Embretson, 1994). The examinee is postulated to mentally overlay two sides of the unfolded stem on the response alternative and then fold down the remaining side. Items vary in the difficulty of the rotation and folding processes, which are reflected, respectively, by (1) the degrees of rotation to mentally attach the stem to the response alternative and (2) the number of surfaces carried in folding the third side. For example, the item shown in Figure 15.1 has 90 degrees of rotation to align the stem and three surfaces to be carried.

Participants

SLAT was administered to 748 Air Force recruits in a computer laboratory at Lackland Air Force base. Data on demographics, as well as scores on the Armed Services Vocational Aptitude Battery (ASVAB), were also available for the sample.

15.1.2 Results

Construct Representation on SLAT

The mixed RM was applied to the SLAT item response data. The number of classes was determined by comparing the data log-likelihood of solutions with varying numbers of latent classes. For model comparisons, the AIC (Akaike, 1973) was used to decide upon the necessary number of latent classes for the mixed Rasch model. The relatively best solution, according to AIC, was the four-class solution, since only a trivial change in the AIC (i.e., 3.22) was observed from the four-class to the five-class solution. Further, the five-class solution had a class with approximately 30 participants, which would be too small to obtain stable estimates of item difficulty.

Thus, the four-class solution was accepted as appropriate for the data, and the proportions in each class were as follows: Class 1, .342; Class 2, .293; Class 3, .205; and Class 4, .160.

The nature of the latent classes was further examined by the psychometric properties of scores. Individuals were assigned to the latent class in which their response pattern had the highest relative likelihood. Table 15.1 shows the mean ability estimates, standard deviations, mean raw scores and reliabilities obtained for each class. The ability estimates differed between classes, which were statistically significant ($F = 225.594, df = 3,744, p < 0.001$). The reliability estimates also differed between classes. Class 1 and Class 4 had reliabilities that exceeded .70, the traditional cutoff for a research instrument. The reliability of Class 2 fell somewhat below .70, while Class 3 had an extremely low reliability. Last, mean item response times (not shown in Table 1) were also available for the four classes. The classes differed significantly on mean item response time ($F_{3,744} = 13.929, p < 0.001$) as well, with Class 3 lower than the other classes. The item-difficulty orders were relatively distinct between classes, since their intercorrelations ranged from .246 to .627.

Table 15.1. Descriptive statistics in four latent classes on SLAT

	Class			
	1	2	3	4
Mean Ability	1.20	.05	−.86	1.14
SD Ability	1.34	.70	.51	1.08
Mean Score	19.48	14.19	8.66	19.54
Reliability	.80	.62	.26	.74

To interpret the meaning of the pattern differences, the linear logistic test model (LLTM; Fischer, 1973) was applied separately within each class, using the two variables that were available to characterize processing on SLAT items, namely, the degrees of rotation of the stem and the number of surfaces carried. In addition to these two variables, their first-order interaction was also included in the LLTM analysis. The results indicated that the cognitive model provided moderately strong prediction of item difficulty for all classes except Class 3, which had a likelihood ratio model fit index (Embretson, 1997) of only .481. This index is similar in magnitude to a multiple correlation. For the other classes the fit indices were moderately high: Class 1, .664; Class 2, .716; and Class 4, .723. The LLTM parameter estimates are shown on Table 15.2.

Table 15.2. LLTM weights, standard errors, and t values for SLAT.

	Class1			Class2			Class3			Class4		
	Weight	SE	t	Weight	SE	t	Weight	SE	t	Weight	SE	t
Surfaces	.80	.04	18.14	.93	.04	22.53	.22	.05	4.51	.70	.06	11.25
Degrees	.01	.04	.24	.09	.04	2.70	.13	.04	3.04	.60	.06	10.77
SurfXDeg	.14	.06	2.43	−.32	.05	−5.88	−.23	.06	−3.70	.49	.08	5.90

For all classes, the weights for the number of surfaces carried and the degrees of rotation were positive. However, their magnitude and significance varied by class. Further, the nature of the interaction varied substantially by class. In Class 3, where the model fit poorly, although all model variables reached statistical significance, the weights were relatively small. A plot of predicted item difficulty by the model revealed that degrees of rotation and surfaces carried mattered only for the easiest items. In Class 1, although the number of surfaces carried and the interaction were significant, the degrees of rotation were not significant. The small positive weight for the interaction indicated a slightly increasing impact of the number of surfaces carried with greater degrees of rotation. In Class 2, all model variables reached significance. The interaction was negative, such that the impact of a model variable (i.e., degrees or surfaces) mattered less with increasing levels of the other variable. Last, in Class 4, all variables in the model had a significant and positive impact on item difficulty. Degrees of rotation had a much larger weight in this class as compared to the other classes. Further, the large positive interaction meant increasing impact of a model variable as the other increased.

Nomothetic Span Analysis of Latent Classes

Demographic data and Armed Services Vocational Aptitude Battery (ASVAB) test scores were available on 702 individuals in the sample. As in other studies in spatial ability, men scored slightly more than a half standard deviation higher than women ($F = 26.55, df = 1,700 p < 0.001$). Mean total response times were equal for men and women, however. Men and women were also differentially represented in the latent classes. A Gender (2) X Class (4) contingency analysis was significant ($\chi^2 = 17.43, df = 3, p < 0.001$), indicating that gender and class were significantly associated. Women were relatively more represented in Class 2 and Class 3.

Class membership was also related to scores on the ASVAB. A multivariate analysis of variance indicated that the four classes differed significantly on the ten subtests of the ASVAB ($F_{Wilks} = 7.13; df = 30, 2005, p < 0.001$). The pattern of differences between classes was consistent with their pattern of differences on SLAT; Class 1 and Class 4 were significantly higher than Class 2 and Class 3, and Class 2 was significantly higher than Class 3.

Structural equation modeling (SEM) was employed to examine the possible differential validity of SLAT for predicting ASVAB scores in the four classes. Moreno et al. (1984) found that four factors adequately reproduce the covariances between the ASVAB subtests, as follows: (1) verbal ability, with loadings for paragraph comprehension, word knowledge and general science; (2) math/reasoning, with loadings for mathematical knowledge, arithmetic reasoning and mechanical comprehension; (3) speed, with loadings for coding speed and numerical operations; and (4) technical, with loadings for mechanical comprehension, electrical information, auto and shop and general science.

With the pattern of factor loadings defined as above, each of the four ASVAB factors was regressed on SLAT in a multisample analyzes defined by the four latent classes. The first SEM was most constrained, with the factor loadings and the regression of the factors on SLAT fully constrained across classes. The covariance matrix of residuals for the ASVAB subtests and the variance of SLAT were free to vary across classes, to allow for the different variances. The model did not fit ($\chi^2 = 320.72, df = 170, p < 0.001$) and the comparative fit index was .920. A second SEM model, with the regression of the factors on SLAT free to vary across classes, led to significantly better fit ($\chi^2 = 39.01, df = 12, p < 0.01$). Although the data still departed significantly from the model ($\chi^2 = 281.71, df = 158, p < 0.001$), the comparative fit index was higher (CFI = .934). Further empirical fitting of the model would have involved changing the factor structure across classes, which would lead to incomparable factors across classes.

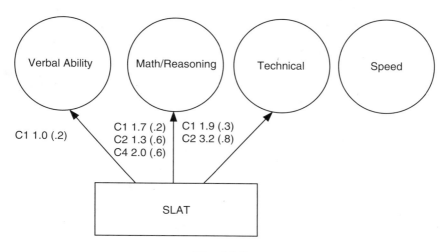

Fig. 15.2.

Figure 15.2 shows the regression of the ASVAB factors on SLAT. In Figure 15.2, the significant unstandardized regression coefficients and their standard errors are shown by class. No paths to the speed factor or from the SLAT scores in Class 3 are shown, since none of these relationships reached significance ($p > 0.05$). SLAT significantly predicted mathematical reasoning in all other classes and the weight was largest for Class 4. However, SLAT in Class 4 was not related to any other ASVAB factor. SLAT was a significant predictor of verbal ability only for Class 1. Last, technical competency was significantly related to SLAT for both Class 1 and Class 2.

15.1.3 Discussion

The mixed RM analysis indicated four large latent classes for SLAT item responses. The item difficulties were only modestly correlated across classes, which indicates substantial differences in response patterns. Most importantly, construct validity also varied by class, since differences for both construct representation and nomothetic span were observed.

The spatial ability construct does not appear to be measured for Class 3 examinees. The low mean on SLAT combined with a low reliability is indicative of random responding. Further, the weak relationships to the cognitive model variables in the LLTM analysis indicates that examinees are performing less systematically on more cognitively challenging items. Further, unlike the other classes, the SLAT scores in Class 3 are unrelated to the external variables, the ASVAB factors.

In contrast, spatial ability appears to be well measured in Class 1 and Class 4. These classes are characterized by high ability and acceptable levels of reliability. However, these classes differ from each other in both construct representation and nomothetic span. In Class 1, the degrees of rotation variable was not significantly related to item difficulty. Instead, item difficulty was related to the number of surfaces carried, where the number of changes in appearance of the markers becoming increasingly complex when folded. These results are consistent with Class 1 as involving verbal-analytic processing. The nomothetic span results are also consistent with verbal-analytic processing for Class 1 examinees. That is, unlike any other class, the SLAT scores in Class 1 were related to verbal ability. In contrast, Class 4 appears to contain individuals who employ analogue spatial processes. The LLTM results indicated that item difficulties were strongly related to both degrees of rotation and the number of surfaces carried, as would be expected in an analogue process. The nomothetic span results were also consistent with analogue processing. Although SLAT scores in Class 4 were unrelated to verbal ability, they were strongly related to mathematical reasoning.

Last, in Class 2, ability is somewhat lower than in Class 1 and Class 4. The LLTM results indicated that although the number of surfaces carried was strongly related to item difficulty, the impact of degrees of rotation was weak. Further, a significant interaction of the model variables indicated that degree of rotation became a weaker predictor with successive number of surfaces carried. Hence, items became more similar in difficulty at two or more surfaces carried. Nomothetic span results indicated that SLAT scores had a relatively weak relationship to mathematical reasoning but a strong relationship to technical ability. The technical-ability subtests on the ASVAB consist of primarily two-dimensional figures and diagrams. The interpretation of the class seems unclear, but it may consist of individuals who employ analogue processing methods successfully only to two-dimensional items.

In summary, the construct validity of the spatial ability scores depended on the latent classes. For one class, spatial ability appeared to be interpretable as spatial analogue processing and was related only to mathematical reasoning. For another class, spatial ability was related to both verbal and mathematical reasoning but was less related to technical competency. The other two classes had yet different patterns of construct representation and nomothetic span. Thus, one must conclude that spatial ability scores are not interpretable without reference to the latent class.

15.2 Abstract Reasoning

Abstract reasoning, also described as fluid intelligence (e.g., Horn & Cattell, 1966), is the ability to make inferences relatively independently of specific knowledge. Matrix-completion problems have a long history in the measurement of abstract reasoning. Raven (1938) introduced the item type early in the history of measurement. Matrix-completion problems were well connected to both Spearman's cognitive theory (1923) and his psychometric theory (1927).

Although Spearman's cognitive theory did not stand the test of time, contemporary approaches in cognitive psychology permit empirical support to establish a theory. Carpenter et al. (1990) developed a theory of abstract reasoning, using the Raven's Advanced Progressive Matrices (APM) as the target task in their studies. They applied a variety of methods to examine the plausibility of their theory, including computer simulation, response-time analysis and eye-tracker studies.

Figure 15.3 shows the stem of a matrix-completion item.

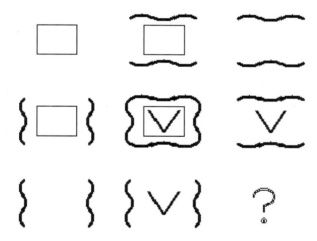

Fig. 15.3. A stem of a matrix-completion item

Carpenter et al. (1990) postulated that rules were attempted successively for each object or attribute that changes in the matrix. Carpenter et al. (1990) postulated a specific order in which various types of rules were attempted by the examinee. Their rule hierarchy consisted of the following relationships: (1) constant in a row, where the same figure appears in every column of a particular row; (2) pairwise progression, where the value of an attribute changes across columns of a particular row; (3) figure addition, where figures are added (or subtracted) across the columns in a particular row; (4) distribution of three, where an object (or attribute) occurs once and only once in each row and column; and (5) distribution of two, where object (or attribute) changes have a null value and hence only two of three appear in the matrix. According to their theory, an examinee attempts to explain changes in the matrix with lower-level rules prior to progressing to higher-level rules. The highest-level rule, distribution of two, demanded the most abstraction. Table 15.3 shows the relationship of item difficulty to the rule hierarchy, based on Embretson's (1998) matrix-completion-item data on the Abstract Reasoning Test (ART).

Table 15.3. Item difficulty by relationship type

	N	Item Difficulty Mean	Std. Deviation
Pairwise	25	−.5154	1.37065
Figure addition	35	−.9201	1.11620
Distribution of three	60	.2132	1.15391
Distribution of two	30	1.5409	.90191
Total	150	.0929	1.41545

Like many contemporary views of intelligence (Ackerman et al., 2005; Kyllonen & Christal, 1990), Carpenter et al.'s (1990) theory gave a primary role to working-memory capacity. The demand of a specific item on working-memory capacity was theorized to result from the number of relationships required to solve it, as well as the position of the relationships in the rule hierarchy. However, to quantify working-memory demand in an item, Carpenter et al. (1990) scored only the number of relationships. The position of the rule in the hierarchy was important in a second aspect of processing, abstraction capacity. The demand for abstraction was primarily defined on the distribution of two relationships.

Embretson (2002) adapted the Carpenter et al. (1990) theory to develop variables for a cognitive model of item difficulty. Embretson (1998, 2002) modeled item difficulty on a large bank of matrix-completion problems. Two models were developed. In both models, variables were added to reflect encoding differences between items. The first model reflected the Carpenter et al. (1990) theory by including their two predictors of rule-processing difficulty, number of relationships and abstraction level, as well as the new encoding variables. A second model was developed to reflect inference difficulty in a single variable: memory load. Embretson (2002) hypothesized that including both the number of rules and the position of the rules in the hierarchy in a single variable would more adequately reflect working-memory demands. Embretson's (1998;

2002) memory-load variable is the sum of the rule positions (i.e., 1 through 5) of all the rules in the problem. Although both models provided the same moderately high prediction of item difficulty, the memory-load variable was the single strongest predictor.

Carpenter et al. (1990) noted an interesting ambiguity in rule hierarchy. Although figure-addition relationships seemed to reflect low-level holistic processes, they also could be solved by high-level analytic relationships, namely, distribution of two. Consider the item in Figure 15.3. It can be solved readily by simply mentally overlaying the elements. Duplicate parts cancel out and unique parts add up. This is the essence of a Figure addition/subtraction relationship. However, it also is a distribution of two relationship because there are two of every unique element in each row and column. Rather than mentally overlaying the objects, one counts up the number of each element.

If some examinees do not apply the figure addition/subtraction relationship in their problem solution, then the much-harder distribution of two rule would be required. Both construct representation and nomothetic span would be impacted for such examinees. For construct representation, the item would be much more difficult, since it would demand high levels of working-memory capacity and abstraction. As a consequence, the estimated abilities for such an examinee would be lowered. For nomothetic span, if scores are artificially lowered, then the test would be expected to be a less-valid predictor.

In this study, the latent class structure of item responses on a matrix-completion test is examined to determine whether figure addition problems are solved by different methods for different examinees. The potential impact of these latent classes on both construct representation and nomothetic span is also examined.

15.2.1 Methods

Participants

The participants were 801 Air Force recruits at Lackland Air Force Base. Data on demographics, as well as scores on the Armed Services Vocational Aptitude Battery (ASVAB), were also available for the sample.

Instruments

A fixed-content form ART (Embretson, 1995b) was administered. The ART consisted of 34 matrix-completion problems (as shown in Figure 15.3), with a multiple-choice format of eight response alternatives. A measure of the big 5 personality factors (see Digman, 1990) was also administered. The big 5 personality factors include neuroticism, extroversion, intellect, agreeableness, and conscientiousness. The test consisted of adjectives in which the examinee evaluated appropriateness in a continuous response format.

Procedure

ART and the big 5 personality factors were administered on Lackland Air Force Base in a large computer laboratory. A laboratory supervisor monitored all examinees.

15.2.2 Results

Construct Representation

The mixed RM was applied to the ART item response data. The data log-likelihoods of solutions with successively larger numbers of classes were compared in the same manner as for Study 1. According to the AIC, the two-class solution fits better than the one-class solution. The AIC index dropped by 328.33. The correlation of item difficulties between the classes was moderate ($r = .737$, $p < .01$), indicating substantial differentiation between the classes. The proportions in each class were .64 for Class 1 and .36 for Class 2. According to the AIC, the three-class solution fit the data better than the two-class solution. Note that the change in AIC was smaller, dropping by 50.70. No further extraction of classes was attempted, since the BIC index increased from the two-class to the three-class solution. The proportions in each class were .365, .323, and .313, respectively, for Class 1, Class 2, and Class 3.

The correlations of item difficulties in the three-class solution are shown in Table 15.4.

Table 15.4. Correlations of item difficulties in two- and three-class solutions

	2-Class Class1	2-Class Class2	3-Class Class1	3-Class Class2	3-Class Class3
2-Class: Class1	1	.737**	.969**	.957**	.693**
2-Class: Class2	.737**	1**	.767**	.678**	.996**
3-Class: Class1	.969**	.767**	1 **	.862**	.736**
3-Class: Class2	.957**	.678**	.862**	1	.622**
2-Class: Class1	.693**	.996**	.736**	.622**	1

**Correlation is significant at the 0.01 level (2-tailed).

Class 1 and Class 2 of the three-class solution had a relatively high correlation and appeared to be a subdivision of Class 1 of the two-class solution, since the intercorrelations were high. A scatter-plot of the regression of Class 2 on Class 1 in the three-class solution revealed that only one item fell outside a 95% confidence interval, namely, an extremely easy item with a large standard error. Thus, the three-class solution, although better in fit by the AIC but not the BIC, led to only trivial pattern differences between two of the

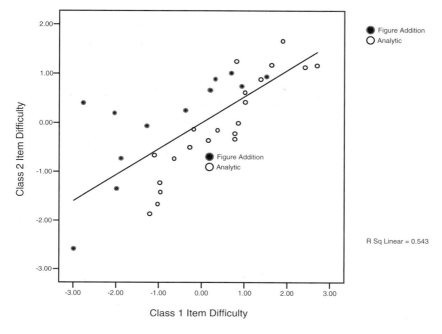

Fig. 15.4.

three classes. Thus, the two-class solution was deemed the most appropriate for the data.

Figure 15.4 is a scatter-plot of the item difficulties in the two-class solution. Items are designated by type of relationship: figure addition/subtraction versus analytic relationships (i.e., all other types). It can be seen that items with figure addition/subtraction relationships are relatively harder in Class 2 than in Class 1.

The latent classes were further studied by examining the psychometric properties of ART scores. Individuals were assigned to the latent class in which their response pattern had the highest relative likelihood. Table 15.5 shows that Class 1 had a substantially higher mean ability than Class 2. This difference was statistically significant ($F = 519.166, df = 1, 799, p < .001$). The internal consistency reliabilities, also shown in Table 15.5, are reasonably high for both latent classes.

Table 15.5 also presents results on response-time differences between classes. Overall response time on the items differed significantly ($F = 73.311, df = 1, 799, p < .001$), with the Class 1 mean higher than the Class 2 mean. However, these results do not necessarily indicate that Class 1 processed the items more slowly, because total response time includes both correct and incorrect items. In fact, examinees with lower ability may spend less time on

Table 15.5. Descriptive statistics for latent classes on the Abstract Reasoning Test

	Class 1	Class 2
Trait Mean	1.17	−.42
Trait SD	.91	.97
Reliability	.77	.84
Total RT Mean	35.01	26.77
Total RD SD	12.36	13.67
Correct RT Mean	28.86	21.23
Correct RT SD	9.98	10.88

difficult items due to the perceived difficulty (Schnipke & Scrams, 1997). Thus, correct response time is a better indicator of processing than total response time. It can be seen in Table 15.5 that correct response time also differed between classes ($F = 95.421, df = 1,799, p < .001$), with the Class 1 mean again higher than the Class 2 mean. However, since Class 1 members solved more items, due to their higher ability, their mean on correct response time is based not only on more items, but on more difficult items than the Class 2 mean. Thus, correct response times were further analyzed by using the number of items solved as a covariate in a repeated-measures ANOVA. A type (figure addition versus analytic items) by class analysis of correct response time was performed with the number of analytic items and the number of figure addition items solved as covariates. The data did not meet the assumption of sphericity ($\chi^2 = 444.649, df = 2, p < .001$), but the use of single-degree-of-freedom tests in the current design minimized the impact of the assumption on error (see Judd & McClelland, 1989). In the repeated-measures ANOVA, the class main effect was not significant ($F = 2.617, df = 1,797, p < .001$), but the interaction of class with type was statistically significant ($F = 4.776, df = 1,797, p < .05$).

Figure 15.5 plots the residualized correct response times by type and class. It can be seen that when residualized, Class 2 had somewhat longer response times than Class 1. Further, although the analytic items differed little between classes, the figure addition items are associated with increased response time for Class 2, which is the basis of the significant interaction.

To further elucidate construct representation, cognitive models were fit separately within each class. Memory load, as defined above, and three encoding variables—distortion, fusion, and number of unique elements—were scored for each item. this variable is the weighted sum of the relationships in an item, where the weights reflect the position of the relationship in the hierarchy described above. Thus, figure-addition relationship were scored with the second-lowest weight, according to the hierarchy, indicating that less memory load was required to process these relationships. LLTM was applied separately within each class, using memory load and three variables to reflect encoding difficulty, distortion, fusion, and number of unique elements in the stem.

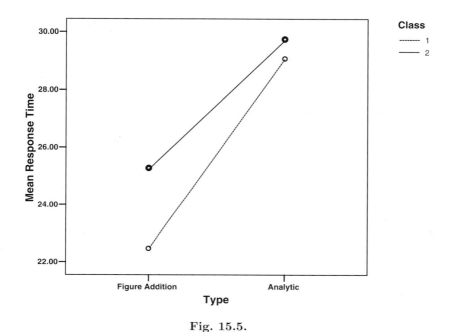

Fig. 15.5.

The LLTM parameter estimates are shown in Table 15.6. The overall model fit was quite similar in the two classes, .681 and .708, respectively in Class 1 and Class 2. Further, in both classes, memory load, distortion, and number of unique elements had positive and significant weights in the cognitive model. However, the weights for two variables differed significantly in magnitude between the classes. Memory load had a significantly smaller weight in Class 2, while number of unique elements had a significantly greater weight in Class 2.

15.2.3 Nomothetic Span

The relationship of ART scores to external variables was examined using SEM. A multisample model was specified for the regression of the ASVAB factors on ART. In the most-constrained model, the regressions of the ASVAB factors on ART were fully constrained across classes. The prediction residual variances for the factors and their intercorrelations were free to vary across classes. The data departed significantly from this model ($\chi^2 = 18.432, df = 4, p < .01$,

Table 15.6. LLTM Weights and standard errors for cognitive models of ART in two latent classes

Variable	Class 1 Weight	Class 1 SE	Class 2 Weight	Class 2 SE	t Value
Memory Load	.197	.004	.119	.007	9.78
Distortion	.115	.052	.233	.073	−1.32
Fusion	−.029	.018	.110	.063	−1.75
Unique Elements	.102	.012	.196	.015	−4.94

CFI $= .929$) and the comparative fit index was moderately high. The Lagrange multiplier test indicated that releasing two constraints across the latent classes would significantly improve fit; namely, the relationship of ART with both verbal reasoning and mathematical reasoning. A second SEM model, with the regression of the factors on ART free to vary across classes, led to significantly better fit ($\chi^2 = 8.792, df = 2, p < .01$). The data did not depart significantly from the model ($\chi^2 = .294, df = 2, p = .863$) and the comparative fit index was at the boundary (CFI $= 1.000$).

Figure 15.6 shows the unstandardized regression coefficients and their standard errors (in parentheses) for the ASVAB factors on ART. All four factors were significantly predicted by ART.

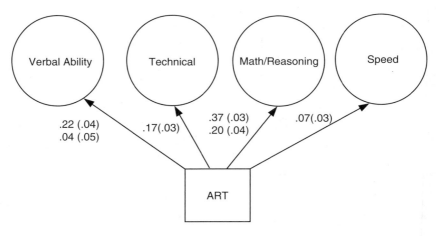

Fig. 15.6.

For the two factors technical and speed, only one set of coefficients is shown since these coefficients did not differ significantly across classes. However, for the other two factors, verbal reasoning and mathematical reasoning, the regression coefficients for both classes, Class 1 followed by Class 2, are shown. For mathematical reasoning, the estimated regression coefficients were .37 and .20, respectively. For verbal reasoning, the estimated regression coefficients were .22 and .04, respectively.

Since the distribution of ART scores in the classes varied substantially, class differences in the regression estimates may have been biased by the scant information at the opposite extremes within the two classes. Thus, for comparison, estimates were obtained by employing a common range on ART for both classes, from -1.00 to 2.00, which resulted in 429 and 197 cases, respectively, available from Class 1 and Class 2. For mathematical reasoning, the estimated regression coefficients were close to the full sample results for both Class 1 ($b = .34$) and for Class 2 ($b = .24$) and within the range of their respective standard errors shown in Figure 15.6. Similarly, for verbal reasoning, the common range on ART yielded regression coefficients of .15 and .03, respectively, for Class 1 and Class 2. The regression coefficient was nearly identical for Class 2, but the regression coefficient for Class 1 appeared to decline. However, the Class 2 regression coefficient was still within two standard-error units of the full class estimate.

The relationship of ART to the personality measures was also examined in a multisample SEM. In the most constrained model, only the regression of the personality factors on ART was fully constrained across classes. The residual variances for the factors and their intercorrelations, as well as the ART variances, were free to vary across classes. The data departed significantly from this model ($\chi^2 = 12.118, df = 5, p < .05$, CFI $= .991$) although the comparative fit index was high. Since the Lagrange multiplier test indicated that releasing the constraint for the regression of intellect on ART would significantly improve fit, a second SEM model, with this constraint released, was run. This model fit significantly better ($\chi^2 = 8.067, df = 1, p < .01$). The data did not depart significantly from the model ($\chi^2 = 3.854, df = 4, p = .426$) and the comparative fit index was at the boundary (CFI $= 1.000$).

Figure 15.7 shows the unstandardized regression coefficients and their standard errors for the two classes. Both neuroticism and intellect were significantly related to ART scores. However, the relationship of intellect varied by class; a strong positive relationship was observed for Class 1, while an insignificant negative relationship was observed for Class 2.

15.2.4 Discussion

The results generally supported the hypothesis that processing differences between examinees in solving abstract reasoning items had impact on the construct validity of scores. Both construct representation and nomothetic span were impacted.

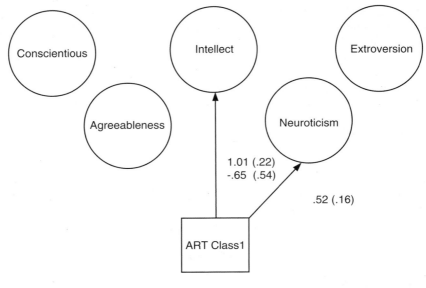

Fig. 15.7.

The rule hierarchy is central to Carpenter et al.'s theory of processing abstract-reasoning items because it determines the working-memory load of a particular item. However, items that involved a low-level holistic relationship, figure addition, also could be solved by a high-level abstract relationship with null values. It was hypothesized that some examinees may not apply the low-level rule and consequently could solve items only by applying the high-level abstract rule. Since presumably easy items become more difficult for these examinees, their estimated abilities would be expected to be lower, since they would be less likely to solve the items. Further, for those items that are solved, more-extended processing time is expected since they must progress up the rule hierarchy to reach the more abstract relationship. Last, the relationship of test scores to other variables is expected to be lowered for these examinees since their processing strategy is artificially lowering their scores.

The diverse results presented above on construct representation supported the hypothesized differences between examinees. First, the application of the mixed RM supported two latent classes. As predicted, these classes were differentiated by the relative difficulty of the items that could be solved by either figure addition or abstract analytic relationships. For the smaller class (Class 2), the items were more difficult. Further, the estimated abilities for Class 2 were substantially lower on average, also as expected. Second, the cognitive modeling of item difficulty within the classes, using LLTM, indicated differential impact of the underlying sources of cognitive complexity. In particular, the weight of memory load in item difficulty was lower in Class 2. This could be expected also, because the memory-load factor depends on the position of the relationships in the rule hierarchy. Some items were inappropriately characterized by the rule hierarchy for Class 2 because they apparently were solved by the abstract high-level rule rather than the simple holistic rule. Third, the results on correct response time indicated that Class 2 spent relatively more time on items that could be solved by simple holistic relationships. That is, Class 2 examinees generally solved only the easiest of these items and when they were solved, they spent longer on the items than did Class 1 examinees.

In conclusion, the impact of the latent classes on both construct representation and nomothetic span indicates that the construct differs qualitatively between classes. In general, the construct appears to be only weakly measured for Class 2 examinees, due to their failure to apply a relatively simple type of relationship to the items. There are several approaches to resolving this issue. One approach would be to include both ability estimates and latent-class membership in the interpretation and use of the ability scores. This approach is certainly feasible, since currently available programs for the mixed RM provides the appropriate indices. However, for this particular source of class differences, there may be a more parsimonious solution. Now that the latent classes have been identified, perhaps some intervention can be undertaken to ensure that the construct is uniform across examinees. Perhaps processing can be equalized for all examinees by more extensive test preparation. It may be only that an example or two of the low-level rule is needed to ensure the appropriate application of it. In any case, however, the utility of the mixed Rasch for construct validity is clearly indicated by the results of this study.

General Conclusion

The applications of the mixed RM to spatial ability and to abstract reasoning indicated that construct validity is impacted by latent classes. Thus, the same construct is not measured uniformly for all examinees and the same interpretations do not apply. This creates a problem for traditional test use, since the interpretations based on a single class are not appropriate for all examinees.

The solution to handling ability tests for multiple latent classes may depend on the particular ability and the nature of the latent classes. For spatial ability, the classes had substantive meaning. Thus, classifying examinees prior to interpreting test results would be appropriate. Then, interpretations could be developed separately for each latent class. For abstract reasoning, however, removing the source of the second class may be more feasible. That is, if the basis of the class differentiation could be removed, application of an easy relationship, a single class may then be appropriate. In any case, further research is needed on other abilities to determine whether uniform construct interpretations are appropriate.

Detecting Response Styles and Faking in Personality and Organizational Assessments by Mixed Rasch Models

Michael Eid[1] and Michael J. Zickar[2]

[1] Free University of Berlin
[2] Bowling Green State University

16.1 Introduction

Mixture IRT models such as the mixed Rasch model (RM) have the potential to illuminate conflicting findings in the analysis of responses to organizational assessments of noncognitive abilities such as personality inventories and attitude assessments. The preponderance of psychometric work (especially in the early history of test analysis) has been done in the realm of cognitive abilities, where data are presumably much more ordered than in the personality or noncognitive ability domains (see Zickar, 2001). One key difference between personality and ability assessment is that in personality measurement, respondents often know what the "correct" or socially desirable answer is even if that answer does not apply to their own personality. Given this, responses to personality items depend not only on the respondent's true personality but also his or her motivation to respond favorably (or unfavorably in certain situations). This can create problems because in a given sample of job applicants there may be a diversity of faking styles present. Some or most respondents may reply honestly out of ethical or religious reasons or for fear of getting caught. Other respondents may feel no compunction about distorting and will choose answers that they believe will result in their best chance of being hired. Finally, others, perhaps worried about getting caught but still motivated to get hired, might slightly exaggerate their personality characteristics to increase their chances of being hired.

Response distortion has been studied extensively throughout the last half-century. Researchers have examined faking positively (McFarland & Ryan, 2000), social desirability (Edwards, 1957; Paulhus, 1984), and even faking negatively or malingering (Gillis et al., 1990; Lim & Butcher, 1996). In addition, others have examined the role of response sets or response tendencies on personality and attitude scales (Graham, 2000; Messick & Jackson, 1961). For example, some respondents may have an acquiescence tendency and agree passively with personality items regardless of the items' content. Other respondents may have a central tendency style and be more likely to choose options that are in the middle of the scale. Moreover, the number of categories that are appropriate for expressing one's opinion might differ between individuals. There might be individuals who prefer simple judgments such as *yes* versus *no* and might be overwhelmed by more response categories, whereas others would prefer a response scale with many categories to express their opinions appropriately and would consider a binary response scale as insufficient. Individual preferences for the number of response categories can produce structural differences in category use if all respondents have to respond to the same response scales (Eid & Rauber, 2000).

Given the diversity of response styles, motivations, and sets, mixed RMs seem particularly appropriate for analyzing data from personality tests and attitude surveys. It seems possible that the complexity of these types of data lends itself well to being modeled by mixture-distribution IRT. In addition, the number and nature of classes may depend on the types of samples that are completing the personality inventory or attitude survey. For example, telling research participants that they should answer as honestly as possible may result in a simpler solution (i.e., fewer classes) than a sample that includes job applicants with a wide variety of motivations. In the case of attitude surveys, having someone sign their name may provide different types of responses than if the survey were anonymous. The aim of this chapter is to illustrate how mixed RMs can be used in personality and organizational research to detect structural differences in response processes that may be caused by response styles, social desirability, faking, and structural differences in the construct under consideration. Moreover, the chapter aims at reviewing the major results of previous studies that have applied mixed Rasch models in this context. Because response scales with two categories differ in many ways from response scales with more than two categories, the topics mentioned above will be discussed separately for binary and polytomous response variables.

16.2 Binary Response Scales

Binary response scales have many advantages. They are simple and economical, and everybody can understand the meaning of response categories such as *yes* and *no*. Binary response scales prevent many of the individual differences in category use that are caused by individual differences in understanding category labels and that are due to response styles such as preferences for the middle category. Nevertheless, binary response scales are prone to response styles (e.g., yea- and nay-saying), faking, and other influences that can cause structural differences between individuals. Some of these response styles and structural differences will be discussed and illustrated in this section.

16.2.1 Yea- and Nay-saying

Classical response styles that are typically discussed when binary response categories are under consideration are *yea-saying* and *nay-saying*. Respondents who have either of these two response styles tend to use one of the two categories regardless of the content of the item. What are the consequences of these response styles for modeling binary item responses, and what are the advantages of mixed modeling in this domain? Response styles such as yea- or nay-saying make it likely that the population consists of latent subpopulations that differ structurally in the item parameters of the IRT model considered. For example, in analyzing a personality inventory consisting of binary items, there may be three separate classes of respondents: a yea-saying class, a nay-saying class, and a class with neither of these tendencies. Mixed RMs can help to detect these subgroups in different ways.

In order to detect yea- and nay-saying, it is important to have positively and negatively keyed items to separate these response patterns from those that can be expected for individuals with high and low trait values. There are at least two ways to detect these response tendencies. First, person-fit indices can be used to detect individuals with unexpected response patterns (e.g., Meijer, 2003; von Davier & Molenaar, 2003). If the items measure a one-dimensional trait, response patterns of yea- and nay-saying are response patterns that are unlikely, and individuals showing these response patterns would be detected as outliers. Consequently, these individuals could be removed from the total sample and treated as a special subsample. HYBRID models (Yamamoto, 1989) would be a model-based alternative to the person-fit approach. If there are yea- and nay-sayers, we would expect two latent classes in addition to a latent Rasch homogeneous class. One class would comprise the yea-sayers with high probabilities for choosing the *yes* category independently of the (positively or negatively keyed) content of the item, and one latent class would consist of nay-sayers with high probabilities for the category *no*. In order to test the existence of yea- and nay-saying response styles, the fit of a HYBRID model with three classes (one Rasch homogeneous class, one yea-saying class, one nay-saying class) can be compared with a one-class RM, and it can be analyzed to determine whether the probabilities of the responses in the latent classes are in line with the expectations.

16.2.2 Social Desirability and Faking

It is more difficult to detect social desirability and faking patterns. Social desirability and faking produce response patterns that are in line with the desirability of specific behavioral acts. If a questionnaire measuring a trait that is socially desirable (e.g., emotional stability) contains both negatively and positively keyed items, a response pattern with high probabilities of the *yes*-categories of positively keyed items and high probabilities of the *no*-categories of the negatively keyed items would be in line with a social desirability pattern. This response pattern would be clearly different from a response pattern of *yea-* and *nay*-saying. However, it would be hard to distinguish a socially desirable or faking response pattern from a pattern produced by an individual with a high trait value who responds honestly or accurately. Even including behavioral acts that are very difficult to show (e.g., items that have very rare frequencies) would not solve this problem perfectly. It seems to be easier to detect the response styles of social desirability and faking with polytomous response categories because it is much more unlikely that individuals always choose the highest categories when items vary in their difficulties and highly difficult items are included. Moreover, it would be important to research the influence of different instructions on item parameter estimates under mixed RMs. We will explain such a research program and its results when we describe models for polytomous items.

16.2.3 Structural Differences in Item Difficulties

One-dimensional IRT models assume that all items can be ordered on a single latent continuum, and that this ordering of items is identical for all individuals. However, this assumption is very restrictive. If the trait of conscientiousness is measured, for example, by items indicating several behavioral acts, it is likely that for some individuals one behavioral act (e.g., to keep to schedule) is easier than another (e.g., always cleaning the recreation room) whereas for others, cleaning the recreation room would be easier than keeping to schedule. If structural differences exist, a one-dimensional model would not fit the data, and the mixed RM allowing structural differences in item parameters between subpopulations and individual differences within subpopulations would be superior (see also Embretson's chapter in this volume).

These structural differences are not due to response styles and faking. Instead, they represent true differences that exist between individuals. That means that the mixed RM not only is useful for detecting response patterns that indicate invalid responses but also enables the researcher to scrutinize valid structural differences between individuals in a more appropriate way.

In empirical applications it is often not known whether there are structural differences between individuals that are due to response styles, faking, or valid differences. In the following section we will present an empirical application of the mixed RM to binary items and we will show how the comparison of different models and the interpretation of the best-fitting model can help one to understand whether structural differences between individuals are valid or caused by response styles or faking.

16.2.4 An Example

In order to illustrate the usefulness of mixed RMs for personality assessment we selected six items from a scale measuring *social orientation*, a subscale of the Freiburg Personality Inventory (Fahrenberg et al., 1984), a widely applied German personality questionnaire. The wording of the six items was translated and is given in Table 16.1.

Table 16.1. Response probabilities and item parameters for the HYBRID model with two Rasch classes and one latent class

Item	Class 1 (size: 41%)		Class 2 (38%)		Class 3 (21%)
	Probabilities	Item Parameters	Probabilities	Item Parameters	Probabilities
The probabilities and item parameters refer to the category *yes*					
1. I often think that I should reduce my spending in order to give it to disadvantaged people	.71	−.08	.14	2.65	.36
2. I often feel guilty when I see how bad off other people are	.81	−.98	.36	1.10	.65
3. I occasionally give money and donations to emergency services, charitable organizations, and other collections.	.42	1.95	.37	1.05	.99
The probabilities and item parameters refer to the category *no*					
4. I think that people in developing countries should first of all help themselves.	.75	−.43	.86	−1.77	.56
5. I think everybody should make sure by him- or herself to have enough	.66	.24	.89	−2.09	.48
6. Because the government provides welfare aid I do not have to care for others in a particular case	.78	−.70	.75	−.94	.66

Each item has to be answered by choosing the response category *yes* or *no*. Three items are positively keyed, and three items are negatively keyed. The negatively keyed items were recoded in order to apply a Rasch model with the computer program WINMIRA (von Davier, 2001). The sample consisted of 500 individuals who responded to the FPI. In order to find the most appropriate model and in order to find out whether there are response styles, we applied several models:

1. The RM that assumes that all items are indicators of one latent variable representing individual differences in social orientation. According to this model all individuals use the items in the same way and there are no structural differences.
2. A HYBRID model with one Rasch homogeneous class and two latent classes comprising yea- and nay-sayers. The basic idea of this model has been described above.

3. A HYBRID model with one Rasch homogeneous class and one latent class. Whereas the Rasch homogeneous class can represent valid individual differences, the latent class could cover a response style such as social desirability (high probabilities for the *yes* categories of the positively keyed items and high probabilities for the *no* categories of the negatively keyed items).

4. Mixed RMs with several latent classes representing the idea that there might be valid structural differences between subgroups. Because we have not a specific hypothesis about the number of the latent classes, we augmented the number of latent classes until the fit of the model could not be improved.

5. Because there could be valid structurally different classes as well as response style classes we also tested a HYBRID model with two Rasch classes and a latent class.

The fit coefficients are given in Table 16.2. The fit of the models can be tested by the Pearson test, the likelihood ratio test, and the Cressie–Read test (von Davier, 2001). All three test statistics show that the RM does not fit the data well but that all extensions of the RM fit the data quite well. To find the (relatively) best fitting model among the ones compared, information indices such as the AIC and CAIC can be used. According to these criteria, the best-fitting model is the model with the lowest value for a particular index. According to the AIC coefficient, the HYBRID model with three classes (two Rasch classes, one latent class) shows the best fit. This model is also quite competitive when one looks at the other fit coefficients. We chose the AIC coefficient for selecting the best model because we have only a small number of possible response patterns ($2^6 = 64$) and a reasonable expected cell count given the sample size compared to table size (Rost, 2004).

The response probabilities characterizing the three classes are given in Table 16.1. These response probabilities describe the classes in general. They are also the individual response probabilities in Class 3 because this is a traditional latent class. The individual response probabilities in the Classes 1 and 2 vary, since an RM explains individual differences in these classes. In the first two classes, item parameters can also be estimated, indicating the location of the items on the latent continuum.

The table shows that the first class may be labeled the "high social orientation class" because the response probabilities of all categories indicating a positive social orientation are high. Members of the second class agree in general that there is a responsibility to care for disadvantaged people but they do not feel guilty, they do not want to change their life and they do not give money to charitable organizations. The differences between the first two classes are also reflected in the item parameters. The item parameters are very different in the two classes. Some items that are rather easy in Class 1 (negative item parameters) are rather difficult in Class 2 (positive item parameters) and vice versa. In Class 1 the item parameters are more homogeneous than in Class

Table 16.2. Goodness-of-fit of different models

Model	AIC	CAIC	df	Pearson	p	Likelihood Ratio	p	Cressie–Read	p
RM	3642.32	3678.82	56	118.86	< .01	108.55	< .01	112.50	< .01
HYBRID models									
2 classes: 1 Rasch class 1 latent class	3611.27	3684.28	49	59.97	.14	63.50	.08	60.20	.08
3 classes: 2 Rasch classes 1 latent class	3601.02	3715.74	41	35.47	.71	37.25	.64	35.33	.72
3 classes: 1 Rasch class 2 latent classes	3606.82	3716.33	42	43.60	.40	45.05	.35	43.25	.42
Mixed RMs									
2 classes	3610.61	3688.83	48	56.68	.18	60.84	.10	57.20	.17
3 classes	3606.39	3726.33	40	37.61	.58	40.62	.44	37.88	.57
4 classes	3609.38	3771.03	32	25.05	.79	27.61	.69	25.29	.79

2. The only item that is comparatively difficult in Class 1 is Item 3 concerning the donation of money. In Class 2, there are stronger differences between the positively and negatively keyed items. In this class, the negatively keyed items, indicating a general responsibility for the disadvantaged, have negative item parameters, indicating that they are more likely to be endorsed, whereas the items measuring individual feelings and behaviors are more difficult and less likely to be endorsed.

In each class the raw score of an individual can be estimated. The raw score is the number of items that has been answered according to social orientation (possible range: 0 to 6). In the first class, the mean score of the raw score is 4.12 and the standard deviations of the raw scores is 1.85, indicating a generally high social orientation in this class but also substantive individual differences. In Class 2, the mean raw score is 3.36 and the standard deviation is 1.29, indicating that the mean social orientation and the degree of individual differences are smaller in the second class. The third class is characterized by a large probability to give money to charitable organizations, whereas all other probabilities vary around .50, particularly considering the negatively keyed items. This means that members of this class give money but they have an uncertain attitude toward the responsibility of supporting disadvantaged people.

What do the results tell us about structural differences between subpopulations and response styles? First of all, the results show that mixture-distribution extensions of the RM are more appropriate than the one-dimensional RM for this sample. The results show that we have not found a model with one latent class of yea-sayers and one latent class of nay-sayers. At first glance, the general response probabilities of the first class is consistent with a social desirability pattern, and the pattern of general response probabilities of the second class resembles a nay-saying response set. However, the two classes are not homogeneous with respect to the response probabilities, since there are individual differences between individuals in each class and the item parameters differ between items. These differences show that there is not a clear homogeneous pattern that would be consistent with yea-saying and nay-saying and social desirability response styles.

In the case of response styles one would have expected classes in which the item parameters do not differ because the response probabilities of all items (and therefore their difficulties) should be the same. Moreover, in the case of response styles the individuals should not differ because each and every individual should have answered all categories with high probabilities. Instead, the different latent classes indicate substantial structural differences in item parameters. There are differences in the difficulties of the item parameters between the first two classes that are reasonable from a substantive point of view. Moreover, the third class includes a group of people that give money, but are generally more uncertain concerning their attitude toward disadvantaged people. These results demonstrate that typological differences have to be taken into consideration if we intend to measure personality traits. The fact that we have not found response style classes might be due to the anonymity of the study and that every participant was free to decide whether to participate.

16.3 Polytomous Response Scales

In addition to research on binary response scales in noncognitive ability assessment, it is important to consider research on polytomous scales, given that many tests include such formats. This section gives an overview of previous studies that have used mixture-distribution IRT to model polytomous data and discusses the implications of these studies for future research.

16.3.1 Analysis of Unmotivated Personality Data (Rost et al., 1997)

Rost et al. (1997) report the analysis of two scales (extraversion and conscientiousness) of a German-language version of the five-factor personality inventory (NEO-FFI; Costa & McRae, 1992). They found that, while a four-class solution fits the extraversion scale, the conscientiousness scale could be fitted with a two-class solution. Even though the four-class solution fit best statistically (using the CAIC criterion), for the extraversion scale they preferred to interpret the two-class solution for both scales, since the two-class solution seemed more interpretable. For the extraversion scale, the two classes corresponded to two subdimensions of the extraversion scale: sociability and impulsivity. The two classes separated the sample into those who were more sociable relative to other components of extraversion, and those who shared all of the extraverted components equally. In a sense, the two-class structure of the extraversion scale is due to construct heterogeneity, not response tendencies.

The different classes in the conscientiousness scale, however, were attributed to different usages of the response scale. Class one had a tendency to extreme ratings (people in that class avoid the middle categories), whereas class two has a tendency for more moderate ratings. Upon further investigation (e.g., they analyzed dimensions of the extraversion scale separately to eliminate construct heterogeneity), Rost et al. (1997) found the same class structure within the extraversion scale in which separate extreme responding and moderate responding classes were identified. They also found moderate concordance between class memberships across scales. Individuals who were in the moderate responding class for the conscientiousness scale were more likely to be in the moderate responding class for the extraversion scale as well.

Rost et al. (1997) point out that by using mixture-distribution IRT to estimate latent traits, there is an automatic correction used to compare people with different response sets. In a sense, people with the same overall score for the scale may get assigned different latent-trait scores if they are in different classes. People in the moderate responding class who receive an overall low score will be assigned a lower latent-trait score compared to those who are in the extreme responding class who receive the same overall score. Of course, there are difficulties in comparing latent-trait scores of individuals from different classes. It is important to ensure that the structure of the traits does not differ substantially across the classes. In this analysis, the main difference, especially for the conscientiousness scale, appears to be in how people react to the response scales. In this case, the comparison seems useful; estimating person parameters within classes may help control for different response styles.

The Rost et al. (1997) analysis provides a useful first step in demonstrating how mixture-distribution IRT can help us to better understand response styles in personality data. However, the respondents from that sample were predominantly students who were filling out the personality inventory for research purposes. It might be expected that the differences in motivation between the respondents would be less than in other scenarios. In the following we summarize three studies applying mixed RMs to nonstudent samples, two from organizational psychology (Eid & Rauber, 2000; Zickar et al., 2004), and one from clinical psychology (Gollwitzer et al., 2005).

16.3.2 Detecting Measurement Invariance in Organizational Assessment: Eid & Rauber (2000)

Eid & Rauber (2000) investigated whether judgments of satisfaction with ones superior can be compared across the divisions of an organization. For example, if one wishes to create a ranking of all superiors of a company with respect to their leadership behavior it is necessary that all employees use the response scales similarly to obtain fair comparisons. Moreover, the benchmarking of different companies is possible only if the employees of the companies do not differ in how they use the categories. Eid & Rauber (2000) applied mixed RMs to six satisfaction ratings with a six-point response scale (not at all true, mainly not true, rather not true, rather true, mainly true, exactly true). Their results revealed that not all employees of the organization used the response scale in the same way. Instead, two latent classes were identified. Threshold parameters are used to model the amount of difficulty of particular options. With scales that are working normally, the least-extreme or easiest option should have a lower threshold compared to an option that is more extreme. In this data set, for the majority of employees (71%) a model with ordered thresholds held, indicating that these employees made use of all response categories in a comparable way using the order implied by the category labels; about one-third of employees preferred the most extreme response categories to express their attitudes. That means that members of the latter group were overwhelmed by a six-point response scale and evaluated their superiors more in a binary way. Most interestingly, class membership differed across job categories and demographic variables (e.g., gender, tenure, and age). Women were more extreme responders compared to men, and those who were in their positions longer and who held leadership positions were more likely to be in the extreme responding class than employees with short tenures and low levels of leadership.

The results of this study show that measurement invariance might not be the rule in organizational surveys, and that the assumption of measurement invariance should be routinely checked in organizational surveys, particularly when different divisions or organizations are to be compared. But even in the case of lack of measurement invariance, ratings can be compared across divisions and companies with the help of mixture-distribution models. Employees can be assigned to the subgroup to which they most likely belong, and the divisions and companies can be compared within each subgroup. Hence, taking class differences into account could be much more informative than ignoring the problems that are caused by measurement invariance in organizational surveys.

16.3.3 Analysis of Faking Data: Zickar et al. (2004)

The motivation to fake may influence the class structure for personality inventories. There has been extensive research to demonstrate that faking influences responses to personality inventories and modifies the factor structure. For example, Schmitt & Ryan (1993) found that the factor structure of a big five personality inventory differed across applicant and nonapplicant samples; in the applicant sample, an additional factor (an "ideal employee" factor) was needed that was not present in the nonapplicant sample. Using traditional IRT methods (the graded response model), Zickar & Robie (1999) also found that the factor structure changed across samples.

Zickar et al. (2004) reanalyzed faking study data from two different samples using a mixture-distribution IRT. The first data set was an experimental faking sample in which some respondents (military recruits) were told to respond honestly whereas other respondents were told to fake positively. There were two conditions within the faking group; the *ad lib faking* group was given no instructions about how to fake, whereas the *coached faking* group was given explicit instructions on how to fake. The other sample had applicants to a middle-management sales position for a large retail organization; another group of job incumbents also completed the inventory. With both of these samples, Zickar et al. (2004) examined the class structure and differences in class membership across context. It should be noted that the personality inventories used in both analyses were different. The inventory used in the experimentally induced faking study was designed by the military as part of its massive personnel research effort Project A (see White et al., 1993). The other inventory used in the analysis of applicants versus incumbents was a proprietary instrument designed by a private consulting company (Personnel Decisions International, 1997).

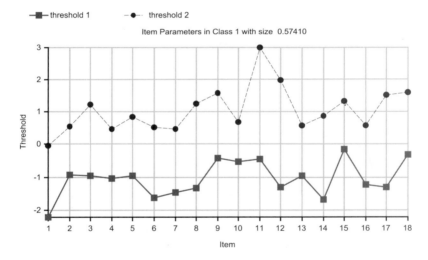

Fig. 16.1. Threshold parameter estimates for the honest class

In the experimentally induced faking samples, a two-class solution fit the data best across five different personality traits (work orientation, conscientiousness, nondelinquency, cooperativeness, and emotional stability). One of the classes appeared to be an honestly responding class, whereas the other appeared to be a faking class. The honestly responding group had much lower item-level scores than the faking class. In addition, the category threshold parameters were ordered properly for the honestly responding class whereas the thresholds were less ordered for the faking class. Figures 16.1 and 16.2 illustrate this effect. The first threshold parameter estimate corresponds to the

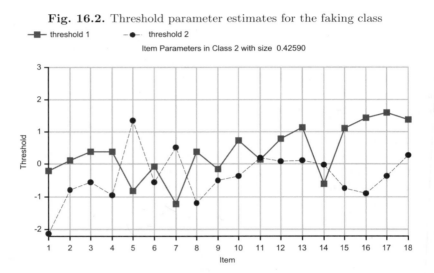

Fig. 16.2. Threshold parameter estimates for the faking class

level of the latent trait at which the probability of choosing option 2 becomes larger than the probability of choosing option 1. The second threshold parameter estimate corresponds to the same probability difference between option 3 and option 2. Therefore, in Figure 16.1, which shows the honest class, it makes sense that the first threshold parameter estimate is lower than the second parameter estimate. In addition, the difference between the two thresholds is roughly equal for most items in the scale. For the faking class, however, the pattern of thresholds is much less orderly. As can be seen in Figure 16.2, the difference between the first threshold estimate and the second threshold is much smaller than the difference for the first class. In addition, for fourteen of the items, the second threshold is lower than the first threshold. This suggests that in the faking class, few individuals choose the first and second options. Similar results were found across all five of the personality traits.

A three-class solution was chosen based on information criteria for the applicant-incumbent sample. Among the three classes, one was labeled an honestly responding class; in that class, thresholds were ordered properly as in Figure 16.1. Another class was identified as a slightly faking class. Item scores were higher than those for the honestly responding group. Thresholds were less orderly than those in Figure 16.1. Finally, the third class appeared to be related to extreme faking.

One of the interesting findings from these analyses was that there was substantial overlap among conditions in class membership. For example, 27.6%

of the applicants were in the extreme faking class for the agreeableness scale, which makes sense since applicants would be motivated to fake their responses to get hired; however, 13.7% of incumbents were also in the extreme faking class. Conversely, 26.5% of the applicants were in the honestly responding class. Similar results were found in the experimental samples. In those samples, some people in the honest responding condition were classified in the faking class, whereas some participants in the faking conditions were also classified in the honest class. Although classification error is a possibility, it is also likely that there was significant overlap across the groups. People who were expected to fake did not necessarily do so.

This mixture-distribution IRT analysis provided several insights into faking on personality inventories. First, much of the research has assumed that there is little variability in types of faking strategies and methods. In the typical applicant-incumbents comparison, it is assumed that applicants are faking and incumbents are responding honestly. This research demonstrated that there is an overlap of strategies and motivations among groups that might have previously been assumed to be distinct. In addition, it has been extremely difficult to ascertain the prevalence of faking using traditional methods (see Donovan et al., 2003). For fear of reprisal, applicants are reluctant to admit that they distorted their responses. Mixture-distribution IRT provides another way to assess the number of individuals who fit the profile of fakers. In short, mixture-distribution IRT can help illuminate faking research.

16.3.4 Analysis of Response Styles in Anger Expression: Gollwitzer et al. (2005)

Detecting response styles and faking with respect to personality question-naires is important not only for organizational but also for clinical psychology. The application of personality questionnaires has a long tradition in clinical psychology. Response tendencies such as the simulation and dissimulation of symptoms are well known (Franke, 2002; Linden et al., 1986). Gollwitzer et al. analyzed the three expression subscales of the State-Trait Anger Expression Inventory (STAXI) in a clinical sample of 4,497 patients with the mixed RM. Their results revealed that there were different response styles that were robust across two randomly selected subsamples of the total sample. They found response styles that reflect psychologically meaningful biases (i.e., social desirability) as well as nonmeaningful response-category preferences. Moreover, they detected gender differences. In the female sample they found three latent classes for anger-in and anger-out, and two latent classes for anger-control. In the male sample, however, a two-class solution was appropriate for each scale. In all samples and gender groups the largest class showed a response pattern with equally distant and ordered thresholds. Individuals with high membership for this first class for one scale also had high membership probabilities for the first class of all other scales. That means that individuals generally differ in the appropriate use of response categories. The second latent class seemed to reflect social desirability. The threshold parameters in this class were partly unordered and narrowly located. Moreover, frankness measured by a subscale of the Freiburg Personality Inventory (Fahrenberg et al., 1984) discriminated between Classes 1 and 2 for anger-in and anger-out. In the third class in the group of women the threshold parameters were ordered in almost all cases, demonstrating the adequate use of response categories. In contrast to the first class, the mean sum scores in this class were elevated, indicating the display of anger-expression styles to a higher degree. The authors of this study found some clues that this pattern might be due to symptom aggravation, and suggested further studies to advance this result. Several personality variables were able to separate the latent classes, but the effect sizes were generally small, showing that response styles have their own quality and structure and cannot be simply explained by personality variables.

16.3.5 Future Research Directions

We believe that mixture-distribution IRT is an important psychometric tool that can help integrate latent-class analysis with item response theory. In each of the research studies presented in this chapter, single-class solutions result in worse fit compared to more-complex solutions. In each of the examples, the explanation given for the additional classes differs. In some cases, the classes can be attributed to yea-saying or nay-saying. Other cases can be attributed to socially desirable responses and structural differences in perceptions of how behavioral acts fit into latent-construct structures. Below are some thoughts that we have on how mixture-distribution IRT can help advance research and practice.

Better Trait Estimation

Mixture-distribution IRT provides the potential for better trait estimation. As Rost et al. (1997) suggest, in certain cases trait estimates from a mixture distribution might be used to correct for response sets or even faking. For the faking research, it may be possible that the latent traits estimated by mixture-distribution IRT are much better estimates of personality traits compared to latent traits estimated by a traditional psychometric technique. In order to determine whether traits estimated using mixture-distribution IRT are indeed more useful statistics, it is important to evaluate the predictive validity of those trait estimates compared to other types of trait estimates.

Better Understanding of Subgroups

Mixed-group IRT is in a way similar to differential item functioning (DIF) methods developed by item response theorists to model how items function across *known* groups (Raju et al., 1995). With mixed-group IRT it is possible to identify groups for which the items function differently; mixture-distribution IRT could be thought of as an exploratory DIF technique.

16.3.6 Limitations of Mixture-Distribution IRT

Reliance on Rasch-Related Models

Mixture-distribution item response theory, as currently operationalized in WINMIRA, relies on item response models derived from the Rasch family. For example, WINMIRA currently allows for estimation of the RM, the partial-credit extension of the RM for ordinal polytomous data (Masters, 1982) and several other Rasch-based models. Although it is beyond the scope of this chapter to reiterate all of the points in support of or against the RM, it is important to note that the item response models currently assume that all items have equal discrimination. This may be an assumption that could be hard to justify in models that allow for differences in discrimination. Note, however, that recently von Davier & Yamamoto (2004b) developed an EM algorithm for estimating more general mixture IRT models, namely the two-parameter logistic model and the generalized partial-mixture IRT models. For researchers who are worried about discriminations, another strategy would be to pay close attention to item-level fit statistics; it may be possible that only one or two items may emerge as misfit by the RM. It could be simple to either eliminate those items or tolerate a small amount of misfit. In Zickar et al.'s (2004) mixed-group IRT analysis, we found that fewer items were misfits than would even be expected given the alpha .05 error rate.

What Do the Groups Mean?

Another challenge associated with mixed-group IRT methods is determining the substantive grounding of individual classes. An analysis may indicate that there is significant statistical evidence to warrant consideration of a latent class; that evidence, however, reveals little about what are the particular characteristics that distinguish that particular class from the other latent classes.

There are several ways to interpret the meaning of class membership. Rost et al. (1997) and Zickar et al. (2004) analyzed the pattern of item (and option) parameter estimates and item scores to gain a better understanding of the meaning of class membership. In Rost et al.'s (1997) analysis, the interpretation based on the dimensionality of the extraversion scale and based on the different threshold parameter estimates allowed them to conclude that some classes related to construct heterogeneity and others related to response sets. In Zickar et al. (2004), a similar analysis of response patterns along with an investigation of how class membership differed across experimental condition and applicant-incumbent status allowed the investigators to establish meaning to the statistical classes.

To better interpret class membership, however, we believe that it is important to consider ancillary information. The studies of Eid & Rauber (2000) and Gollwitzer et al. (2005) showed how ancillary information can be used to learn more about the differences between classes. Also, Gibby (2004) used ancillary information to better understand some of the faking research findings previously discussed. In a student sample, he found two classes that corresponded to the honestly responding class and the slightly faking class found in Zickar et al. (2004). Respondents in the faking class had higher social intelligence scores (i.e., a higher skill for faking) and also reported at a higher rate after the experiment that they had indeed faked their responses.

16.3.7 Conclusions

We believe that mixture-distribution IRT has a great potential for personality assessment and its application in several fields of applied psychology such as organizational and clinical psychology. The mixture-distribution approach in general, and the development of further mixture-distribution IRT models overcoming some limits of the mixed RM will have a strong impact on personality assessment. This approach allows a more complete view of structural differences that can be caused by interindividual differences in item difficulties but also by response styles and distortions due to faking, simulation, and dissimulation. Several empirical applications reviewed in this chapter demonstrated the power of this modeling approach for psychological assessment.

Application of Multivariate Rasch Models in International Large-Scale Educational Assessments

Raymond J. Adams[1], Margaret L. Wu[1], and Claus H. Carstensen[2]

[1] University of Melbourne
[2] Leibniz Institute for Science Education, Kiel

17.1 Introduction

In large-scale educational assessments, such as the Programme for International Student Assessment (PISA) and the Trends in Mathematics and Science Study (TIMSS), a primary concern is with the estimation of the population-level characteristics of a number of latent variables and the relationships between latent variables and other variables. Typically these studies are undertaken in contexts in which there are constraints on sample size and individual student response time, yet there are high expectations with regard to the breadth of content coverage. These demands and constraints have resulted in such studies using rotated-booklet designs, with each student responding to a limited number of items on each of a number of scales. This paper describes the techniques that have been employed in such studies to enable the reliable estimation of population characteristics when there is considerable unreliability at the student level. It also discusses the methodology that is used to make the data sets produced in such studies amenable for use by data analysts undertaking secondary analyses using standard analytic tools.

A primary concern in large-scale educational assessments is with the estimation of the population-level characteristics of a number of latent variables and their relationships with other variables. Such characteristics are, for example, the mean, variance, and percentiles of latent-ability distributions; correlations between latent variables; the relative performances of subpopulations (e.g., males and females); correlations between latent variables and other variables (e.g., indices of socioeconomic status); and variance decompositions such as the relative proportions of within- and between-school variance in latent variables. This interest in population characteristics is in contrast to many other educational measurement contexts in which the primary concern is the reliable measurement of the abilities of individual students.

Large-scale assessments also have a number of other distinguishing, if not unique, features. Due to a desire to meet the needs of many stakeholders, they typically attempt to simultaneously assess a large number of latent variables. Second, they need to report their results as simple, summarized outcomes, and third, they need to produce data products that can be used in secondary analyses using standard statistical software tools such as SPSS (2003) or SAS (The SAS Institute, 2002).

At the same time, such studies have to deal with a range of constraints. First, there are cost-imposed limits on the student and school sample size. Second, there are limits to the amount of testing time that is available for each sampled student. The consequences of a desire to cover many latent variables with a limited sample and a limited amount of testing time are complexity in the study design and in the analytic techniques that are necessary to analyze the data, summarize the data, and prepare a database suitable for secondary analyses using standard tools.

In the following, we use PISA as an example to show how these demands and constraints have resulted in such studies using rotated booklet designs, with each student responding to a limited number of items on each of a number of scales. The chapter then describes the techniques that have been employed in such studies to enable the reliable estimation of the population characteristics when there is considerable unreliability at the student level. It also discusses the methodology that is used to make the data sets produced in such studies amenable for use by data analysts undertaking secondary analyses using standard analytic tools.

17.2 The PISA Design

PISA is a cyclical study with data collections occurring every three years (OECD, 2001, 2004). Here we discuss the second cycle of PISA: PISA 2003. In PISA 2003, four subject domains were tested, with mathematics as the major domain, and reading, science and cross-curricular problem solving competencies as minor domains. Student achievement in mathematics was assessed using 85 test items representing approximately 210 minutes of testing time. The problem-solving assessment consisted of 19 items, the reading assessment consisted of 28 items, and the science assessment consisted of 35 items, representing approximately 60 minutes of testing time for each of the minor domains.

The major domain of mathematics was made up of four subscales: space and shape, quantity, change and relationships, and uncertainty. In total, therefore, PISA 2003 used seven latent reporting scales.

The 167 main study items were arranged into thirteen item clusters (seven mathematics clusters, and two clusters in each of the other domains), with each cluster representing 30 minutes of test time. The items were presented to students in thirteen test booklets, with each booklet being composed of four clusters according to the rotation design shown in Table 17.1. M1 to M7 denote the mathematics clusters, R1 and R2 denote the reading clusters, S1 and S2 denote the science clusters, and PS1 and PS2 denote the problem-solving clusters. Each cluster appears in each of the four possible positions within a booklet exactly once and each cluster occurs once in conjunction with each other cluster. Each test item, therefore, appeared in four of the test booklets. This linked design enabled standard measurement techniques to be applied to the resulting student response data to estimate item difficulties and student abilities (OECD, 2004).

The sampled students were randomly assigned one of the booklets, which meant that each student undertook two hours of testing.

Table 17.1. Cluster rotation design used to form test booklets for PISA 2003

Booklet	Block 1	Block 2	Block 3	Block 4
1	M1	M2	M4	R1
2	M2	M3	M5	R2
3	M3	M4	M6	PS1
4	M4	M5	M7	PS2
5	M5	M6	S1	M1
6	M6	M7	S2	M2
7	M7	S1	R1	M3
8	S1	S2	R2	M4
9	S2	R1	PS1	M5
10	R1	R2	PS2	M6
11	R2	PS1	M1	M7
12	PS1	PS2	M2	S1
13	PS2	M1	M3	S2

The two-hour test booklets were arranged in two one-hour parts, each made up of two of the 30-minute time blocks from the columns in Table 17.1. PISA's procedures provided for a short break one hour after the start of the test, and a longer break to be taken between administration of the test and a student questionnaire.

17.3 Steps in Scaling the Data

The PISA data were scaled with the mixed-coefficients multinomial logit (MCML) model as described by Adams, Wilson and Wang (1997) and Adams and Wu (Chapter 4 in this volume). The scaling was undertaken using the ConQuest software (Wu et al., 1997).

A total of 42 countries participated in PISA 2003. The first step in the scaling was to undertake a set of separate national calibrations. The outcomes of the national calibrations were used to make a decision about how to treat each item in each country. The possible treatments of items were as follows: an item may be deleted from PISA altogether if it has poor psychometric characteristics in more than ten countries (a *dodgy item*); it may be regarded as not administered in particular countries if it has poor psychometric characteristics in those countries but functions well in the vast majority of others; or an item with sound characteristics in each country but that shows substantial item-by-country interactions may be regarded as a different item (for scaling purposes) in each country (or in some subset of countries), that is, the difficulty parameter will be free to vary across countries.

In reviewing the national calibrations, particular attention was paid to the fit of the items to the scaling model, item discrimination, and item-by-country interactions (see OECD, 2004).

17.3.1 International Calibration

International item parameters were set by applying the MCML model, to a subsample of 15,000 students. The model was specified so that dichotomously scored items were scaled with Rasch's simple logistic model (Rasch, 1960) and items with multiple score categories were scaled with Masters's partial-credit model (Masters, 1982). This subsample of students, referred to as the international calibration sample, consisted of 15,000 students comprising 500 students drawn at random from each of the 30 participating OECD countries.[3]

17.3.2 Student Score Generation

As with all item response scaling models, student *proficiencies* (or measures) are not observed; they are missing data that must be inferred from the observed item responses. There are several possible alternative approaches for making this inference.

Plausible Values

PISA uses the imputation methodology usually referred to as plausible values (PVs). It is very important to recognize that plausible values are *not* test scores and should not be treated as such. They are random numbers drawn from the distribution of scores that could be reasonably assigned to each individual. As such, plausible values contain random-error variance components and are not optimal as scores for individuals. Plausible values, as a set, are better suited to describing the performance of the population. This approach, developed by Mislevy & Sheehan (1989) and based on the imputation theory of Rubin (1987), produces consistent estimators of population parameters. Plausible values are perhaps best viewed as intermediate values that are provided to obtain consistent estimates of population parameters using standard

---

[3] While 42 countries participated in PISA 2003, 30 of them were OECD member countries and data from the OECD countries were used in the calibration sample.

statistical analysis software such as SPSS and SAS. As an alternative, some analyses can be completed using ConQuest (Wu et al., 1997).

Using the notation of Adams and Wu (this volume), Equation 17.1 gives the posterior distribution from which the plausible values are drawn as

$$h_\theta \left(\theta_n; \mathbf{W}_n, x, \gamma, \Sigma | \mathbf{x}_n \right) = \frac{f_\mathbf{x} \left(\mathbf{x}_n; x | \theta_n \right) \, f_\theta \left(\theta_n; \mathbf{W}_n, \gamma, \Sigma \right)}{f_\mathbf{x} \left(\mathbf{x}_n; \mathbf{W}_n, x, \gamma, \Sigma \right)}, \qquad (17.1)$$

where the vector θ_n is the (multidimensional) latent ability for student n, ξ is a vector of estimated item response parameters, $\mathbf{W}_n$ is a set of background characteristics for student n, γ are the estimated regression coefficients of θ_n onto $\mathbf{W}_n$, and Σ is the estimated conditional covariance matrix. $f_\mathbf{x} \left(\mathbf{x}_n; \xi | \theta_n \right)$, is the conditional item response model, $f_\theta \left(\theta_n; \mathbf{W}_n, \gamma, \Sigma \right)$ is distribution of the latent variables (see Equations 4.2 and 4.16 in Adams & Wu, this volume) and $f_\mathbf{x} \left(\mathbf{x}_n; \mathbf{W}_n, \xi, \gamma, \Sigma \right)$ is the marginal item response model (see (4.17) in Adams & Wu, this volume).

In PISA, the plausible values are drawn from the marginal posterior distribution (17.1) as follows:

M vector-valued random deviates, are drawn at random from $\{\varphi_{mn}\}_{m=1}^M$, the multivariate normal distribution, $f_\theta \left(\theta_n; \mathbf{W}_n, \gamma, \Sigma \right)$, for each case n.[4] These vectors are used to approximate the integral in the denominator of (17.1), using the Monte Carlo integration

$$\int_\theta f_\mathbf{x} \left(\mathbf{x}; \xi | \theta \right) f_\theta \left(\theta, \gamma, \Sigma \right) d\theta \approx \frac{1}{M} \sum_{m=1}^M f_\mathbf{x}(\mathbf{x}; \xi | \varphi_{mn}) \equiv \Im. \qquad (17.2)$$

At the same time, the values

$$p_{mn} \quad = \quad f_\mathbf{x} \left(\mathbf{x}_n; \xi | \varphi_{mn} \right) \, f_\theta \left(\varphi_{mn}; \mathbf{W}_n, \gamma, \Sigma \right) \qquad (17.3)$$

are calculated, so that the set of pairs $(\varphi_{mn}, \, p_{mn}/\Im)_{m=1}^M$, which can be used as an approximation of the posterior density (17.1) is obtained; and the probability that φ_{nj} could be drawn from this density is given by

$$q_{nj} \quad = \quad \frac{p_{mn}}{\sum\limits_{m=1}^M p_{mn}}. \qquad (17.4)$$

At this point, L uniformly distributed random numbers $\{\eta_i\}_{i=1}^L$ are generated, and for each random draw, the vector φ_{ni_0} that satisfies the condition

$$\sum_{s=1}^{i_0-1} q_{sn} < \eta_i \leq \sum_{s=1}^{i_0} q_{sn} \qquad (17.5)$$

---

[4] The value M should be large. For PISA, $M = 2000$.

is selected as a plausible vector.

Note, importantly, that this procedure does not assume normality of the marginal posterior (17.1), as is the case for the procedures that have been applied in the U.S. National Assessment of Educational Progress (NAEP) (Beaton, 1987; Mislevy, Beaton, Kaplan, & Sheehan 1992).

Model Estimation

Before the plausible values can be drawn from the estimated marginal posterior distributions it is first necessary to estimate the regression parameters γ and Σ for each country. This is done by fitting the MCML model on a country-by-country basis with the item parameters anchored at the values that were estimated in the international calibration.

Before this model can be estimated it is also necessary to select the fixed $\mathbf{W}_n$ variables that will be used in each country. In NAEP and PISA, these variables are referred to as conditioning variables. The steps used to prepare the conditioning variables are based on those used in NAEP (Beaton, 1987) and in TIMSS (Macaskill et al., 1998). The steps involved in this process are as follows:

- *Step 1.* Five variables (booklet ID, gender, mother's occupation, father's occupation, and school mean mathematics score) were prepared to be directly used as conditioning variables. For mother's and father's occupation, the SEI index was used. For each student the mean mathematics achievement for that student's school was estimated using the mean of weighted likelihood estimates for mathematics for each of the students that also attended that student's school.
- *Step 2.* Each variable in the student questionnaire was dummy coded. The details of this dummy coding are provided in the PISA 2003 Technical Report (OECD, 2005).
- *Step 3.* For each country, a principal-components analysis of the dummy-coded variables was performed, and component scores were produced for each student (a sufficient number of components to account for 95 per cent of the variance in the original variables).
- *Step 4.* The item response model was fit to each national data set and the national population parameters were estimated using item parameters anchored at their international location and conditioning variables derived from the national principal-components analysis and from *Step 1*.
- *Step 5.* Five vectors of plausible values were drawn using the method described above. The vectors were of length seven, one for each of the PISA 2003 reporting scales.

Weighted Likelihood Estimates

The PISA 2003 study did not provide maximum likelihood estimates of students' proficiencies. For the purposes of this study, in which we wish to illustrate the differences between results obtained from the analysis of plausible values and point estimates, such as maximum likelihood estimates, we have rescaled the original PISA data for one country (Australia) and produced weighted likelihood estimates (WLEs; Warm, 1989; Adams & Wu, this volume).

17.4 Analysis of PISA 2003 Plausible Values

To illustrate the use of plausible values, we now report the results of several analyses of the Australian PISA 2003 data set (PISA, 2003) using both plausible values and weighted maximum likelihood estimates.

Note that in the estimation of all of the following models, a number of procedures had to be implemented. First, all of the results are based on weighted data, using the replicate student weights provided in the PISA database. Second, the balanced repeated replication BRR method had to be used (Judkins, 1990) to estimate the sampling variance of the various parameter estimates. Third, in the case of plausible values, the analysis had to be computed five times—once using each plausible vector—and then aggregated to obtain the various parameter estimates. Finally, in the case of plausible values, the sampling variances had to be enlarged to incorporate the presence of measurement error. The procedures involved in each of these steps are described in the PISA technical reports (Adams & Wu, 2002; OECD, 2005).

Regression Results

Table 17.2 shows the results of a regression of mathematics achievement onto the PISA socioeconomic status index ESCS. The estimates of the constant are very similar, but note that the slope estimate for the WLE is less than that for the plausible value. This is to be expected, since the WLE estimate is attenuated by the unreliability of the mathematics scale.

Table 17.2. Regression of Mathematics Achievement onto socioeconomic Status[*]

Regression Parameter	Plausible Value-Based Estimate and Standard Error	WLE-Based Estimate and Standard Error
Constant	515.58 (2.0)	513.99 (2.0)
Slope	42.50 (2.2)	38.29 (2.0)
R-squared	13.7	10.9

[*] The socioeconomic status index used was ESCS (OECD, 2005)

Correlations Between the Mathematics Subscales

The estimates of the correlation between the four mathematics domains are shown in Table 17.3. The values above the diagonal are estimates that are based on plausible values and the values below the diagonal are based on the weighted likelihood estimates. The correlations estimated with the WLEs are substantially less than those estimated with the plausible values. The WLE-based estimates are biased toward zero due to unreliability. Later we shall show that this bias can be corrected for by means of reliability estimates.

Table 17.3. Estimated correlations between mathematics subscales: plausible-values based estimates above the diagonal and WLE-based estimates below the diagonal

	Space & Shape	Change & Relationships	Uncertainty	Quantity
Space & Shape		0.90 (.003)	0.89 (.004)	0.91 (.003)
Change &Relationships	0.54 (.010)		0.95 (.002)	0.93 (.002)
Uncertainty	0.53 (.009)	0.60 (.009)		0.93 (.002)
Quantity	0.53 (.008)	0.58 (.009)	0.55 (.007)	

To illustrate the bias in correlations computed using WLEs, the results of a simulation study are shown. Table 17.4 shows the correlations from two-dimensional models, generated with 15 dichotomous items for each dimension and 500 subjects. Two hundred data sets were generated according to a set of generated *true* person abilities for each row of the table. The correlations printed in the table are from the generated abilities and averaged over the replications for WLEs, for disattenuated WLE correlations and for the average of five plausible values. The disattenution was computed by dividing the correlation by the square roots of the reliabilities, which were estimated as the ratio of the variance of the plausible values (an estimate for the true variance) divided by the variance of the WLEs (see the observed measures; Walter, 2005; Wang, 1999).

From the results it is apparent that the uncorrected WLE-based correlations are biased toward zero, due to measurement error. Correcting the WLE correlations seem to solve the measurement-error question quite well except for very high true correlations.

Regression of SES and Gender onto the Mathematics Subscales

In the case of multiple regression, it is well known that simple disattenuation formulae are not available to correct for the bias in regression-parameter estimates and R-squared estimates that is caused by unreliability (Fuller, 1987).

In Table 17.5, we show the results of four multiple regressions that were undertaken with plausible values and WLEs. In each case the ESCS effect

Table 17.4. Mean correlation estimates from simulated data, $n = 1000$, 200 replications, two subscales with 15 dichotomous items each

Generating Value	WLE-Based Estimate and Standard Error	Wle-Based Corrected Estimate and Standard Error	Plausible Value-Based Estimate and Standard Error
0.52	0.37 (0.02)	0.51 (0.03)	0.52 (0.03)
0.61	0.44 (0.02)	0.61 (0.03)	0.62 (0.03)
0.71	0.51 (0.02)	0.71 (0.03)	0.71 (0.03)
0.81	0.58 (0.02)	0.80 (0.03)	0.81 (0.03)
0.90	0.63 (0.03)	0.81 (0.05)	0.90 (0.02)

estimated with plausible values exceeds the same value when estimated with WLEs. The gender differences, however, are not consistently higher or lower in one analysis when compared to the other. A variety of simulations that show the superiority of the estimates derived using plausible values are shown in Monseur & Adams (2002) and Wu & Adams (2002).

Table 17.5. Regression of SES and gender onto the mathematic subscales, based on plausible values and WLEs

	PV-Based Estimates			WLE-Based Estimates		
	Constant	ESCS	Gender	Constant	ESCS	Gender
Space & Shape	518 (2.8)	43 (2.2)	−12.1 (2.9)	514 (2.2)	34 (1.5)	−8.9 (2.7)
Change & Relationships	519 (2.9)	42 (2.3)	−4.7 (3.0)	520 (2.8)	35 (2.1)	−4.9 (3.0)
Uncertainty	525 (2.6)	47 (2.2)	−7.6 (2.8)	523 (2.4)	36 (2.3)	−3.3 (3.0)
Quantitiy	510 (2.5)	40 (2.1)	−1.6 (2.8)	504 (2.3)	31 (2.0)	−1.8 (2.7)

17.5 Conclusion

Large-scale assessment studies focus on population-level results rather than on individual-level results. Due to constraints on testing time and content coverage, individual-level results might not be reliable enough for reporting. We have shown how multidimensional item response models and latent regression may be used to provide estimates of population parameters even when individuals cannot be measured reliably.

Ideally this would be achieved by estimating population characteristics directly from student responses to items via an appropriate multilevel item response model. See, for example, Adams, Wilson, & Wu (1997) and Goldstein et al. (2005). In the absence, however, of readily accessible software and methods for easily estimating a full range of population parameters; an alternative is to provide the secondary data analyst, with imputations for the missing student abilities, so-called plausible values. Plausible values are best viewed as intermediate values that are provided to obtain estimates of population parameters using standard statistical-analysis software such as SPSS and SAS.

The key advantage of the plausible-values methodology is that it enables secondary analysts to use widely available tools to replicate the results that would be obtained from the use of more-sophisticated direct-estimation tools. The disadvantage is that plausible values are imputed on the basis of certain modeling assumptions, and if the imputation model assumptions are different from the analytic model assumptions then the results may be misleading.

There are a number of common differences between the imputation model and analytic model. One is that the current imputation models do not take into account the often hierarchical structure of educational data. Some methods for dealing with this and their effectiveness are discussed by Monseur & Adams (2002). Second, secondary analysts are from time to time interested in using variables in their models that were not used in the imputation model. Third, the assumption of conditional multivariate normality for the latent variables may not hold. These issues and the biases that may result are discussed by Thomas (2000). In general, it appears that the bias introduced by differences between the imputation and analysis are deemed to be of less concern than the bias that would be otherwise introduced if likelihood-based ability estimates were used and measurement error were ignored.

Studying Development via Item Response Models: A Wide Range of Potential Uses

Judith Glück and Christiane Spiel

Faculty of Psychology, University of Vienna

18.1 Introduction

In this chapter, we illustrate the spectrum of developmental questions that can be investigated using Rasch models (RMs). We structure the chapter by different types of developmental research questions. RMs are recommended as method of choice (1) for cross-sectional as well as longitudinal designs, and (2) for exploratory as well as theory-guided research questions. All aspects are illustrated by examples from a variety of constructs and life phases. At the end, we discuss the advantages and limitations of Rasch-based approaches for studying development. We hope to show that the focus of these models on the item level allows for a highly differentiated, substantively informative perspective on change.

18.1.1 Methods of Studying Development

There are several ways of studying psychological development, and several issues that researchers need to consider. We structure our exposition according to two aspects: cross-sectional vs. longitudinal designs and exploratory vs. hypothesis-testing research.

Methodologically, developmental psychologists distinguish cross-sectional and longitudinal studies. While longitudinal studies are clearly superior to cross-sectional studies when individual trajectories of change are of interest, and when cohort effects are likely, systematic dropout may make interpretations difficult, and effort and time required are clearly larger than in cross-sectional designs. A special type of longitudinal designs are intervention studies with pre- and posttest designs. RMs are available both for comparing age groups in cross-sectional designs and for analyzing change in longitudinal designs. Of course, they are also applicable to more complex cohort-sequential designs that allow for controlling some of the problems in cross-sectional and longitudinal studies.

A more conceptual distinction is between different levels of "theory-guidedness" in developmental research. In some cases, researchers have clear hypotheses about the changes they expect to occur. In the most differentiated case, these hypotheses are formulated on the item level. For example, a researcher may assume that acquisition of a new strategy increases participants' probability to solve one particular type of test items, but not the other items. In other cases, researchers expect changes in sum scores on the scale level, and want to test if these changes generalize across all items. In the most exploratory case, researchers may just generally want to know whether there are subgroups of individuals with different item difficulties in the sample, and they want to test whether subgroup membership is related to age (in cross-sectional designs) or time point (in longitudinal designs). RMs can be used for all these types of research questions. It is important to distinguish between the degree of theory-guidedness of a researcher's hypotheses and the degree of theory-guidedness that a particular statistical model requires. For example, classical Mixed RMs are exploratory in that number of latent classes, class membership probabilities, and class-specific item and person parameters are all determined from the data. In some applications, however, such as the one we present below, researchers have relatively clear ideas about which latent classes they expect.

This chapter is structured according to the degrees of theory-guidedness of the statistical models we use. We give examples of the use of RMs, first, for cross-sectional designs, and then for longitudinal designs. Within each section, we start from the exploratory case where subgroups of participants are to be identified. Then, we present methods for testing the generalizability of scale-level hypotheses across items, and then, methods for testing item-level hypotheses. For reasons of simplicity, we limit our presentation to applications to dichotomous data. However, models for polytomous indicators are available for all approaches presented.

18.2 Rasch-Based Methods for Cross-Sectional Designs

Technically, the application of RMs in cross-sectional designs is straightforward, as any standard methods that identify or compare subsamples of participants can be used to compare age groups.

18.2.1 Exploratory Research Questions

The most exploratory case of using RMs in cross-sectional research is the following: a researcher has tested a group of participants heterogeneous in age with a set of items, and wants to test whether there are subgroups of participants with different item difficulty patterns. If such subgroups exist, she could then test whether subgroup membership probability is related to age.

Mixed RMs (Rost, 1990, 1991, 1996; Rost & von Davier, 1995; see also von Davier & Yamamoto, this volume) can be used to identify such subgroups, and group membership can later be related to age. For example, Spiel et al. (2001, 2004); see also Spiel et al. (1997), presented students aged 12 to 18 years with a set of 24 syllogism items measuring deductive reasoning. Each item consisted of a premise and a question (inference), followed by three possible answers: "yes" (correct answer for modus ponens items), "no" (correct answer for modus tollens items), or "maybe" (correct answer for negation of antecedent and affirmation of consequent items). Table 18.1 gives examples of all item types.

Table 18.1. Illustration of four syllogistic item types (concrete content)

Premise: *If the sun shines, Tina wears a red skirt.*

Item Type	Example	Correct Solution	Biconditional Response
Affirmation of Antecedent	The sun is shining. Is Tina wearing a red skirt?	Yes	Yes
Affirmation of Consequent	Tina is wearing a red skirt. Is the sun shining?	Maybe	Yes
Negation of Antecedent	It is raining. Is Tina wearing a red skirt?	Maybe	No
Negation of Consequent	Tina is wearing a blue skirt. Is the sun shining?	No	No

The 24 items of the scale were developed according to construction rules. There were six different premises. The premises differed in *content* (concrete, abstract, and counterfactual), and in whether the premise contained a *negation* or not. For each premise, there were four items corresponding to the four *item types* in Table 18.1. Based on theory and on previous studies, we expected concrete-content items to be easier than abstract or counterfactual items, and we expected those items whose solution was "maybe" to be more difficult than the others. The typical mistake in these items (also referred to as "fallacies") is to draw a biconditional conclusion, that is, to assume that "if A, then B" implies "if B, then A" (see Table 18.1).

We collected data from a total of 418 7th- to 12th-grade students (39% were females). Applying Mixed RMs, we used the BIC to determine the number of latent classes that best described the data following a recommendation by Rost (1996). Both the BIC and the CAIC had a minimum for the three-classes solution, so we settled for three classes. (Bootstrap analyses will be reported by Spiel, Gössler, & Glück, in preparation.). Figure 18.1 illustrates the solution frequencies for the different types of items in the three classes.

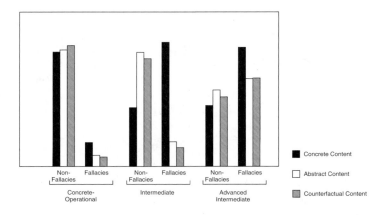

Fig. 18.1. Solution frequencies in three latent classes by syllogism item type

The three classes correspond quite well to theories about the development of deductive reasoning. We have labeled them concrete operational, intermediate, and advanced intermediate. Concrete-operational participants generally drew biconditional conclusions. Thus, these participants had a high probability to solve the nonfallacies, but systematically gave incorrect responses to the fallacies. Intermediate participants showed a similar response pattern for the abstract and the counterfactual tasks, but for the concrete items, they showed a higher probability to solve the fallacies than the nonfallacies. Advanced intermediate participants generally performed better in the fallacies than in the nonfallacies. There were a few participants in the sample who had almost perfect scores, that is, who had reached the formal-operational stage, but they were too few to form a latent class of their own.

Do these latent classes really reflect different stages of development? In addition to the theoretical plausibility of this interpretation, the classes differ significantly in average age, F $(2, 415) = 9.021$, $p < .001$. There is, however, considerable overlap of the three classes with respect to age: 18% of the concrete operational, but also 12% of the advanced intermediate participants were only 12 years old. At the other end of the age range, 14% of the concrete-operational and 32% of the advanced intermediate participants were at least 17 years old. Thus, deductive-reasoning performance is only partly age-dependent.

This example shows how development can manifest in qualitative changes in the pattern of item difficulties within a scale. Interestingly, while for the fallacy items, correct responses were more probable in the more advanced latent classes, the nonfallacies were actually more difficult. This makes sense as participants in the more advanced classes probably think about the items in a more complex way. Thus, they have a larger probability to commit errors in those items that are actually relatively easy.

More conceptually, the syllogistic-reasoning data are a good illustration of qualitative changes in the structure of a scale. As the scale is measuring substantively different latent dimensions in the different latent classes, it makes no sense to quantitatively compare sum scores of participants in different latent classes. Such qualitative changes in scale meaning may be a frequent phenomenon that is not necessarily reflected in classical measures such as reliability (see, e.g., Glück & Indurkhya, 2001).

18.2.2 Scale-Level Hypotheses

Very often, substantive researchers assume age group differences on the scale level without looking into such differences at the item level. Scale-level changes (or stability) can, however, be largely meaningless if they are the result of subgroups of items changing in different ways. For example, if one part of the items becomes easier while others become more difficult, the overall result would be "no change," which would not be true for a single item of the scale. Differences between items can be relevant for the interpretation of age group differences, and they can provide interesting substantive information. Test developers quite routinely test for such differential item functioning (DIF) across age groups, but, for example, attitude or personality questionnaires are seldom evaluated using Rasch-based methods such as mixed RMs.

The question whether age differences are the same across all items can routinely be tested using Andersen's (1973c) likelihood ratio test, a goodness-of-fit test for the RM that examines whether item difficulty patterns differ across groups of participants. The following example illustrates the procedure.

The European Study of Adult Well-Being (ESAW) is a cross-sectional study of individuals aged 50 to 90 years that was conducted in six European countries, involving representative samples of around 2000 participants per country (see *http://www.bangor.ac.uk/esaw*). The main goal was to study the influences of five factors—material resources, health, social support, activity, and self variables—on well-being. In the self-variables section, among other scales, participants filled out Paulhus' (1983) personal-control scale. For reliability issues, only five of the originally ten items of this scale were used in the data analyses.

For the analyses presented here, data from the Austrian ESAW sample (Weber et al., 2005) were used. Participants were divided into two age groups: 50 to 69 ($N = 1516$) and 70 to 90 years ($N = 599$). On the scale level, the younger age group had a significantly higher mean in personal control ($M = .68$ on a 0-to-1 scale, $SD = .29$) than the older age group ($M = .60$, $SD = .30$), $t(2102) = 5.897$, $p < .001$. To test whether this result really reflects quantitative overall changes, we compared the item difficulty patterns in the two age groups using Andersen's test. The original item responses were recoded from a seven-point scale to a dichotomous format. As is typical with control scales, agreement rates to the items were quite high. Therefore, categories 1 to 5 ("strongly disagree" to "slightly agree" were coded as 0), and only categories

6 and 7 ("agree" and "strongly agree") were coded as 1. Note, however, that such post-hoc reductions of response categories have been critically discussed in the literature (Andrich, 1995b,a; Andrich et al., 1997; P. G. W. Jansen & Roskam, 1986; Müller, 1995; Roskam, 1995; Roskam & Jansen, 1989). For a complete analysis of polytomous data, RMs for polytomous item responses such as the partial-credit model or the rating-scale model should additionally be used in order to identify potential (age) group differences in use of the response categories. Such analyses were difficult to perform with the present data because of the unequal response distributions.

In our analysis, the Andersen likelihood ratio test was significant, χ^2 (4) = 65.97, $p < .001$. Figure 18.2 shows the agreement frequencies for each item in the two age groups. The items are sorted by size of age difference.

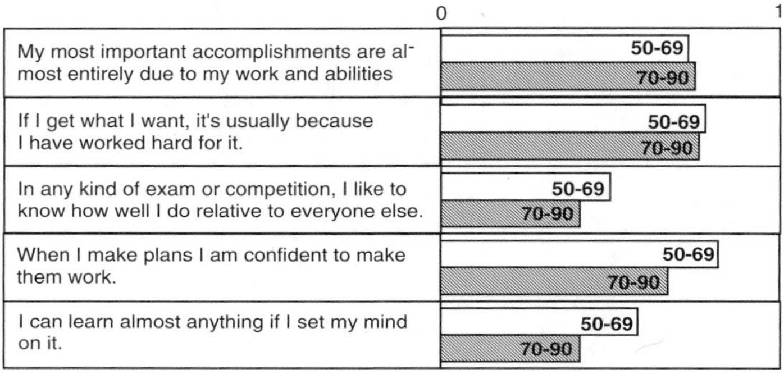

Fig. 18.2. Age-group differences in agreement frequencies in the ESAW control scale

As the figure shows, the first two items show almost no age differences in agreement rates. The first item clearly refers to past accomplishments, the second can also be interpreted as past-related. The next three items are more future-oriented—knowing ones standing in a competition is useful mostly for future instances, making plans confidently and learning things are clearly oriented towards improving ones future. It makes sense that the older participants show less agreement to these items.

What do such results mean substantively? If a 60-year-old has agreed to one item in this scale, it most likely was "When I make plans, I am confident to make them work." An 80-year-old with the same score has more probably agreed to "My most important accomplishments are almost entirely due to my work and abilities." Thus, though numerically identical, these two scores reflect different views about control. It would be incorrect to say that the two participants do not differ in perceived personal control, and the same goes for any other numerical score. As a basic assumption of the RM states, score comparisons make conceptual sense only if there are no (age) differences in item difficulty patterns. In addition to this "technical" issue, however, the pattern reflected in these data is substantively interesting. Older participants show the same level of agreement as younger ones to items that refer to the past, and lower levels of agreement with respect to current and future-related control. This result speaks to the necessity of differential analyses of relationships of these two control aspects to other variables.

18.2.3 Item-Level Hypotheses

In some cases, researchers have clear hypotheses about age differences in different item types. For example, Draney and Wilson (see chapter 7 in this volume) report a study on using the saltus model (Wilson, 1989) to study children's propositional reasoning. The items used in this study were systematically constructed so as to reflect different levels of cognitive development: On each level, children should be able to solve a new type of items and all items from previous levels. The results, obtained by using constrained versions of mixture RMs, largely confirmed the expectations. As in the syllogisms example given above, class membership was related to age. Other applications of the saltus model were reported by Demetriou et al. (1993), with respect to the development of causal experimental thought in adolescence, and by Wilson (1989).

In other cases, a researcher may want to directly test hypotheses about differences between specific age groups in item difficulty patterns. Such hypotheses about age group differences in certain items or groups of items can be directly tested using a new nonparametric family of RM tests (Ponocny, 2001), or by using multidimensional models such as MULTIRA (Carstensen & Rost, 2001) or the multidimensional random coefficient multinomial logit model (Adams, Wilson, & Wang, 1997) with the corresponding software Conquest (Wu et al., 1997).

18.3 Longitudinal Designs

18.3.1 Data Structures

Longitudinal designs have the clear advantage that changes in item difficulty can be observed within the same sample of individuals over time. Technically, the situation is somewhat complicated by the fact that the underlying structure of the data is three-dimensional (n participants by k items by t time points) while common item response models are designed for two-dimensional participants by items matrices. Various ways of dealing with this problem have been suggested. One is to treat the different time points as independent data, thus obtaining a data set that has t x n virtual persons (Rost, 1989; Rost & Spada, 1983; Spada & McGaw, 1985). Especially when using mixture models, this approach has the advantage that sample size is technically increased, and class membership probabilities for each individual at each time point can be directly estimated. Therefore, changes in class membership are easy to analyze (see, e.g., Glück & Spiel, 1997). The disadvantage of this method is that local dependencies between responses to the same item are ignored, which violates a basic assumption of the RM. The effect of this violation in practice has not yet been systematically studied.

A second way of dealing with three-dimensional data structures is treating each item as a test of its own, with t virtual items reflecting participants' item responses to the test at each time point. This approach is used in the linear logistic model with relaxed assumptions (Fischer, 1976, 1983, 1989, 1995d,b; Fischer & Formann, 1982). This model can be used in a very flexible way because it allows researchers to test hypotheses about differences in changes between items as well as between individuals (see below). Meiser et al. (1995) used a longitudinal mixture RM on this type of data structure, thus directly identifying subgroups of participants with different trajectories of change.

The third possibility is to treat the data from each time point as different items in one long test. Thus, the data set has N persons and t x k items. Because of the increased number of items, this approach can run into technical problems with larger sets of items, and restrictions are necessary for parameter estimations: item parameters from later time points are modeled as item parameters from t1 plus some change parameters that can be specific to person and item groups. Fischer's linear logistic test model for longitudinal data (see, e.g., Fischer, 1995d,b) as well as related models such as Andersen's (1985; 1991) model and Embretson's (1991) model fall into this category. The one practical disadvantage of this approach is that it requires that the RM holds for the pretest data, which is often not the case.

Loglinear representations of RMs for longitudinal data (Meiser, this volume; see also Meiser, 1996) use the same data structure, but are more flexible in the hypotheses they can test. This very general approach incorporates all hypothesis-testing approaches that we describe in this chapter and allows for flexible modeling of many types of hypotheses about change. Its only disadvantages are the size and complexity of the design matrices that need to be specified and, in longitudinal cases, the above mentioned sample size issue.

Exploratory Research Questions

A typical exploratory case would be a researcher who, similar to the case for cross-sectional data, is interested in whether there are subgroups of participants in a sample that differ in item difficulty patterns. As the data are longitudinal, one interesting question is whether subgroup membership is constant over time, and if not, whether changes in membership are systematic. Meiser (this volume) gives an example of a mover-stayer mixed RM formulated and tested in the longitudinal mixed RM context; the analysis is described in more detail by Meiser et al. (1998).

Another example is the following. Glück et al. (2002) studied the effects of a mental rotation training on solution strategies in a cube comparison test (IST). A total of 205 participants, divided into a control group and a training group, participated; the training group had about five hours of training between pre- and posttest. Previous studies had identified three types of cube comparison items in the IST: (1) items that could be solved using a non-spatial strategy (i.e., assuming that two cubes are identical if they show the same three patterns on their faces, independent of the patterns' positions), (2) items that could be solved by this strategy plus additional considerations to decide between two remaining distractors, and (3) items that required spatial cognition. In addition to testing specific hypotheses about item-level changes (which will be described below), we used mixed RMs to test for the presence of distinguishable subgroups of participants at pretest. As the sample was relatively small, we only analyzed the responses to a subset of five items, which contained at least one item of each type. In addition, we evaluated the stability of our solution using bootstrap analyses.

Both information criteria and chi-square statistics suggested that the two-classes solution fit the pretest data best. One class had a very high solution probability for the items that did not require spatial cognition. For items that did require spatial cognition, solution probabilities were relatively low. Thus, we assumed that these participants indeed used a nonspatial strategy. The other class had intermediate solution probabilities for both types of items, and we assumed that they used spatial cognition for all items. The question now was whether the same two classes would be found after the training, and if yes, whether training participants had predominantly shifted from the nonspatial to the spatial strategy. However, the posttest data were better described by a one-class solution than by two classes. The item difficulties in the one-class model were similar, but not identical, to those of the second latent class at pretest. Thus, the data suggested that independent of training, most participants had shifted to the spatial-cognition strategy. However, the result was not quite convincing because the posttest item difficulties were not identical to those at pretest. We then used a direct theory-guided class assignment to clarify this question: In other cases, however, restricted-mixture models, directly testing whether the same latent classes hold across time points, may be more useful.

As mentioned above, another exploratory approach is to directly look for subgroups showing different longitudinal patterns within items. Meiser et al. (1998) analyzed such longitudinal trajectories for two personality variables (activity and adjustment) measured in about 600 children when they were 10, 11, and 12 years old. Mixed rating scale models resulted in two classes for both variables: one class with largely stable responses, the other class showing a peak at the second time point. With respect to activity, there was a tendency for boys to be more often in the latter class than girls, and with respect to adjustment, there was a significant effect in the opposite direction.

A different exploratory approach could directly look for differences in the amount of change between items. In such a case, a linear logistic model with relaxed assumptions (LLRA) could be specified that assumes one change parameter per item and (if necessary) per predefined person group. Such models are often used as base models against which more restricted models can be tested (see below for an example). However, in some cases (and with sufficiently large samples) it may make sense to directly interpret the item-specific change parameters. To check whether two parameters are significantly different, a more restricted model in which the two parameters are set equal can be tested. Glück & Spiel (in press) present an analysis of changes in personality scales in very old age using a more exploratory approach.

Scale-Level Hypotheses

There are two types of hypotheses in this group. On the one hand, a researcher may want to test whether longitudinal changes in scores are generalizable across all items. The most straightforward test of this assumption is using the linear logistic model with relaxed assumptions (LLRA).

Glück & Indurkhya (2001) used the LLRA to analyze changes and potential gender differences in aggressive behavior in children. A total of 219 children were rated by their teachers with respect to aggressive behavior when they were 8, 10, and 13 years old. An Andersen test comparing boys and girls at $t1$ showed that there might be a dissociation between physical (e.g., harming others, fighting) and nonphysical (e.g., being stubborn, teasing classmates) aggressive behaviors. The former was more frequent in boys, the latter in girls. Thus, we tested a series of LLRA models starting from a quasi-saturated model distinguishing the two types of aggressive behavior, boys, girls, and $t1$-$t2$ and $t2$-$t3$ changes. We then tested a number of more restrictive models against this base model. None of these more restrictive models—assuming equal changes in the two groups of items, assuming equal changes across boys and girls—fit the data. Thus, the first model provided the relatively best data description. Physical aggression decreased in both boys and girls from age 8 to 10, and increased again afterward in girls; nonphysically aggressive behavior increased in boys between age 10 and 13. This example again shows that in order to interpret a change in scores as a change in the underlying dimension, the stability of item difficulty patterns needs to be proved: Even if a child's score in the aggression scale stays the same over time, the child's way of expressing aggression may have dramatically changed.

On the other hand, there are cases where the RM holds for a test or questionnaire, and the researcher does not expect differences between groups of items, but wants to test whether predefined subgroups of participants differ in change, e.g., due to some interventions. For example, Gittler & Glück (1998) used the linear logistic test model to analyze changes in spatial ability in secondary school students who took descriptive geometry (DG) classes. They used the three-dimensional cubes test (3DC), a spatial ability test that had been constructed using the RM (Gittler, 1990). Over a period of about 20 months, a control group who did not take DG classes did not show any changes in 3DC performance, but DG participants improved significantly, and girls improved more than boys.

Other examples of this type come from Embretson's (1991; 1995a; 2000) work on dynamic testing. In these approaches, items are presented to participants under different conditions (e.g., before vs. after an intervention, under presence vs. absence of stressors). Performance levels in the different conditions are compared using RMs. These methods allow for quantifying the effects of different conditions on performance both on the group and on the individual level. These approaches are interesting in the context of developmental research because they may allow for examining the "limits" of a person's current performance level, in the sense of Wygotsky's zone of proximal development (see Embretson, 2000).

Item-Level Hypotheses

Researchers may have explicit hypotheses about differences in change between different types of items. In the training study on spatial ability by Glück et al. (2002) described above, we derived specific hypotheses about change for the three item types of the IST. Used the LLRA, we tested a number of models against a "quasi-saturated" model containing two parameters per item: one for the control group and one for the training group. Models assuming no differences in change between control and training group and no differences across items were rejected. A model assuming no change in the control group and item-type-specific change in the training group fit the data well, and even better when only two item types were distinguished: items requiring and not requiring spatial cognition. Both change parameters in the training group were significantly different from zero, but the training effect for the items requiring spatial cognition was three times as large as for the other items.

18.4 Discussion and Conclusions

The main aim of this chapter was to show the wide spectrum of possible applications of Rasch-based methods in developmental psychology. We consider the use of this methodology to be an important and informative tool. In our view, any cross-sectional or longitudinal comparison of test scores should be accompanied by tests of equivalence of item difficulty patterns, for example by means of analyses with longitudinal versions of the mixed RM. If there is no such equivalence, comparison of scores is misleading.

As this type of equivalence is hardly ever tested, an interesting question is how often such a lack of equivalence would occur. Fischer (2003) stated that such changes should be an exception because tests should be constructed so as to measure the same latent trait for anybody. Our own experience shows that violations of item difficulty invariance occurs relatively often both in intelligence tests, especially if they were not constructed using IRT or RMs, and in questionnaires (which are hardly ever IRT-based). While completely agreeing with Fischer that the careful construction of tests is very important to guarantee test fairness, we also want to emphasize that age differences in item difficulty patterns may be more than just "noise" that needs to be removed in test development. They may reflect interesting processes of change that can contribute to our understanding of development. In the current, computer-based version of the syllogism test that was described above (Spiel et al., 2001, 2004), examinees are not just described by a score, but their response patterns are used to assign them to one of the latent classes described above. Thus, their current qualitative level of development, as well as their quantitative standing within that level, can be diagnosed. Similarly, it may make sense to compare a 60-year-old's response pattern in a questionnaire to those of 60-, 70-, and 80-year-olds—if he or she responds more like an 80-year-old, this is of importance and of potential diagnostic value.

18.4.1 Potential Problems

Although extensions of RMs for longitudinal data allow for important insights about the substantive nature of change, practical problems may sometimes limit their applicability. One important problem with longitudinal approaches is that no good way of dealing with missing values has been developed yet (see, however, von Davier & Yamamoto, 2004b). In most cases, analyses are limited to participants with complete data, thus, when study dropout is systematically related to variables of interest, these analyses will be biased (as are any other analyses that require complete data).

Another potential problem is that RMs require relatively large sample sizes. This is especially problematic in longitudinal approaches that model t x k items, and less of a problem in those approaches that model t virtual items (i.e., each item as a test of its own). As the problems result from the number of possible response patterns, they are the more severe the larger the number of items, the larger the number of categories, and the smaller the sample. Therefore, selecting representative items and recoding to a smaller number of categories may sometimes help. Some software programs, such as WINMIRA (von Davier, 2001), allow for bootstrap analyses of goodness of fit statistics to evaluate the stability of results in smaller samples.

A third issue concerns the exploratory models we have presented. As with any exploratory approach, especially when patterns are identified, cross-validation is very important, but not always easy to accomplish. Softwares that allow for setting restrictions in mixture models are very helpful here.

In spite of these difficulties, which will hopefully be overcome by future software generations, we hope to have shown that RMs are an important tool for developmental research. Analyses on the item level may help to explain many seemingly surprising findings on the scale level.

A Comparison of the Rasch Model and Constrained Item Response Theory Models for Pertinent Psychological Test Data

Klaus D. Kubinger[1] and Clemens Draxler[2]

[1] Vienna University
[2] Leibniz Institute for Science Education, Kiel

19.1 Introduction

This paper provides an application of a generalization of the dichotomous Rasch model (RM) to the study of guessing behavior of respondents to typical achievement tests. One of the models applied is a constrained version of the 3PL model where a lower asymptote parameter is assumed in order to account for guessing behavior, but no variation of item discrimination is modeled. In addition, an application of mixture-distribution RMs aimed at modeling guessing effects and a comparison of the two approaches is presented. If such a constrained 3PL model is applied, in particular, to tests consisting of multiple-choice formatted items, the lower asymptote parameter can be interpreted as a guessing parameter. Therefore, the model is called the difficulty plus guessing PL (DGPL) model. An empirical example shows that a multiple-choice item pool only fits the Rasch model after a large number of items have been deleted, while the DGPL model can save most of those deleted items as it takes the severe but item-specific guessing effects into consideration. Furthermore, multiclass mixed RM analyses show — in comparison to the Rasch model — a good fit of the data and confirm item-specific guessing effects.

Since the first publication of the model now known as the Rasch model in 1960 (cf. Rasch, 1980; often called 1PL model — PL for parameter logistic), several psychological tests have been constructed using this model. Although there are various concurrent IRT (item response theory) models, the RM is often — in particular, for European applications — preferred for two reasons. Firstly due to the simplicity of the model. As it is based on just a single item parameter, the parameter estimation doesn't need as large sample sizes as is necessary for the well-known 2PL or 3PL model (Birnbaum, 1968). Furthermore, we have simple sufficient statistics and the possibility of a specific objective parameter estimation, which is the well-known conditional maximum likelihood method (CML). Thus, we can carry out a conditional likelihood ratio test (Andersen, 1973c) to check the model assumption of statistically equal item-parameter estimates obtained from different subpopulations. Secondly, a mathematical proof (cf. Fischer, 1995a) shows that the RM has a particularly useful property. An examinees number of correct responses to a set of items can be considered as a sufficient statistic for a latent trait parameter (person parameter), which is an adequate and fair representation of the empirical relations of proficiency of this examinees of test performance and any other examinees', if and only if the dichotomous RM or a monotone transformation of it) holds for the set of items under consideration.

Perhaps the best known psychological tests calibrated according to the RM are the BAS II (*British Ability Scales II*; Elliot et al., 1996) and its American edition DAS (*Differential Ability Scales*; Elliot, 1990), the K-ABC (*Kaufman Assessment-Battery for children*; Kaufman & Kaufman, 1983), and, within German speaking countries, the AID 2 (*Adaptive Intelligence Diagnosticum — version 2.1*; Kubinger & Wurst, 2000).

There are several tests that have been constructed using the RM, even though they are administered in a multiple-choice format. In such a case, the examinees guessing strategies have to be taken into account. All the tests cited above, however, use a free response format. In the case of multiple-choice responses, an RM fit seems less likely for an item pool because the model obviously postulates the probability of a correct response of examinee v on item i depending on the person parameter θ_v of v and an item-difficulty parameter β_i of i. The lower asymptote of the item-characteristic curve approaches zero for $\theta_v \rightarrow -\infty$. Thus, there is no effect modeled to (lucky or systematic) guessing. Therefore, if such tests are found to fit the RM, it might be due to two reasons — in case the actual severe guessing effects are not all exactly the same: There are either enough distractors and, thus, guessing effects are almost negligible or, a lot of items have been deleted as pertinent model checks have proved that they explicitly do not fit the RM. Those items probably consist of distractors of number or content, which establish severe guessing effects.

In this paper, we analyze an example of such a test with respect to the problem of misfit due to guessing. The question is whether it is possible to retain items that would have otherwise been deleted in an RM analysis by applying a more general model with an additional item-guessing parameter or a mixture-distribution model. Such a model can also be used as a tool to detect items where guessing occurs in order to give the researcher an indication as to which item and/or which distractors of the multiple-choice format need to be modified. Although a number of alternative models for guessing do exist, we propose to consider a model for the construction of multiple-choice tests as a special case of the 3PL model, where the item discrimination parameter is set to be equal for all items. In addition, we will compare the proposed constrained 3PL to two alternative models further on in this paper, which provide us with the opportunity to model the existence of guessing, but to us seem less suitable for constructing unidimensional psychological measures.

These are the mixed RM (Rost, 1990) and a HYBRID model (Yamamoto, 1989).

19.2 Birnbaum's 3PL Model

As it is well-known, the 3PL model provides, in addition to the real valued person parameter θ_v of examinee v and the real valued item-difficulty parameter β_i of item i, a positive real valued item discrimination parameter α_i and an item-guessing parameter c_i of item i. Let X_{vi} be a Bernoulli distributed response variable with realizations $X_{vi} = x_{vi} = 1$ for a correct response of v to item i and $X_{vi} = x_{vi} = 0$ for an incorrect response. According to the model, the probability of a correct response to item i for examinee v amounts to

$$P(X_{vi} = 1 | \theta_v; \alpha_i, \beta_i, c_i) = c_i + (1 - c_i) \frac{\exp[\alpha_i(\theta_v - \beta_i)]}{1 + \exp[\alpha_i(\theta_v - \beta_i)]} \qquad (19.1)$$

with $\alpha_i > 0$ and $0 \leq c_i \leq 1$.

The probability of an incorrect response decreases with c_i, that is, $\lim_{\theta \to -\infty} P(X_{vi} = 0/\theta_v; \alpha_i, \beta_i, c_i) = 1 - c_i$.

In the case that all $c_i = 0$ the model is reduced to the 2PL model. When, in addition, all α_i are set to be equal, the RM (1PL model) is obtained. What is of interest now, however, is the case where all α_i are set to be equal but the c_i are not constrained to zero. This results in a model that, like the RM, assumes equal discrimination for all items.

However, by introducing a guessing parameter, we get rid of all the convenient properties of the RM. No sufficient statistic for the person parameter exists any more. Hence, we forsake the possibility of separating the parameters and applying the CML method. Consequently, we cannot assess the goodness of fit of the model with Andersen's conditional likelihood ratio test. Loosely speaking, these statistical properties are the justification for talking about "Rasch models." Thus, it would probably be better not to call this model a "RM with a guessing parameter" (cf. Puchhammer, 1989). We prefer to call the model "difficulty plus guessing PL model" (DGPL). Although such a model sounds trivial, it has hardly ever been taken into account before.

19.3 Parameter Estimation in the Difficulty Plus Guessing PL Model

Because a sufficient statistic does not exist for the DGPL model and thus the CML method is not applicable, the model parameters have to be estimated either jointly (JML) or by the marginal maximum likelihood method (MML). As far as the former is concerned, there are relevant results from simulation studies conducted by Puchhammer (1989). He showed that the estimation of the item-guessing parameters becomes rather inaccurate when the number of examinees is less than 500. In such a case, even the item-difficulty parameters are biased. Furthermore, the distribution of the person parameters has to be of a great variance otherwise item-parameter estimates will not be accurate enough. At any rate, the person parameter estimation becomes less reliable as the ability of the testees decreases. As a matter of fact, Puchhammer (1989) also showed that item pools that have been simulated according to the difficulty plus guessing 1PL model do not actually fit the RM.

More generally, for instance, Andersen (1971, 1973a) and Haberman (1977b) have shown that JML estimates are inconsistent for the number of fixed items k but $n \to \cdot \infty$. This is because the incidental person parameters cannot be conditioned out of the likelihood function and the number of person parameters increases with $n \to \infty$. However, to achieve consistency of ML (maximum likelihood) estimates the number of unknown parameters must be finite when $n \to \infty$ (cf. Fischer, 1974). This is obviously not the case concerning the person parameters. Due to the inconsistency of the parameter estimates and the results of the simulation studies from Puchhammer (1989) as well as the fact that most computer programs use the MML method (e.g., BILOG-MG 3, Zimowski et al. (2003) — which is also used for our analyses), we will avoid the JML method.

The MML method (Bock & Aitkin, 1981), however, requires the estimation or an assumption of the form of the latent trait distribution, that is the distribution of the θ_v. It is assumed that the sample of examinees is randomly drawn from this distribution. For this it is convenient to write our DGPL model as a continuous mixture-distribution model with θ as the (continuous) mixing variable (see von Davier & Rost, 1995). When doing so the unconditional or marginal probability of an observed response vector $\boldsymbol{x}_v = (x_{v1}, \dots, x_{vi}, \dots, x_{vk})$ is given by

$$P(\boldsymbol{X}_v = \boldsymbol{x}_v / \phi(\theta); \boldsymbol{\beta}, \boldsymbol{c}) = \int_{-\infty}^{+\infty} \prod_{i=1}^{k} f_i(\theta)^{x_{vi}} [1 - f_i(\theta)]^{1-x_{vi}} \phi(\theta) d\theta,$$

where

$$f_i(\theta) = \frac{c_i + \exp(\theta - \beta_i)}{1 + \exp(\theta - \beta_i)}. \tag{19.2}$$

$\phi(\theta)$ is the probability distribution of the latent variable θ. β and c are the vectors of the difficulty and guessing parameters, respectively. The observed stochastic response variable X_{vi} is described by conditional probability functions, whereby the variable on which the probabilities are conditioned is the mixing variable θ. In other words, the probability of a correct response to item i is considered under the condition (of all values) of the density of the latent trait, $\phi(\theta)$.

The marginal likelihood of a response pattern x_{v1} is obtained by integrating the conditional pattern probability over the ability distribution $\phi(\theta)$. The total likelihood of the the data is obtained by assuming independence of observations and multiplying the marginal response patterns across all examinees. Equation 19.2 is a function of the item parameters (β_i, c_i) only and of the parameters of the assumed latent density $\phi(\theta)$. Often, a normal distribution of the latent trait θ is assumed and its parameters, the mean and variance, are estimated jointly with the item parameters. This ensures that the number of unknown parameters is fixed when $n \to \infty$ so that the statistical information for an accurate estimation of those parameters can arbitrarily be increased. For more details for the MML method and the numerical solutions for the MML equations by appropriate algorithms, such as the Newton–Raphson procedure or the EM-algorithm, see Andersen (1977), Sanathanan & Blumenthal (1978), and Bock & Aitkin (1981).

In the program BILOG MG 3, the Gaussian quadrature formula is applied to approximate the marginal probability 19.2 as accurately as required (see Zimowski et al., 2003). Thus, the integral structure is reduced to a sum whereby the number of summands or quadrature points has to be specified by the user.

It is well known that the scales of the parameters of IRT models are, in the first instance, undetermined. The unit and the origin of the scale have to be fixed by appropriate constraints. In the RM, the indeterminacy of the model parameters (in the case of CML estimation) is solved by restricting the item-difficulty parameters to the sum of zero — and to set the item discrimination parameter α_i in 19.1 as equal to one for all items. For our DGPL model, however, we use another widely accepted approach. Due to the fact that the MML estimation requires an assumption of the latent trait distribution, we fix the location of the scale by setting the mean of the latent distribution to zero and we also fix the unit of the scale by setting the standard deviation as equal to one. In this case the common discrimination of all items amounts to $\alpha_i = \alpha$ for $i = 1, \ldots k$, (which is referred to as the scale parameter) and has to be estimated additionally to the item difficulty and the item-guessing parameters. Thus, the marginal probability 19.2 is a function of the item parameters only.

However, in order to achieve a simpler model the scale parameter may also be fixed at an arbitrary value. In order to obtain a concrete value for the common discrimination of all items (which can then be fixed for the DGPL model analyses) one can use the mean of the unconstrained estimated item discrimination parameters of the 3PL model.

Finally, we will also place a constraint distribution on one set of item parameters. For keeping the item-guessing parameter estimates within the admissible interval $0 \leq c_i \leq 1$ BILOG MG 3 assumes a beta prior distribution for the c_i. The choice of the parameters of the assumed beta distribution depends on the number of response alternatives of the (multiple-choice formatted) items. For more details, see Zimowski et al. (2003).

The disadvantage of the MML method is, however, that it does not provide estimates for the person parameters θ_v. Perhaps the most promising method for obtaining these estimates is the Bayes or EAP (expected a posteriori) estimator (see Bock & Aitkin, 1981), which is, amongst another Bayes and a ML estimator, also implemented in BILOG MG 3.

19.4 Method

In order to calibrate a given item pool, we use the following strategy:

Firstly, we analyze the item pool using the RM by applying the software LPCM-WIN 1.0 (Fischer & Ponocny-Seliger, 1998). The CML method will be applied in order to obtain item-difficulty parameter estimates and a model fit will be assessed using Andersen's conditional likelihood ratio test.[1] The partition of the sample will be carried out with respect to three criteria: "examinees with low *vs.* high score"; "male *vs.* female examinees"; "younger *vs.* older examinees." We are aware of a higher factual than nominal type-I-risk in doing so, therefore we use a nominal type-I-risk of $\alpha = 0.01$. We are aware that the quite large sample ($n = 4153$) is an advantage for parameter estimation but at the same time a disadvantage for testing the goodness of fit of the model. Because the power of a statistical test increases with sample size, even irrelevant differences of item-parameter estimates in the two subsamples may become significant when applying a likelihood ratio test. However, the chosen significance level of $\alpha = 0.01$ is a way to counteract that effect, at least to some degree. The decision as to which items are to be deleted is based on Rasch's graphical model check, whereby item-parameter estimates of the first subsample of examinees are contrasted to item-parameter estimates from the second subsample, as well as on the z_i-values from Fischer & Scheiblechner (1970), where the difference of the item-parameter estimates (per item) obtained from two subsamples is divided by the square root of the sum of the error variances from the corresponding parameter estimates. The latter yields an asymptotically normally distributed test statistic. Items are deleted stepwise until we obtain insignificant likelihood ratio test with respect to all partition criteria or until certain fit indices disclose a satisfying model fit. The statistic that will be applied is the conditional item fit index (Q-index) from Rost & von Davier (1994).

Secondly, we analyze the item pool according to the DGPL model using BILOG MG 3 (Zimowski et al., 2003). To assess model fit we apply a likelihood ratio χ^2-fit statistic for every item that is incorporated in BILOG MG 3. The significance level will again be $\alpha = 0.01$. To compute this statistic the latent

---

[1] Since the very beginning of RM applications and the establishment of Andersen's LRT, many different model checks have been proposed. Kubinger (1989), as well as Glas & Verhelst (1995), give an overview; for more recent ones see Waldherr (2001). From the latter, the model check from Verguts & De Boeck (2001), a generalization of the Mantel–Haenszel χ^2-statistic, is of major importance because it offers the possibility of testing several more RM presuppositions other than those discussed in this paper.

continuum is divided into a number of intervals. Each examinee is assigned to an interval on the basis of the EAP estimates of the person parameters θ_v. The following statistic may be used to compare the observed frequency r_{hi} of correct responses to item i in interval h with the probability or expected proportion $P_i(\bar{\theta}_h)$ of correct responses to i at the point $\bar{\theta}_h$, which is the average ability of examinees belonging to interval h:

$$G_i^2 = 2 \sum_{h=1}^{n_g} \left[r_{hi} \ln \frac{r_{hi}}{N_h P_i(\bar{\theta}_h)} + (N_h - r_{hi}) \ln \frac{N_h - r_{hi}}{N_h [1 - P_i(\bar{\theta}_h)]} \right], \qquad (19.3)$$

where n_g is the number of intervals and N_h is the number of examinees assigned to interval h. If necessary, adjacent intervals are merged to avoid expected values $N_h \cdot P_i(\bar{\theta}_h)$ less than 5. The number of degrees of freedom is equal to the number of remaining intervals. Unfortunately, an overall goodness of fit test is only available for very short tests ($k \leq 10$; cf. Zimowski et al., 2003) with the presupposition that (nearly) all 2^k possible response patterns have been observed — and this requires large sample sizes.

Thirdly, we have to decide whether the DGPL model does indeed explain the data better than the RM. For this, we proceed with the following two stages. If the model fit according to the fit statistics is almost equal for both models then, the first stage involves the question as to whether more items fit the DGPL model than the RM. The second stage only concerns the items that fit the RM. We apply a likelihood ratio test based on the maxima of the marginal likelihoods of the data X for both models

$$G^2 = -2 \ln \frac{mL(\hat{\alpha}, \hat{\boldsymbol{\beta}}, \mu, \sigma; \boldsymbol{X})}{mL(\hat{\alpha}, \hat{\boldsymbol{\beta}}, \hat{\boldsymbol{c}}, \mu, \sigma; \boldsymbol{X})}, \qquad (19.4)$$

where $\hat{\boldsymbol{\beta}} = (\hat{\beta}_1, ... \hat{\beta}_i, ... \hat{\beta}_k)$ and $\hat{\boldsymbol{c}} = (\hat{c}_1, ... \hat{c}_i, ... \hat{c}_k)$ are the vectors of the ML estimates of the item-difficulty and item-guessing parameters, and $\hat{\alpha}$ is the estimate of the scale parameter or the common discrimination of all items.[2] As mentioned above, $\mu = 0$ and $\sigma = 1$ are the parameters of the assumed (standard) normal density. The null hypothesis of the validity of the RM can be tested against the more general alternative of the DGPL model, if the latter model is assumed to be true. Although no formal proof exists of the distributional properties of the test statistic (19.4) of this special likelihood ratio test under the null hypothesis, we assume an asymptotic χ^2-distribution (cf. Glas & Verhelst, 1995, p. 86, and the references there) with degrees of freedom equal to the difference of the number of parameters estimated in the

---

[2] The scale parameter α must be estimated for the RM if using a prior standard normal density for θ. Thus, the number of independent parameters is equal to k+1. In the DGPL model, we set α equal to the mean of the estimated discrimination parameters of an unconstrained 3PL model. The number of estimated or independent parameters will then be equal to $2k$ (the sum of the number of item-difficulty and item-guessing parameters).

DGPL model and the number of estimated parameters in the RM. The aim of this likelihood ratio test is to decide whether the DGPL model can explain the data based on the Rasch conform items even (significantly) better than the RM itself. If this happens to be true, it would imply that scoring according to the RM would no longer be the most proper measurement of a examinee's ability.

Fourthly, we carry out the same procedure, that being the application of the likelihood ratio test (Equation 19.4) with respect to those items that fit the DGPL model — in the case that there are actually more items that fit the DGPL model than the RM. If the likelihood ratio test (19.4) then indicates that the DGPL model can (significantly) explain the data better than the RM, then the guessing effect is confirmed: the item pool is not sufficiently utilized by the RM with regard to the item pool's psychometric potential.

Lastly, as already indicated we estimate alternative models, namely extensions of the RM that provide an alternative for modeling the existence of guessing. That is to say, we use the mixed RM and a HYBRID model, both of which can be estimated using the software WINMIRA (von Davier, 2001).

19.5 Applications

To illustrate an application of the DGPL model, we analyze data from 4153 examinees who took an intelligence test battery.[3] For our analyses we chose the first subtest (verbal comprehension), which consists of 20 items. The response format is multiple choice with 5 response alternatives (the correct answer plus 4 distractors).

Some results from the Rasch analyses of the 20 items are given in Table 19.1. Andersen's likelihood ratio test with a partition of the sample according to the criterion "examinees with low $vs.$ high score" is significant ($\chi^2 = 318.8071, df = 19$; the critical χ^2 at $\alpha = 0.01$ is 36.216). The likelihood ratio test carried out with respect to the criteria "male $vs.$ female examinees" and "younger $vs.$ older examinees" are also significant. After the stepwise deletion of 9 misfitting items according to Rasch's graphical model check and the described z_i-values, we obtained an insignificant likelihood ratio test with respect to the criterion score ($\chi^2 = 21.9095, df = 10$; the critical χ^2 at $\alpha = 0.01$ is 23.239). However, the two likelihood ratio test with respect to the criteria gender and age are still significant (gender: $\chi^2 = 46.3723, df = 10$; age: $\chi^2 = 211.3766, df = 10$). Of course, this indicates, in the first instance, some amount of differential item functioning, but in view of the large sample size and particularly in view of the graphical model check (see Figure 19.1),

---

[3] We want to thank *Harcourt Test Services* and its general manager, Dr. Ralf Horn, for placing the data at our disposal. The test battery has been in practical use for years but was removed from the market because of issues regarding item copyright. However, the data copyright is by *Harcourt Test Services*.

we conclude that the 9 item reduced data set fits the RM well enough — the graphical model check discloses that differences of item-parameter estimates in the two respective subgroups are rather negligible. Moreover, the conditional item fit statistic from Rost and von Davier (1994; Q_i-index) also discloses an acceptable fit of the reduced item pool (cf. Table 19.2). The 9 deleted items may, therefore, establish either severe guessing effects or discrimination effects.

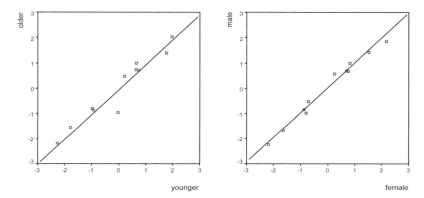

Fig. 19.1. Graphical goodness-of-fit tests of the reduced item set for the two external partition criteria age and gender

The results of the analyses of the total data set with the DGPL model are as follows. The fixed scale parameter resulted as $\alpha = 1.427$. The estimates of the item-difficulty and the item-guessing parameters as well as the special likelihood ratio test χ^2 fit statistics are given in Table 19.3. Unfortunately, a global goodness of fit test is not possible because the number of unobserved response patterns is too high, even though the sample size is quite large.

Both the special likelihood ratio test χ^2 statistics based on 15 ability intervals (given in the Table 19.3) and the z_i-values computed for the criterion score (given in the Tables 19.1 and 19.2) are sensitive to differences of the observed and the expected proportions of correct responses — expected in the sense that the respective model is assumed to be valid. If, for instance, the number of correct responses for an item i is higher than expected in the low-scoring group — as happens when guessing effects occur — this item will be easier than in the high-scoring group: That is to say, a negative z_i-value has resulted.[4] Table 19.1 shows that every item with a large negative z_i-value

---

[4] Note that another reason for a negative z_i-value of an item might simply be a too low discriminatory power of the item. The number of correct responses is higher than expected in the low-scoring group and thus the item-parameter estimate is smaller than for the total sample, whereas in the high-scoring group, the number .

Table 19.1. CML item-parameter estimates (and standard errors in parenthesis) of the RM for the total of 20 items and the total sample of $n = 4153$ examinees, the (according to the score median) low-scoring sample $n = 1811$, the high-scoring sample $n = 2342$; the corresponding z_i-values are given as well. Significant values at the level $\alpha = 0.01$ are typed in bold.

Item No.	Cml Estimates Total Sample	Cml Estimates Low Scorer	Cml Estimates High Scorer	z_i-Values
1	-2.4016 (0.0587)	-2.2998 (0.0634)	-2.7762 (0.1539)	**2.8625**
2	-1.3078 (0.0401)	-1.2905 (0.0343)	-1.3034 (0.0780)	0.1504
3	-1.8299 (0.0490)	-1.7024 (0.0383)	-2.2334 (0.1166)	**4.3267**
4	-0.5578 (0.0191)	-0.5553 (0.0282)	-0.5229 (0.0349)	-0.7209
5	-0.9173 (0.0232)	-0.9797 (0.0333)	-0.7650 (0.0391)	**-4.1786**
6	-0.9029 (0.0230)	-0.9947 (0.0336)	-0.7033 (0.0416)	**-5.4440**
7	-0.5817 (0.0191)	-0.5599 (0.0283)	-0.5768 (0.0321)	0.3948
8	-0.4641 (0.0189)	-0.3346 (0.0289)	-0.6253 (0.0364)	**6.2593**
9	-0.7456 (0.0202)	-0.6927 (0.0302)	-0.7991 (0.0517)	1.7777
10	-0.3506 (0.0187)	-0.3713 (0.0267)	-0.2859 (0.0459)	-1.6070
11	-0.2648 (0.0191)	-0.1501 (0.0357)	-0.3788 (0.0409)	**4.2138**
12	-0.2035 (0.0198)	-0.5137 (0.0266)	0.1752 (0.0432)	**-13.5735**
13	0.2742 (0.0223)	0.0741 (0.0372)	0.4800 (0.0319)	**-8.2832**
14	0.7005 (0.0182)	0.9525 (0.0460)	0.5810 (0.0325)	**6.5924**
15	0.5694 (0.0170)	0.4361 (0.0441)	0.6966 (0.0304)	**-4.8614**
16	0.9506 (0.0222)	1.0638 (0.0570)	0.9245 (0.0375)	2.0416
17	0.9326 (0.0220)	1.1996 (0.0592)	0.8315 (0.0303)	**5.5366**
18	1.6757 (0.0301)	1.8186 (0.0763)	1.6627 (0.0415)	1.7951
19	2.1979 (0.0338)	2.3448 (0.0929)	2.1955 (0.0430)	1.4591
20	3.2269 (0.0552)	2.5551 (0.1013)	3.4232 (0.0522)	**-7.6149**

Table 19.2. CML item-parameter estimates (and standard errors in parenthesis) of the RM for the 9 item reduced test; the Q_i-indices as well as their corresponding standard normal distributed test statistic Z_Q

Item No.	CML Estimates Total Sample	Q_i-Indices	Z_Q
2	-1.4791 (0.0416)	0.1723	0.9310
3	-2.0150 (0.0484)	0.1225	-1.7936
4	-0.7042 (0.0275)	0.1715	1.5160
7	-0.7290 (0.0263)	0.1624	0.7872
9	-0.8989 (0.0284)	0.1578	0.1233
11	-0.3992 (0.0307)	0.1470	-0.3423
14	0.6156 (0.0204)	0.1491	-0.1775
16	0.8807 (0.0227)	0.1472	0.0574
17	0.8616 (0.0225)	0.1329	-1.2898
18	1.6536 (0.0352)	0.1488	-0.0517
19	2.2139 (0.0421)	0.1609	0.2111

Table 19.3. MML estimates of item-difficulty and item-guessing parameters (and standard errors in parenthesis) of the DGPL model for the total of 20 items and the total sample of 4153 examinees; the χ^2 fit statistics based on 15 ability intervals with corresponding degrees of freedom and the p-values are given as well

Item No.	Item-Difficulty Parameters	Item-Guessing Parameters	χ^2	df	p-Values
1	−2.202 (0.123)	0.156 (0.072)	15.2	11.0	0.1727
2	−1.186 (0.109)	0.158 (0.063)	17.1	12.0	0.1444
3	−1.641 (0.101)	0.122 (0.057)	**35.0**	**12.0**	**0.0005**
4	−0.827 (0.106)	0.165 (0.058)	16.9	14.0	0.2614
5	−0.831 (0.128)	0.273 (0.066)	20.0	14.0	0.1316
6	−0.696 (0.131)	0.305 (0.063)	19.1	14.0	0.1600
7	−0.745 (0.125)	0.255 (0.064)	8.2	14.0	0.8812
8	−0.624 (0.078)	0.081 (0.035)	**33.7**	**14.0**	**0.0023**
9	−0.860 (0.105)	0.164 (0.058)	8.4	14.0	0.8672
10	−0.495 (0.092)	0.129 (0.045)	29.6	15.0	0.0135
11	−0.462 (0.080)	0.088 (0.036)	23.7	15.0	0.0703
12	0.493 (0.144)	0.433 (0.035)	13.6	14.0	0.4818
13	0.289 (0.103)	0.209 (0.036)	19.1	15.0	0.2097
14	0.394 (0.078)	0.079 (0.024)	**32.3**	**15.0**	**0.0058**
15	0.554 (0.096)	0.146 (0.030)	16.1	15.0	0.3768
16	0.557 (0.079)	0.069 (0.022)	19.3	13.0	0.1130
17	0.571 (0.066)	0.036 (0.016)	**29.9**	**12.0**	**0.0029**
18	1.132 (0.087)	0.058 (0.017)	24.4	13.0	0.0277
19	1.401 (0.089)	0.051 (0.014)	25.6	13.0	0.0195
20	2.918 (0.224)	0.064 (0.011)	11.7	12.0	0.4709

— that therefore does not fit the RM (especially the items number 5, 6, 12, 13, 15, and 20) — can actually be fitted using the DGPL model: as is seen, insignificant χ^2 statistics were obtained. The estimated guessing parameters of the items under consideration, except item 20, disclose that high-guessing effects occur especially with these items in particular. Thus, one of the most likely reasons for a nonfit to the RM is indeed guessing effects.

On the other hand, the items that do not even fit the DGPL model (items 3, 8, 14, and 17 — according to the χ^2 statistic) are not affected by guessing. Their estimated item-guessing parameters are barely higher than zero. The z_i-values of these items, with respect to the RM, are high, but positive, which may indicate a discriminatory power that is too high. This is because in the low-score group the number of correct responses is even lower than expected according to the estimated item-difficulty parameters from the RM, whereas in the high-score group this number is higher than expected. At least, this is

---

of correct responses is lower than expected and thus the item-parameter estimate is larger than for the total sample. This result may also be due to the case that the item-characteristic curve is very flat.

a good explanation for the fact that those items do not fit either the DGPL model nor the RM.

The result creates the a posteriori hypothesis of an even more general model, that being the unconstrained 3PL model.[5] However, there are only 4 out of 20 items that indicate a different discrimination parameter. This should be interpreted here as a matter of chance; of course, the 3PL model is always applicable for dichotomously scored items. This paper, however, aims to highlight a valid approach for saving an item pool that is designed to fit the RM but suffers from guessing effects caused by the multiple-choice format. Because the model fit analyses disclose that both models, the RM and the DGPL model cannot explain the data sufficiently enough as a whole, a comparison of the two models by means of the special likelihood ratio test (19.4) does not really pay off. Of course, if the more general model does not fit, then an insignificant result from a likelihood ratio test will not support a more restrictive model. On the other hand, there is the chance of a significant result in favor of the DGPL model. Therefore, we have computed the respective test χ^2 statistic (19.4) for just this reason: Indeed, the result is significant ($\chi^2 = 83.8502, df = 19$) and thus indicates once more a superior fit of the DGPL model in comparison to the RM.

Furthermore, a comparison of the goodness of model fit of these two models can be carried out by using the information criterion AIC (Akaike information criterion; Akaike, 1973). For this, the logarithmic function of the respective marginal likelihood times -2 and plus twice the number of estimated parameters has to be calculated. Table 19.4 gives the results. The AIC for the DGPL model is lower than the AIC for the RM. Hence, the additional item-guessing parameter of the DGPL model contributes to a descriptively important increase of the likelihood in comparison to the RM. This again confirms the superiority of the DGPL model for the given item pool as a whole.

Table 19.4. Comparison of the goodness of model fit for the RM and the DGPL (D+G PL) model

Model	Log Marginal Likelihood	Number of Parameter Estimates	AIC
RM	-12751.5672	21	25545.13
D+G PL model	-12709.6421	40	25499.28

The χ^2-fit statistics of the items 3, 8, 14, and 17 indicate an unacceptable fit with respect to the difficulty plus guessing PL model. We have concluded above that these items may discriminate too much in contrast to the rest of items because their estimated guessing parameter is negligibly low and be-

---

[5] Although this is beyond the focus of this paper, an analysis of the data according to the 3PL model indeed showed an acceptable fit with respect to all items.

cause of the positive sign of the z_i-values in Table 19.1 with respect to the RM. The items with a high negative z_i-value in Table 19.1, on the other hand, fit the DGPL model because obviously these items are affected by guessing. Thus, a comparison of the goodness of fit of the two models in question with respect to the reduced item set, where items 3, 8, 14, and 17 have been discarded, may confirm our conclusions above. With this in mind, we have computed the likelihood ratio test statistic (19.4). The logarithmic function of the marginal likelihood of the RM (log mL $= -10303.28$) is lower than the logarithmic function of the marginal likelihood of the difficulty plus guessing PL model (log mL $= -10281.87$). The difference according to the likelihood ratio test (19.4) is significant ($\chi^2 = 42.83, df = 15$; the critical χ^2 at $\alpha = 0.01$ is 30.58) and thus clearly shows a better fit of the DGPL model for the reduced item pool under consideration.

There still remains the question as to whether the DGPL model explains the data, with respect to the 11 RM fitting items, even significantly better than the RM itself. In order to answer this question, we again used the special likelihood ratio test (19.4). Therefore, we have to estimate the item parameters of the RM applying the MML method once more as described above (cf. footnote 4): In particular, the common discrimination of all items α has to be estimated in addition to the item-difficulty parameters. The logarithmic function of the marginal likelihood of the DGPL model (log mL $= -7181.0895$) is now just slightly higher than the logarithmic function of the marginal likelihood of the RM (log mL $= -7183.6911$) so that the difference is, according to the χ^2 statistic (19.4), not statistically significant ($\chi^2 = 5.2032, df = 10$). That is to say, the 11 items in question not only fit the RM to a satisfactory extent but also do not need an additional guessing parameter in order to improve the fitting of the data.

Although the application of the DGPL model saves most of the items that would have otherwise been deleted using the RM, obviously because of guessing effects (at least for some items), there are a number of other possibilities of modeling such a data structure. In the following, we will consider extensions of the RM to discrete mixture-distribution models, that being the mixed RM and a HYBRID model. The hypothesis might arise that guessing leads to random responses to some or even all items for a subgroup of examinees, for instance, for examinees with low proficiency. Then the data would consist of a mixture of persons who respond according to an item response model such as the RM and another subgroup that displays a random response behavior to some or all items, so that no item response model would actually provide an adequate explanation of the data. Thus we would have to assume an unrestricted multinomial distribution for this subgroup's responses. Such assumptions can be specified using a HYBRID model where one latent class assumes the RM and the other class a one-class latent-class model. Another possibility of untangling different kinds of mixture distributions and thus identifying latent subgroups of examinees for whom different item-difficulty parameters exist is the application of the mixed RM. Different subgroups of examinees that show different intensities of guessing may be reflected in different but class specific item-parameter estimations. To compare the goodness of fit of the competing models with each other and with the RM, we again use the AIC and a likelihood ratio test that is based on a marginal form of the conditional likelihood. Following Rost (2004) we call it the "score distribution likelihood" because the conditional response patterns are multiplied by their corresponding "score parameters," that is to say, the relative frequencies with which the different scores are observed in the sample of examinees. However, the estimation equations are equivalent to the CML method because the score parameters appear as additive constants in the *log likelihood* and thus become zero when taking the partial derivatives with respect to the difficulty parameters. Table 19.5 summarizes the results. It shows the logarithmic function of the score distribution likelihoods and the AIC indices for the RM, for the 2- and 3-class solution of the mixed RM as well as for a 2- and 3-class HYBRID model. The HYBRID models have been specified in each case with one of the classes so as to fit the RM.

Table 19.5. Comparison of the goodness of fit of the 2- and 3-class solution of the mixed RM (MRM), of the 2- and 3-class HYBRID model, and of the RM

	Rasch Model	2-Class MRM	3-Class MRM	2-Class HYBRID	3-Class HYBRID
Log Likelihood	−43563.3	−43347.2	−43218.9	−43419.6	−43298.9
AIC	87204.6	86848.5	86667.1	86959.2	86759.8

It is not surprising that all the models discussed here show a better fit to the data than the RM. According to the AIC, the 3-class mixed RM has the best relative fit.

The likelihood ratio test confirms the superior fit of the 3-class solution in comparison to the RM ($\chi^2 = 688.7, df = 76$) as well as in comparison to the 2-class mixed RM ($\chi^2 = 256.52, df = 38$). Furthermore, the likelihood ratio test comparing the RM with the 2-class model is also significant ($\chi^2 = 432.18, df = 38$) and thus indicates that a parameter restriction that yields the RM is statistically not admissible. (For all tests we have chosen a significance level of $\alpha = 0.01$, again).

Although the two HYBRID models also show a better fit in comparison to the RM they are clearly empirically inferior to the respective solutions of the mixed RM. This is the reason why we will not take these models into further consideration. Instead, we take a closer look at the two mixed-RM solutions.

First, let us consider the 2-class solution. According to the Q-index, which assesses the fit of the items within a latent class, the following occurs: The examinees of the first latent class, consisting of approximately half of the total number of examinees (48.98%), exhibit an RM conform response behavior. Thus, we will consequently call it the Rasch class. The other latent class reflects a response behavior that deviates from the RM, according to the Q-index. Because we have shown that by analyzing the data with the DGPL model severe guessing effects occur, it is plausible to conclude that this class consists of examinees that, to a certain extent, use guessing as their predominant response strategy. We will refer to this class as the guessing class. Another reliable indicator for the plausibility of the above interpretation is the fact that the Rasch class more or less consists solely of examinees with a high score whereas the guessing class is predominantly constituted by low scorers. And of course, it is highly feasible that people with a low-test performance are more likely to guess when responding to the items.

The results of the analyses with the DGPL model disclosed severe guessing effects especially with regard to item number 5, 6, 12, 13, and 15. As can be seen in Figure 19.2, these items in particular are clearly easier in the guessing class of the 2-class mixed RM than in the Rasch class, whereas for most of the other items it is the other way round — or they have approximately the same difficulty estimation in both classes. Given the fit of the DGPL model, in relation to the RM — irrespective of the more discriminating powerful four items — this is exactly what we would have to expect if a subgroup of guessing examinees actually exists. A constant guessing parameter for all examinees and a valid partition into two subgroups of examinees is only possible if the partition takes place according to the level of performance. That is to say, the chance of guessing is of almost no relevance for the high scorer, but actually is of relevance for low scorers, especially with regard to those items that are easier than others to guess correctly.

When considering the 3-class solution of the mixed RM, the above conclusions can be retained. The Rasch class of the 2-class solution is maintained. The class size is nearly exactly the same as in the 2-class model (48.189%) and the Pearson correlation of the two sets of parameter estimations is 0.999. The other two classes, with class sizes 29.61% and 22.20% respectively, have been split from the guessing class of the 2-class model and can be interpreted as a kind of differentiation among the guessing examinees with respect to their intensity of guessing; in other words, one class with a high level of guessing and the other with a lower level. Once again, both guessing classes show that items 5, 6, 12, 13, and 15 are easier than in the Rasch class.

19.6 Discussion

Although our results are not really surprising, they definitely contribute to the practice of test calibration. The DGPL model discussed here is a special case of the 3PL model that has so far not been applied frequently. However, as demonstrated here, it is indeed of practical importance. If a multiple-choice response format is used, often with five response choices, of which only one represents a correct response to the item, then conventional RM analyses may actually be carried out — after deleting some of the items — with a

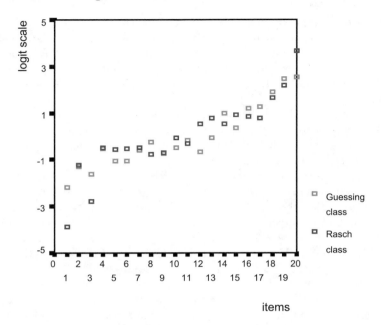

Fig. 19.2. Item-parameter patterns of the 2-class solution of the mixed RM

reduced item pool where the RM holds. However, more items can most likely be retained if an additional item-guessing parameter is taken into account. From a certain point of view, this is of great importance.

There is no doubt that using an additional item-guessing parameter entails severe measurement and psychometric problems as one is not only faced with the problems of parameter estimation, but also with the loss of specific objectivity and the lack of a variety of powerful methods for model checks available for Rasch-based models (see, for example the chapter by Glas in this volume). Above all, choosing the DGPL model involves the loss of the existence of a sufficient statistic for the person parameter sought after. One could argue that because all these psychometric problems arise, would it not be more preferable to use an additional item discrimination parameter, that being the 3PL model, or to use an additional parameter right from the beginning instead of an additional guessing parameter, that being the 2PL model. This argument is of course justified from a psychometric point of view — although three types of item parameters mean additional problems for parameter estimation than only two types. This argument, however, goes beyond practical requirements. Even if test calibration in practice does not favor estimating the person parameter instead of calculating the score as a respectively sufficient statistic, analyses according to the DGPL model would almost always disclose that some of the items show unacceptably high-guessing effects — which could ultimately be repaired by altering the distractors or the like. We doubt that every test that fits the RM and that uses a multiple-choice response format is actually free from (item-specific) guessing effects. And if indeed so, any such effects would probably have occurred before the respective items were deleted. Our empirical example proves this suggestion: The stepwise deletion of items within the RM analysis leads to a reduced item pool in which there was no item that had an item-guessing parameter of relevance; however, there were an additional 5 items from the total of 16 items that fitted the DGPL model that could have been used for the final test. As that amounts to more than 31%, using the RM to fit this data is obviously not very economical.

From a methodological point of view, we conclude that the mixed RM serves not only to check the RM fit of an item pool but can also give an indication of guessing effects. The latter being in the case that at least two classes split the examinees into high and low scorers and furthermore discloses lower item-parameter estimations for the low scorers in comparison to the high scorers for some of the items. However, from a test-construction point of view, the DGPL model seems preferable for establishing a psychometrically sound instrument for pertinent psychological assessment: Examinees' ability can then be estimated in a comparable fashion for all respondents as they are characterized by one ability estimate only, and not by different types of guessing behavior in addition to an ability estimate.

Latent-Response Rasch Models for Strategy Shifts in Problem-Solving Processes

Carl P. M. Rijkes[1] and Henk Kelderman[2]

[1] University of Twente
[2] Vrije Universiteit Amsterdam

20.1 Introduction

In this chapter, the problem of strategy shifts in problem-solving is discussed within the framework an extended Rasch model (RM) theory. A strategy-shift model is formulated that is similar to the (generalized) solution-error response-error model of Westers & Kelderman (1991). Modeling of strategy shifts is illustrated by means of the balance-beam task of Siegler (1981), which was administered to 484 Dutch 12-to-13-year-old children. Different hypotheses regarding the strategy shifts of subjects based on Siegler's theory concerning the balance task are specified and empirically tested.

We present ways to deal with testing hypotheses on strategy shifts in problem-solving processes within the framework of loglinear RMs. Strategy shift is a phenomenon that frequently occurs when subjects solve test items. Siegler (1991) reports multiple-strategy use by children in domains such as arithmetic, causal reasoning, judgments of plausibility, reading and spelling, referential communications, serial recall, and spatial reasoning. Also, Siegler (1987) and Siegler & McGilly (1989) report frequent strategy shifts when children are presented identical problems on two successive days. In a study of spatial intelligence, Kyllonen, Lohman, and Woltz found that different subjects used different strategies for accomplishing the same goal in various spatial tasks, and that subjects shifted strategies depending on the demands of the task. The phenomenon of strategy shift seems to be an important aspect of intelligent behavior. It enables a person to " ...flexibly adapt to problems to maximize performance" (Kyllonen, Lohman, & Woltz, 1984, p. 1343). Siegler & Campbell (1989) noted that:

> Good reasons exist for us to know and to use multiple strategies. Strategies differ in their accuracy, in the amounts of time needed for execution, in their memory demands, and in the range of problems to which they apply. Strategy choices involve trade-offs among these properties; people try to choose strategies that enable them to cope

with cognitive and situational constraints. The broader the range of strategies we know, the more we can shape our approaches to the demands of particular circumstances.

Two kinds of strategy shifts can be distinguished in problem-solving: (1) shifts that primarily originate in the person, and (2) strategy shifts that are induced by the items. A strategy shift originates primarily in the person when the task characteristics of the items do not influence the strategy shift. For example, when a subject shifts strategy between two parallel items with the same difficulty, this is a person-dependent strategy shift. A strategy shift between two items is item-induced when the strategy shift depends only on task characteristics and is independent of the ability of the subjects. This would, for example, probably be the case when all subjects in a population solve one item using strategy 1 and solve an other item using strategy 2.

Usually, a person-dependent strategy shift cannot be distinguished from an item-induced strategy shift when they both can occur at the same time. The strategy-shift model that is presented in this paper can distinguish between the two types of shifts only on the basis of additional theory. The theory should describe which items have identical task characteristics. Item-induced strategy shifts are not expected to occur between structurally parallel items with the same difficulty, and the strategy-shift model of this paper can test this assumption.

In cognitive psychology, linear regression models were used to study strategy shifts of subjects in problem-solving by Ippel & Beem (1987) and Kyllonen, Lohman, & Woltz (1984). In IRT, a number of psychometric models have been formulated that can account for different strategies. Important references are Embretson et al. (1986), Kelderman & Macready (1990), Kelderman & Rijkes (1994), Mislevy & Verhelst (1990), Paulson (1986), Rost (1990), Samejima (1983), Tatsuoka et al. (1988), and Wilson (1989). However, most of these models focus on the case of consistent strategy use of subjects during the test and do not take strategy shifts into account.

In this chapter, the use of a strategy-shift model will be illustrated by means of its application to the balance (beam) task of Inhelder & Piaget (1958). The balance task is well known in developmental psychology, e.g., Case (1985), Inhelder & Piaget (1958), Klahr (1978), Siegler (1981), Wilkening & Anderson (1982). The task is used in this field to assess the knowledge structures and solution strategies of children in the context of a stagewise cognitive development. In this paper, a specific version of the balance task of Siegler (1981) will be used.

A number of measurement models have been formulated to model the subject's response behavior on the balance task (Mislevy, Yamamoto, & Anacker, 1992; Kempf, 1983; Spada & Kluwe, 1980; van Maanen et al., 1989; Wilson, 1989). The balance task is an intriguing problem for psychometricians due to a number of characteristics revealed in Siegler's theory (Mislevy, Yamamoto, & Anacker, 1992). First of all, according to Siegler, differences in understanding of the balance beam will lead to different strategy use of the subjects. Second, the response patterns of the various solution strategies differ from those normally expected on the basis of a latent-trait model. And third, the probability of a correct response is not monotone increasing with the latent ability of the subjects due to the fact that subjects with little understanding of the behavior of the balance task may arrive at the correct response category for a wrong reason, whereas subjects of a higher ability may arrive at an incorrect response category for the same item. This chapter focuses on the strategy shifts of subjects in the balance task, based on Siegler's theory. In the next section, a short description of the balance task and the theoretical assumptions by Siegler will be given. Following this section, a strategy-shift model will be discussed and hypotheses regarding the strategy shifts of subjects in the balance task formulated. In the last part of this paper, the hypotheses will be formalized using an IRT model and then empirically tested.

20.2 The Balance Task

The balance task was used by Inhelder & Piaget (1958) to investigate the proportional reasoning ability of children. There are a number of variants of the balance task, and one example of a task using the balance scale apparatus can be seen in Figure 20.1.

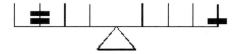

Fig. 20.1. An example of a balance scale

In the balance task, a number of disks of the same weight are placed on two sides of the balance beam, and subjects have to predict on which side the balance beam will fall. Possible responses are left down, balance, and right down. To make the scoring procedures objective, Siegler (1981) used a forced-choice version of the balance-scale task.

The behavior of the balance beam can be explained by the concept of torque. Torque is the outcome of total weight times the distance of the weights to the tilting point. The balance beam will stay in balance when for each side the products are equal, or else fall to the side with the greater torque.

According to Siegler there are four strategies (or "rules") that subjects use to solve the balance task. In the following, strategies will be indicated by the random variable C taking values $c \in M_c$. Although Siegler describes the strategies using a decision tree, in essence they correspond with the descriptions below.

The first strategy is random guessing ($c = 1$). This strategy is used by children who do not know how to solve the problem. The second strategy of a child is to focus only on weight ($c = 2$), and respond by stating that the side with the greater amount of weight will go down. In the third strategy a child focuses on weight and distance ($c = 3$). If the distance of the weights to the tilting point is the same on both sides, then the side with the greater amount of weight will go down. If the weights are equal, then the side will go down where the weights are farther away from the tilting point. The last strategy consists in computing the torques ($c = 4$), where the side with the greater torque is reported to fall down.

To detect the different strategies, Siegler classified different balance tasks in a number of problem types according to dimensional changes. "Balance" items are problems in which there is no difference in the weight and distance dimension. "Weight" items only differ in the weight dimension. "Distance" items only differ in the distance dimension. "Conflict" items have two conflicting dimensions because there is more weight on one side but more distance on the other side. The relation between the different solution strategies and problem types is specified in Table 20.1, where $(3{:}2){\leftarrow}{\rightarrow}(1{:}3)$ means that there are two weights at the third position of the left arm and three weights at the first position of the right arm. For example, the balance in Figure 20.1 is represented by $(3{:}2){\leftarrow}{\rightarrow}(4{:}1)$ in this notation.

According to Siegler, when there are no conflicting dimensions, only the first three strategies specified in Table 20.1 will be used. That is, subjects will compute the torques only when there is no other way of solving the item. When there are conflicting dimensions, the weight-and-distance strategy ($c = 2$) cannot be applied to solve the item, and according to Siegler this strategy will not be used by subjects for conflict items.

Siegler makes the strong assumption that the concept of understanding the balance task develops along a number of progressive stages, where the level of understanding is related to the age of the subject. In the first stage, subjects do not focus on any relevant problem dimension; they will guess at random. In the second stage, subjects focus only on the weight dimension. In the third stage, subjects focus also on the distance dimension, but only when there is no difference in the weight dimension (thus only for the distance item types). So these subjects switch from the weight-and-distance strategy ($c = 3$) for the distance items to the weight strategy ($c = 2$) on conflict items. In the fourth stage subjects always focus on the weight and distance dimension, but they do not know the right rule. These subjects will shift their weight-and-distance strategy ($c = 3$) on the no-conflict items to the random-guessing strategy ($c = 1$) on the conflict items. In the last stage, subjects always focus on both dimensions and apply the multiplicative rule of computing torques. These subjects will switch their weight-and-distance strategy ($c = 3$) for the no-conflict items to the torques strategy ($c = 4$) for the conflict items.

Table 20.1. Theoretical Probabilities of the Different Strategies for the Response Alternatives L, B, R, of the Different Problem Types

Item	Problem	Response	Guessing	Weight	Weight and Dist.	Torques	Buggy Rule
	Balance	L	0.33	0.00	0.00	-	-
1	(3:3)←→(3:3)	B	0.33	1.00	1.00	-	-
		R	0.33	0.00	0.00	-	-
	Weight	L	0.33	1.00	1.00	-	-
2	(3:3)←→(3:1)	B	0.33	0.00	0.00	-	-
		R	0.33	0.00	0.00	-	-
	Distance	L	0.33	0.00	1.00	-	-
3	(3:3)←→(2:3)	B	0.33	1.00	0.00	-	-
		R	0.33	0.00	0.00	-	-
	Conflict Weight	L	0.33	1.00	-	1.00	0.00
4	(3:2)←→(4:1)	B	0.33	0.00	-	0.00	1.00
		R	0.33	0.00	-	0.00	0.00
	Conflict Distance	L	0.33	0.00	-	1.00	0.00
5	(2:2)←→(1:3)	B	0.33	0.00	-	0.00	1.00
		R	0.33	1.00	-	0.00	0.00
	Conflict Balance	L	0.33	0.00	-	0.00	0.00
6	(3:2)←→(2:3)	B	0.33	0.00	-	1.00	1.00
		R	0.33	1.00	-	0.00	0.00

van Maanen et al. (1989) found another strategy that subjects applied in solving conflict items, and called it a buggy rule in the tradition of "mind bugs" of Brown & van Lehn (1980). The rule is described as follows:

If side X has more weights and the weights of side X have the smaller distance to the tilting point then shift the weights on side X away from the tilting point until the distances on both sides are equal and remove for every shift on side X one weight on side X (van Maanen et al., 1989, p. 272).

The relation between the buggy-rule strategy ($c = 5$) and item types is specified in the last column of Table 20.1.

Wilkening & Anderson (1982) criticized Siegler's work for its lack of theory on response error. The conditional probabilities in Table 20.1 between item types and solution strategies assume that subjects make no errors in applying a solution strategy. In the next section, a measurement model is described that takes this concern into account and allows for response errors in the balance task. First the model is described and then an example is given to illustrate the model. The section ends with the formulation of testable hypotheses on strategy shifts in the balance task.

20.3 A Strategy-Shift Model

The strategy-shift model of this paper consists of two connected parts describing two sequential processes in problem-solving. In the first process, a subject chooses a solution strategy from a number of available strategies to solve the problem. In the second process, a subject executes the chosen solution strategy and arrives at an observed response category.

In the first process, the relation between ability and solution strategies is described by an RM. In this model, both the latent ability of a person and the easiness of solving an item with a certain strategy determines the probability that an available strategy is chosen to solve a given item. For a given problem, each strategy has a certain probability of occurring. The same type of strategy may be more readily employed in one item than in another. Different subjects may use different strategies for accomplishing the same goal in various tasks, and subjects may shift strategies depending on the demands of the task.

In describing the strategy-shift model, let an item be indicated by i ($i = 1, \ldots, I$), and let θ be the value that describes the subject's proportional-reasoning ability. Let $M_{c_i} \subseteq \{1, 2, 3, 4, 5\}$ be the set of strategies that can be applied to item i, let $c_i \in M_{c_i}$ be the strategy the subject uses for solving item i, and let $\mathbf{c} = (c_1, \ldots, c_I)$ be the subject's strategy vector for the complete test. Note that the set M_{c_i} of possible strategies for solving item i may vary for different types of items. The first part of the strategy-shift model describes the probability that a subject uses strategy c_i for item i given his subject parameter θ:

$$P(c_i|\theta) = \frac{\exp(\theta s_{ic_i} + \phi_{ic_i})}{\sum_{c \in M_{c_i}} \exp(\theta s_{ic} + \phi_{ic})}, \qquad (20.1)$$

where s_{ic_i} is a strategy-weight specifying the relation between strategy c_i and ability θ, and ϕ_{ic_i} a location parameter describing the easiness of strategy c_i for item i. In solving the items of a test, it is assumed that the strategies c_i of the subjects are locally independent given ability θ. This assumption holds if the process of strategy choice for an item is not influenced by the choices made on previous items.

The second process describes the execution of the chosen solution strategy and arrival at an observed response category by conditional probabilities. If a certain strategy can yield a particular response, the corresponding conditional probability of that response under that strategy is larger than zero. These probabilities may be known or estimated from the data. This part of the model can account for response errors, by allowing for deviations from the ideal conditional probabilities, as for example given in Table 20.1. The second part of the strategy-shift model describes the probability of a response x_i given the latent strategy c_i for item i as

$$P(x_i|c_i) = \pi_{x_i c_i}^{X_i C_i}.$$ (20.2)

Model (20.2) assumes that the conditional probabilities of an observed response x_i are the same for all subjects using the same latent strategy c_i.

Combining (20.1) and (20.2) under the assumption that x_i depends only on c_i, and c_i only on θ, gives

$$P(x_i|\theta) = \sum_{c_i \in M_{c_i}} \pi_{x_i c_i}^{X_i C_i} \frac{\exp(\theta s_{ic_i} + \phi_{ic_i})}{\sum_{c \in M_{c_i}} \exp(\theta s_{ic} + \phi_{ic})}.$$ (20.3)

Model (20.3) is similar in structure to the (generalized) solution-error response-error (GSERE) model of Kelderman (1988) and Westers & Kelderman (1991). The general structure of this model is that of a discrete mixture of conditional strategy-specific response probabilities over the set of available strategies for a particular item. The main difference between the strategy-shift model and the GSERE model is the interpretation of the model parameters. Also, in this study different constraints are imposed on the model parameters.

20.3.1 An Example

A key assumption of the strategy-shift model is that there is a relation between the strategy a subject uses and the subject's latent ability. In the strategy-shift model, this relation is described by the strategy-weights (s_{ic_i}) in (20.3). These strategy-weights are constants that must be specified before the model is fitted. No a priori rules are given for specifying the strategy-weights.

If we assume that older or smarter children use better strategies than younger or less-intelligent children, the solution strategies of the balance task can be scored using strategy-weights expressing a monotonically increasing relation between the strategies and θ. For example, in scoring the solution strategies for a distance item, a strategy-weight specification could be as follows: random guessing ($c = 1$) gets a strategy-weight of 0 and serves as the reference strategy. The weight strategy ($c = 2$) gets a strategy-weight of 1, and the weight-and-distance strategy ($c = 3$) a strategy-weight of 2. In this specification, it is assumed that subjects applying the weight-and-distance strategy tend to have a higher proportional-reasoning ability than subjects applying the weight strategy or random guessers. And also, subjects applying the weight strategy have in general a higher ability than random guessers. Note that for other items, other strategy-weights can be specified, depending on the relation between ability and the solution strategies. Substituting the strategy-weights (ϕ_{ic}) as specified above in (20.1) gives the following model equations for a conflict item:

$$P(c_i = 2|\theta) = c_i^{-1} \exp(\theta + \phi_{i2}),$$
$$P(c_i = 3|\theta) = c_i^{-1} \exp(2\theta + \phi_{i3}), \qquad (20.4)$$
$$P(c_i = 1\theta) = [1 + \exp(\theta + \phi_{i2}) + \exp(2\theta + \phi_{i3})]^{-1} = c_i^{-1}.$$

In these equations, the location parameter ϕ_{i1} for the weight strategy is fixed at zero as a reference point. If, for example, the strategy-location parameters have the values $\phi_{i2} = -1.5$ and $\phi_{i3} = -4$, the item-characteristic curves for the strategies will look like the ones in Figure 20.2.

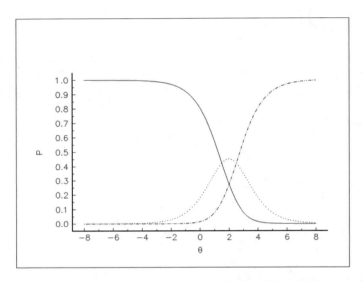

Fig. 20.2. Estimated item-characteristic curve of conflict weight item (20.4)

In Figure 20.2, the probability of applying a strategy changes with different values of θ. The probability of using the strategy random guessing (the solid line in Figure 20.2) decreases as θ increases. The probability of using the weight-and-distance strategy (the line of dots and bars) increases as θ increases. The probability of using the weight strategy (the dotted line) first increases and then decreases as θ increases.

The points in Figure 20.2 where the item-characteristic curves intersect can be called "strategy-shift" points. At these points, the probability of applying one strategy equals the probability of applying the other strategy. So, for example in Figure 20.2, the probability of using the random guessing strategy equals the probability of using the weight strategy at strategy-shift point $\theta = 1.5$.

Notice that when the value of ϕ_i varies between items, then, given a fixed value of θ, the probability of applying a given strategy will also vary. So subjects may shift their strategies depending on the easiness of applying available strategies in a given task. Notice also that the probability of applying a strategy can be influenced by the strategy-weights, which may vary for different items.

20.3.2 Hypotheses

Four hypotheses will be specified with regard to the problem-solving processes in the balance task. They will be denoted by, for example, H10 and H1A standing for the first null and alternative hypotheses, respectively.

The first hypothesis is on the relation between the latent ability θ and the solution strategies. Siegler (1981) assumes that proportional-reasoning ability develops along a number of progressive stages, where each stage has a different relation with the solution strategies, as described in the balance-task section. However, Siegler's theory does not say anything about the relation between the buggy-rule strategy and the latent ability θ. On the basis of Siegler's theory it seems plausible that subjects who only randomly guess on conflict items have approximately the same developmental level as subjects using the buggy-rule strategy. In that case, giving both strategies an equal strategy-weight would be appropriate. Therefore, the null hypothesis H10 assumes that the slopes of the regression function of the buggy-rule strategy ($c = 5$) and random guessing ($c = 1$) on the latent ability are the same on conflict items. The null hypothesis will be compared with the alternative hypothesis H1A, which assumes that the slopes of the regression functions of the two strategies on the latent ability are different.

The next two hypotheses are on strategy shifts in the balance task. According to Siegler, the easiness of applying a strategy for solving an item does not change within an item of the same type. This implies that between items of the same type, there will only be person-dependent strategy shifts. The null hypothesis H20 therefore assumes that the location parameters of strategies for solving items of the same type are equal, and will be compared with the alternative hypothesis H2A stating that they differ.

The third hypothesis concerns strategy shifts in conflict-weight, conflict-distance, and conflict-balance items. According to Siegler, the easiness of applying a strategy to solve an item does not change within the set of conflict items. This fact implies also for conflict items that there will only be person-dependent strategy shifts. For this reason, the null hypothesis H30 postulates that the location parameters of the strategies on conflict items are equal, and will be compared with the alternative hypothesis H3A, stating that they differ.

The fourth hypothesis deals with the conditional probabilities in the second part of the model. The conditional probabilities in the strategy-shift model are specified on the basis of Siegler's theory. The fourth null hypothesis H40 assumes that the conditional probabilities as specified in Siegler's theory lead to an adequate fit of the strategy-shift model to the data. This hypothesis will be tested against the alternative hypothesis H4A stating that a fitting strategy-shift model cannot be found. Because Siegler's work lacks a theory on response errors, a small arbitrary response-error value of 0.05 is chosen. In testing hypothesis H40 this value was allowed to vary between 0.00 and 0.10.

In the next section it will be described how the different hypotheses were tested for an empirical data set.

20.4 Method

20.4.1 Subjects

In this study, an empirical data set from (van Maanen et al., 1989) was used. The sample consisted of 235 children in grade seven and 249 children in grade eight about 12–13 years old. In total, there were 484 children from twelve primary schools in the northern region of the Netherlands participating in the study.

20.4.2 Instruments

(van Maanen et al., 1989)constructed a paper-and-pencil version of Siegler's balance task consisting of five weight items, five distance items, five conflict-weight items, five conflict-distance items, and five conflict-balance items (see Table 20.1). The 25 items were presented in random order to each subject, to prevent systematic learning and fatiguing effects from occurring across subjects. The items were scored dichotomously in correct and incorrect responses. Unfortunately, the original data on the trichotomous responses were lost, so that the dichotomous responses were used in this study. The computer program LEM of Vermunt (1997a) was used to fit the models. The estimation procedure of LEM is based on maximum likelihood.

20.4.3 Analysis

In this study, a subset of items of the test of (van Maanen et al., 1989) was reanalyzed. Their findings, based on cluster analysis, suggested that in their sample only the following four of the five strategies specified in Table 20.1 were used: random guessing ($c = 1$), the weight strategy ($c = 2$), the weight-and-distance strategy ($c = 3$), and the buggy-rule strategy ($c = 5$). They also found that random guessing occurred only at conflict items. The fact that random guessing did not occur at no-conflict items, and that the torque strategy ($c = 4$) was not used, might be caused by a restriction of range in ability levels; only subjects in the age range of about 12–13 years old participated in the study. The item analysis of van Maanen et al. showed that the items of the balance test did not conform to an RM. After the data set was divided into four separate strategy-homogeneous populations, a linear logistic test model (Fischer, 1973; Scheiblechner, 1972) fitting the data matrix of one of the subpopulations was found.

In the following, it was assumed that only the four strategies found by (van Maanen et al., 1989) occurred in the sample. In this study, two parallel subsets of four items were selected from the test of van Maanen et al., each consisting of two distance items (items 1 and 2), one conflict weight item (item 3), and one conflict-balance item (item 4). Differences in predicted conditional probabilities between the strategies of van Maanen et al. (all strategies in Table 20.1 except torques) made it possible to distinguish the strategies from one another.

Two distance items were included in each subset of items to allow for testing hypothesis H2 on strategy shifts between items of the same type.

The first subset of four items was used to test the different specified hypotheses. The second parallel subset of four items was used to cross-validate the best-fitting model.

Standard errors for model parameters were computed using a bootstrap procedure described by Efron (1982). In this procedure, the empirical data set of this study was used as an estimate of an unknown empirical distribution. Given the empirical data, 250 bootstrap samples were drawn. In each sample drawn, the model parameters were estimated. An estimate of the standard errors was then obtained by computing the standard deviation of the estimated model parameters over the 250 data sets.

In the GSERE model, which is similar in structure to the strategy-shift model, there is a trade-off between the item parameters in the first and second layers of the model, which leads to unstable parameter estimates (Verhelst, 1992). The instability of the parameter estimates due to this trade-off can be removed by fixing the conditional probabilities in the second layer of the strategy-shift model. In this study, the conditional probabilities were fixed to values corresponding with Siegler's theory (see Table 20.1).

Note that the conditional probabilities of Siegler given in Table 20.1 do not take response errors into account. Response errors refer to random deviations from the ideal strategy response due to interfering factors in the response process such as loss of concentration, ambient noise, and casual writing errors. In the following, it was assumed that the probabilities of response errors were equal for the different strategies and did not vary across items. Because the actual tendency to produce response errors in solving balance-task items was unknown, a small value equal to 0.05 was chosen. This meant that, on average, once in every twenty times a random deviance of the ideal strategy response would be ascribed to response errors. In Table 20.2, the values at which the conditional probabilities were fixed for three items of the first item set are given. In Table 20.2, the correct response is indicated as 1 and the incorrect as 0. In Table 20.2, only the four strategies that occurred in the sample of (van Maanen et al., 1989) are described.

To test the hypotheses, different models were compared for goodness of fit. When models were nested, the likelihood-ratio statistic (L^2) was used. The difference between the likelihood-ratio statistics related to two nested models is asymptotically chi-square distributed, with degrees of freedom equal to

Table 20.2. Predicted probabilities of the different strategies c for the response alternatives X (1=correct, 2=incorrect) for problem types of the empirical data set

Problem	Response	Guessing	Weight	Weight and Dist.	Buggy Rule
Distance	1	-	0.05	0.95	-
$(3:3)\leftarrow\rightarrow(2:3)$	0	-	0.95	0.05	-
Conflict Weight	1	0.33	0.95	-	0.05
$(3:2)\leftarrow\rightarrow(4:1)$	0	0.66	0.05	-	0.95
Conflict Balance	1	0.33	0.05	-	0.95
$(3:2)\leftarrow\rightarrow(2:3)$	0	0.66	0.95	-	0.05

(header spanning "Guessing Weight Weight and Dist. Buggy Rule" is under "Strategies")

the difference in numbers of linearly independent parameters between both models (e.g., Fienberg, 1980). When models were not nested, the Bayesian information criterion (Schwarz, 1978, BIC) was used. The overall goodness of fit of a model was determined by means of Pearson's chi-square statistic (X^2) and standardized residuals (STR).

To identify the specified models, the strategy-location parameters of the weight strategy ($c = 2$), and the first category of the weight-sum parameter of the proportional-reasoning ability θ were fixed at zero. Furthermore, the strategy-location parameter of the weight-and-distance strategy ($c = 3$) was fixed at zero.

20.4.4 Specification of Hypotheses Using Probability Models

Hypotheses H1 through H4 were tested by the fit of the corresponding strategy-shift model to the data. The first hypothesis, H10, states that the slopes of the regression functions of the buggy-rule strategy ($c = 5$) and random guessing ($c = 1$) on the latent ability are the same on conflict items. To test this hypothesis, the following values for the weights were specified for the strategies of Table 20.2: the weight strategy ($c = 2$) 0, the weight-and-distance strategy ($c = 3$) 1, random guessing ($c = 1$) 1, and the buggy rule ($c = 5$) 1. These s_{ic} weights result for the distance items in a decrease in probability of choosing the weight strategy, and an increase in probability of choosing the weight-and-distance strategy, when θ increases. These s_{ic} weights result for the conflict items in a decrease in probability of choosing the weight strategy, and an increase in probability of choosing the strategies random guessing and the buggy rule, when θ increases. The probability for a correct and incorrect response, respectively, for a distance item is given by

$$P(x_i = 1|\theta) = 0.05c_i^{-1} + 0.95c_i^{-1}\exp(\theta + \phi_{i3}),$$
$$P(x_i = 0|\theta) = 0.95c_i^{-1} + 0.05c_i^{-1}\exp(\theta + \phi_{i3}),$$

where $c_i^{-1} = 1 + \exp(\theta + \phi_{i3})^{-1}$, for a conflict-weight item by

$$P(x_i = 1|\theta) = 0.95c_i^{-1} + 0.33c_i^{-1}\exp(\theta + \phi_{i1}) + 0.05c_i^{-1}\exp(\theta + \phi_{i5}),$$
$$P(x_i = 0|\theta) = 0.05c_i^{-1} + 0.66c_i^{-1}\exp(\theta + \phi_{i1}) + 0.95c_i^{-1}\exp(\theta + \phi_{i5}),$$

where $c_i^{-1} = 1 + \exp(\theta + \phi_{i1}) + \exp(\theta + \phi_{i5})^{-1}$, and for a conflict-balance item by

$$P(x_i = 1|\theta) = 0.05c_i^{-1} + 0.33c_i^{-1}\exp(\theta + \phi_{i1}) + 0.95c_i^{-1}\exp(\theta + \phi_{i5}),$$
$$P(x_i = 0|\theta) = 0.95c_i^{-1} + 0.66c_i^{-1}\exp(\theta + \phi_{i1}) + 0.05c_i^{-1}\exp(\theta + \phi_{i5}),$$

where $c_i^{-1} = 1 + \exp(\theta + \phi_{i1}) + \exp(\theta + \phi_{i5})^{-1}$. The above model equations were obtained by substituting the strategy probabilities of Table 20.2 in Equation 20.3, where for each response category a sum of the strategies is given. The terms of the sum in the model equations for a conflict-balance item, for example, are related to the weight, the random-guessing, and the buggy-rule strategies, respectively.

The above model equations of equal strategy-weights for random guessing and the buggy rule (model a), were compared with the following two weight specifications: (1) random guessing 1 and the buggy rule 2 (model b); and (2) random guessing 2 and the buggy rule 1 (model c). In model b, the slope of the regression function for the buggy rule is steeper than for random guessing, where for model c the reverse is true. These strategy-weight specifications are likely to be more appropriate when subjects differ in developmental ability levels.

The second hypothesis, H20, assumes that the location parameters of the strategies for solving items of the same type do not differ. This hypothesis was tested by restricting the strategy-location parameters ϕ_{ic} for the distance items in the above model equations to be equal (model d).

The third hypothesis, H30, assumes that the location parameters of the strategies on conflict items do not differ. This hypothesis was tested by restricting the strategy-location parameter ϕ_{ic} to be equal in the above model equations for the conflict items (model e).

The fourth null hypothesis, H40, assumes that the conditional probabilities as specified in Siegler's theory lead to an adequate fit of the strategy-shift model to the data. This hypothesis was tested by considering the overall goodness of fit of the best-fitting model. If a fitting strategy-shift model could be found, then hypothesis H40 would not be rejected.

20.5 Results

Table 20.3 lists the number of model parameters (NPAR), the degrees of freedom (DF), and the values of goodness-of-fit statistics for the different models. In model a in Table 20.3, the strategies random guessing and the buggy rule get an equal strategy-weight of 1, whereas in models b and c the strategy-weights differ (model b: random guessing 1, buggy rule 2; model c:

random guessing 2' buggy rule 1). The BIC values of the non-nested models a, b, and c showed that model a fits better than models b and c. Therefore, the null hypothesis H10 could not be rejected. The null hypothesis H10 postulated that the slopes of the regression functions of the buggy-rule strategy ($c = 5$) and random guessing ($c = 1$) on the latent ability are the same on conflict items.

Table 20.3. Values of goodness-of-fit statistics for different models of balance problems

	NPAR	DF	L^2	X^2	BIC
a	10.00	6.00	14.89	14.07	34.89
b	12.00	4.00	14.84	13.92	38.84
c	12.00	4.00	14.91	14.22	38.91
d	9.00	7.00	15.90	14.30	33.90
e	7.00	9.00	-	-	-
d3	9.00	7.00	12.91	13.19	30.91
d3	9.00	7.00	9.27	9.42	27.27

Model d in Table 20.3 is a special case of model a, in which the strategy-location parameter for the weight-and-distance strategy ($c = 3$) are constrained to be equal. Model d has therefore one degree of freedom more than model a. The difference between the values of the likelihood-ratio statistics of models a and d indicate that the constrained model d fits not significantly worse than model a ($\triangle L_1^2 = 1.01, p = 0.31$). The null hypothesis H20 can therefore not be rejected, and we assume that the location parameter of the strategies to solve a problem do not differ within the set of distance items.

Model e is a constrained version of model d in which the strategy-location parameters for random guessing and the buggy-rule strategies are constrained to be equal for items 3 and 4. So model e has two free parameters fewer than model d. In the estimation process, model e did not converge, and we must conclude that model e is not a good representation of the empirical data set. The null hypothesis H30 is tentatively rejected in favor of the alternative hypothesis H3A of varying strategy difficulties in the conflict items.

The goodness-of-fit statistics of models a through d indicate a bad fit to the data. In columns four through seven in Table 20.4, the observed ($f_\mathbf{x}$) and expected ($F_\mathbf{x}$) frequencies, and standardized residuals (STR) of model d indicate that frequency cell $\mathbf{x} = (1, 1, 2, 2)$ is not fitting very well (STR $= -2.00, p = 0.046$). There are fewer subjects than expected with item responses x_1 and x_2 wrong and x_3 and x_4 right.

The expected cell frequency of cell $\mathbf{x} = (1, 1, 2, 2)$ can be changed by means of adjusting the conditional probabilities of a strategy that is involved in all the items, namely the weight strategy ($c = 2$). If the conditional probabilities for a correct response for the weight strategy are increased for items 1 and 2

Table 20.4. Observed and expected cell frequencies and standardized residuals for item set 1 and 2 of balance problems

Response					Item Set 1				Item Set 2		
Pattern					Model d		Model d3		Model d3		
x1	x2	x3	x4	$f_{\mathbf{x}}$	$F_{\mathbf{x}}$	STR.	$F_{\mathbf{x}}$	STR.	f_x	$F_{\mathbf{x}}$	STR.
1	1	1	1	6	6.45	−0.18	9.53	−1.14	13	8.60	1.50
1	1	1	2	2	0.76	1.43	0.66	1.66	1	0.55	0.61
1	1	2	1	104	99.87	0.41	100.23	0.38	90	94.03	−0.42
1	1	2	2	1	5.83	−2.00	2.64	−1.01	2	2.23	−0.16
1	2	1	1	10	8.66	0.46	8.57	0.49	4	6.25	−0.90
1	2	1	2	4	6.09	−0.85	6.10	−0.85	7	6.27	0.29
1	2	2	1	13	19.28	−1.43	19.08	−1.39	11	17.53	−1.56
1	2	2	2	6	3.74	1.17	3.95	1.03	4	3.51	0.26
2	1	1	1	7	8.66	−0.56	8.57	−0.54	8	6.25	0.70
2	1	1	2	5	6.09	−0.44	6.10	−0.45	5	6.27	−0.51
2	1	2	1	26	19.28	1.53	19.08	1.58	24	17.53	1.55
2	1	2	2	2	3.74	−0.90	3.95	−0.98	3	3.51	−0.27
2	2	1	1	97	96.79	0.02	96.87	0.01	62	61.83	0.02
2	2	1	2	113	110.47	0.24	110.52	0.24	114	113.74	0.02
2	2	2	1	63	63.22	−0.03	63.17	−0.02	106	105.90	0.01
2	2	2	2	25	25.08	−0.02	25.00	0.00	30	29.98	0.00

(distance) and decreased for items 3 (conflict weight) and 4 (conflict balance), then the expected frequency of items 1 and 2 incorrect and items 3 and 4 correct will decrease.

In Table 20.5, the goodness-of-fit statistics of different models are depicted in which the conditional probabilities for model d are slightly changed. Notice that now the assumption of constant-response errors over the items and the strategies is dropped for the weight strategy. The value 0.05 of the response errors also changes. Model d3 in Table 20.4 has the lowest BIC value, and should be preferred. The standardized residual (STR) for cell $\mathbf{x} = (1, 1, 2, 2)$ has dropped from −2.00 to −1.01, and the standardized residuals for the other cells in the frequency table (see Table 20.4) show no misfit. The Pearson X^2-statistic shows that model d3 fits at a right-tail significance level of 0.05 under a chi-square distribution. It must therefore be concluded that the overall goodness of fit of model d3 is satisfactory. Therefore, the null hypothesis H40, stating that the conditional probabilities as specified in Siegler's theory lead to an adequate fit of the strategy-shift model to the data, cannot be rejected.

20.5.1 Results from Cross Validation

Model d3 was cross-validated using a parallel set of four items. Pearson's X^2-statistic in Table 20.3 showed a good fit for model d3, and also the standardized residuals (STR) in Table 20.4 showed no signs of misfit for model d3. It might be concluded therefore that model d3 was rightly accepted as a well-fitting model. A peculiar fact was that model d3 of the parallel set of items seemed to fit even better than in the original set of items. The reason for this fact is unknown to the authors, and is ascribed to chance.

20.5.2 Estimated Model Parameters

In Table 20.5, the estimated location parameter for the following four strategies are given: weight $(c = 2)$, weight and distance $(c = 3)$, random guessing $(c = 1)$, and buggy rule $(c = 5)$. as a reference point, the parameters for the weight strategy were constrained to a value of zero. To fix the scale, the parameter of item 1 for the weight-and distance strategy was fixed at zero. Because the parameters of items 1 and 2 were constrained to be equal for the weight-and-distance strategy, the parameter for the weight-and distance strategy was also equal to zero.

Table 20.5. Estimated values of strategy-location parameters and standard errors (S.E.) for model d3 of first item set of balance problems

		Strategy		
Item	Weight	Weight and Dist.	Guessing	Buggy Rule
1	0.00*	0.00*		
2	0.00*	0.00*		
3	0.00*		−43.63 (0.98)	−43.42 (0.62)
4	0.00*		−42.67 (0.81)	−43.33 (0.60)

In Figure 20.3, a plot of the item-characteristic curve of the conflict-weight item 3 is depicted. The solid line describes the probability that a subject with proportional reasoning ability θ applies the weight strategy. The line with bars and dots indicates the probability of applying the buggy-rule, and the dotted line the probability of applying the random-guessing strategy. Because the curves of the buggy-rule and random-guessing strategies do not intersect, there were only two strategy-shift points: at $\theta = 3.42$, the probability of applying the weight strategy equaled the probability of applying the buggy-rule strategy, and at $\theta = 3.63$, the probability of applying the weight strategy equaled the probability of applying the random-guessing strategy. In general, the probability of using the weight strategy for item 3 was high for low values of θ, and decreased for high values of θ. The probability of using the random-guessing or buggy-rule strategy was low for low values of θ, and increased for high values of θ.

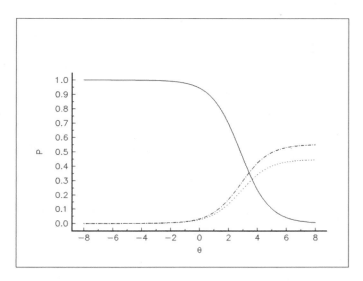

Fig. 20.3. Estimated item-characteristic curve of conflict weight item 3

In Figure 20.4, the estimated frequency distribution of the sum of the strategy-weights is depicted. Although in the strategy-shift model a subject might choose between the available strategies at a every ability level, Figure 20.4 suggests a stagewise development as predicted by Siegler's theory.

20.5.3 Conclusion

The aim of this study was to illustrate the use of a strategy-shift model, and how the model could be used to formalize existing theories of cognitive development. As an example, Siegler's theory of the balance task was used. By formalizing Siegler's methodology within an IRT framework, criticism of Wilkening & Anderson (1982) regarding the lack of handling response error in Siegler's theory was removed. Within the IRT framework different hypotheses regarding the strategy shifts of subjects in the balance task could be tested. Strategy shifts that are induced by the items could be distinguished from person-dependent strategy shifts. Furthermore, a fitting strategy-shift model could be found in correspondence with the specified probabilities of Siegler's theory.

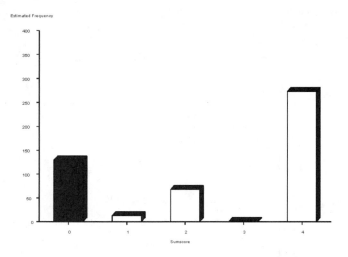

Fig. 20.4. Estimated distribution of the score variable

20.5.4 Discussion

Siegler made the assumption that for a given developmental level, a subject consistently sticks to a certain solution strategy, and switches to another only on the basis of task characteristics. That is, according to Siegler, no person-dependent strategy shifts occur in solving the balance task. This assumption is inconsistent with the strategy-shift model in Equation 20.3, because for any level of θ, a subject has a probability of choosing between various strategies. The fact that a fitting strategy-shift model was found showed that problem-solving is probably not the fixed process Siegler originally assumed, and that his theory might need some modifications. Siegler's later work, as mentioned in the first section, confirms this point. Still, it might be very useful to consider the development of proportional reasoning as a stagewise process, but in a less-rigid way than first considered: "In the process of acquiring a more sophisticated rule individuals use the sophisticated rule they are acquiring and the set of rules they previously mastered alternately in an unpredictable way" (van Maanen et al., 1989, p. 270).

Finally, two points with respect to modeling problem-solving with the strategy-shift model can be made. The strategy-shift model in this paper describes only strategy shifting between items. Strategy shifting within items is not allowed for, although it is likely that these also occur in problem-solving. The second point regards the relation between the conditional probabilities and the latent ability θ in the strategy-shift model. In the strategy-shift model, the conditional probabilities are specified independent of the abilities of the subjects. A model in which the conditional probabilities depend on the latent ability θ seems more realistic.

Validity and Objectivity in Health-Related Scales: Analysis by Graphical Loglinear Rasch Models

Svend Kreiner[1] and Karl Bang Christensen[2]

[1] Department of Biostatistics, University of Copenhagen
[2] Institute of Occupational Health

21.1 Introduction

The total score of items fitting a Rasch model (RM) satisfies assumptions relating to validity and a number of technical requirements. For this reason, the RM is often used as a "gold standard" expressing ideal measurement requirements.

Most summated rating scales in health research that we have worked with have shown evidence of differential item functioning (DIF) and local dependence (LD), thus violating the assumptions of the RM, even though items appear to be face valid. In this situation, Rasch analysis is a destructive process: a large number of face valid items are rejected in order to obtain fit to the model. This can seem unacceptable when items are face valid. Data from a large health survey in Copenhagen County in 1995 is used for illustration focusing on responses to items measuring physical functioning in the SF-36 questionnaire (Ware Jr. et al., 1993).

This chapter views Rasch analysis as an examination of the items given the requirements of ideal measurements, yielding a summary of problems and an evaluation of their relevance. Graphical loglinear RMs (GLLRM) incorporating uniform DIF and uniform LD (Kreiner & Christensen, 2002, 2004) are used for this. This leads to reflection on measurement requirements: We suggest that DIF is more serious than LD, and that sufficiency and reliability are more important than specific objectivity. Items fitting a GLLRM provide measurement that is essentially valid and objective and the total score is sufficient.

Section 21.2 describes the PF subscale of the SF-36. Section 21.3 describes conditional-independence and chain-graph models and their global Markov properties. Section 21.4 introduces Criterion-related construct validity. Section 21.5 defines graphical RMs (Kreiner & Christensen, 2002) describing the latent-trait variable, the set of items, and the exogenous variables in the framework of graphical models (Lauritzen, 1996). Section 21.6 extends these by allowing uniform DIF and uniform LD in the well-known manner of loglinear RMs (Kelderman, 1984, 1992, 1995). This yields graphical loglinear RMs (GLLRM). Section 21.7 presents the analysis of the SF-36 data and the measurement implications of the departures from the RM. Section 21.8 discusses essential objectivity and validity, and section 21.9 presents a summary and discussion.

Items are denoted by $Y=(Y_1,\ldots,Y_k)$, the total score by $S = \sum_i Y_i$, the latent variable by Θ, and exogenous variables by $X=(X_1,\ldots,X_m)$. We assume, without loss of generality, that all items have c+1 ordinal categories coded 0,1, ... , c. Exogenous variables may include response variables depending on Θ, criterion variables known to be monotonously related to Θ, covariates with a potential effect on Θ or simply variables that may be associated with Θ and/or items.

21.2 The Physical Functioning SubScale of the SF-36

The SF-36 (Ware Jr. et al., 1993) is a widely used questionnaire measuring aspects of general health status. It contains 36 items summarized into eight subscales. The physical functioning (PF) subscale summarizes responses to ten items under the common heading "Does your health now limit you in these activities? If so, how much?"

- Vigorous activities, e.g., running, heavy lifting, strenuous sport (PF1)
- Moderate activities (PF2)
- Lifting or carrying groceries (PF3)
- Climbing several fligths of stairs (PF4)
- Climbing one flight of stairs (PF5)
- Bending, kneeling, or stooping (PF6)
- Walking more than a mile (PF7)
- Walking several blocks (PF8)
- Walking one block (PF9)
- Bathing or dressing yourself (PF10)

Three ordinal response categories ("Not limited," "Limited a little," "Limited a lot") are used. The developers claim that "Studies to date have yielded content, concurrent, criterion, construct, and predictive evidence of validity" (Ware, J.E. (undated): SF-36® Health Survey Update. http://www.sf-36.org/tools/sf36.shtml). Scrutinizing the items will show that LD between PF4 and PF5 and between PF7, PF8, and PF9 must be expected if responses are rational and consistent. Whether the reported analyses of construct validity may have overlooked this is not the focus of the present chapter. Problems of this kind are not unusual in health scales, often while items are highly face valid.

21.3 Conditional-Independence and Chain-Graph Models

Conditional independence is the unifying concept of importance for item response models and chain-graph models. We write $X \perp Y|Z$ to indicate that two sets of variables, $X = (X_1, \ldots, X_a)$ and $Y = (Y_1, \ldots, Y_b)$, are conditionally independent given a third set, $Z = (Z_1, \ldots, Z_c)$, in the sense that $P(X|Y,Z) = P(X|Z)$. Chain-graph models are multidimensional block recursive statistical models defined by pairwise conditional independence of variables in the following way. Let $V = \bigcup_i V_i$ be a partitioning of the variables into ordered subsets, $V_1 \leftarrow \cdots \leftarrow V_r$ defining a block recursive statistical model $P(V) = \prod_i P(V_i|V_{i+1}, \ldots, V_r)$. Assume that X and Y are variables belonging to block numbers a and b, respectively, where a$\leq$b. Set $Z_{rest}(X, Y) = \bigcup_{i=a}^{r} V_i \backslash \{X, Y\}$ such that $Z_{rest}(X,Y)$ contains all variables that are concurrent or prior to X according to the recursive structure of the model. A chain-graph model is defined by a set of assumptions concerning pairwise conditional independence, $\{X_i \perp Y_i | Z_{rest}(X_i, Y_i) : i = 1, \ldots, m\}$.

Graphical models are characterized by Markov independence graphs: networks where variables are represented by nodes. Nodes are disconnected if the variables are conditionally independent given all concurrent or prior variables Variables in the same recursive block are connected by undirected edges, whereas variables in different blocks are connected by arrows representing temporal and/or causal direction. The Markov graphs of graphical models are used both as visual diagrams illustrating the structure of the statistical model and as mathematical models—mathematical graphs—where mathematical graph theory may reveal properties of the statistical model that may be helpful both during the analysis of data and for interpretation of what the model conveys about the distribution of the variables. Examples of Markov graphs are shown in Figures 21.1 to 21.4 below. A comprehensive introduction to the theory of graphical models and the way the properties of the Markov graphs correspond to properties of the statistical model may be found in Lauritzen (1996).

21.3.1 Global Markov Properties of Chain-Graph Models

The global Markov properties of chain-graph models are of particular interest here. The global Markov properties tells us that conditional independence between two variables, X and Y, in a chain-graph model sometimes applies under conditioning with respect to subsets of $Z_{rest}(X, Y)$. To find such subsets, we have to examine the moral graph defined by replacing arrows by (undirected) edges and linking "parents" (see Figure 21.4).

The global Markov properties are linked to the concept of separation in undirected graphs. To subsets, A and B, of nodes in an undirected graph are separated by a subset of nodes, S, if every path from a node in A to a node in B contains at least on node in S. The global Markov property of chain-graph models (Lauritzen, 1996, p. 55) implies that two set of variables, A and B, in a chain-graph model are conditionally independent given any subset of variables, S, that separates A and B in the moral graph.

21.4 Criterion-Related Construct Validity

Criterion-related construct validity requires unidimensionality, monotonicity, local independence, and the absence of DIF (Rosenbaum, 1989). The last assumption requires the relation between the latent trait and the items to be the same in any subpopulation and implies criterion validity, which thus is a necessary, but not sufficient condition for construct validity. These assumptions also define nonparametric item response models (Sijtsma & Molenaar, 2002).

The requirement of no DIF in this definition is somewhat vague. We assume that it refers to meaningful and relevant partitions of the persons defined by an exogenous variable, but notice that in most studies a limited number of such variables will be available. Absence of DIF can be stated as the requirement, $Y \perp X \mid \Theta$, of conditional independence and because local independence implies pairwise conditional independence criterion-related construct validity defines a chain-graph model.

21.5 Graphical Rasch Models

The RM for ordinal items (Andersen, 1977; Andrich, 1978; Masters, 1982)

$$P(Y_i = y | \Theta = \theta) = \exp(\alpha_{i0} + \theta y + \alpha_{iy}) \tag{21.1}$$

where $\alpha_{i0} = -\ln \left(\sum_{y=0}^{c} \exp(\theta y + \alpha_{iy}) \right)$ satisfies the first three requirements of criterion related construct validity. The joint conditional distribution

$$P(Y_1 = y_1, \ldots, Y_k = y_k | \Theta = \theta) = \exp \left(\alpha_0 + \sum_{i=1}^{k} (\theta y_i + \alpha_{iy_i}) \right) \tag{21.2}$$

is a loglinear model for a multivariate contingency table with main effects depending on the latent variable and no interaction parameters. Restrictions are needed for parameters to be identifiable. These are imposed by setting $\alpha_{i0} = 0$ for all items and $\sum_i \alpha_{ic} = 0$.

Different data generating processes may lead to this model. Reparameterization replacing item parameters with thresholds, $\tau_{ij} = \alpha_{i(j-1)} - \alpha_{ij}$, yielding a partial credit interpretation (Masters, 1982) where $P(Y_i = y | \Theta = \theta) =$

$\exp(\sum_{j=1}^{y} (\theta - \tau_{ij})) / \Gamma_i$ can be useful, even though it may not be a valid description of the response behavior to the type of questions included in SF-36.

The total score, $S = \sum_i Y_i$, is sufficient for θ in the conditional distribution of items given $\Theta = \theta$ This implies Bayesian sufficiency, (Kolmogoroff, 1942; Arnold, 1988) and conditional independence of items and Θ given S.

The distribution of S is given by

$$P(S = s | \Theta = \theta) = \frac{\exp(\theta s + \varphi_s)}{\Phi} \qquad (21.3)$$

where $\gamma_s = \exp(\varphi_s)$ are referred to as elementary symmetric functions (Andersen, 1973, Fischer, 1974; 1995). We refer to the φ-parameters in (21.3) as score parameters. The probabilities (21.3) can be expressed in terms of threshold parameters in the same way as (21.1).

The RM satisfies construct validity requirements and provides objective measurement by sufficient raw scores. DIF and criterion validity can not be addressed in formal terms within the framework of RMs, but in a larger framework including exogenous variables. One way to do this is to assume that the joint distribution of $(Y_1, \ldots, Y_k, \Theta, X_1, \ldots, X_m)$ is a graphical RM.

A graphical RM is a chain-graph model characterized by two Markov graphs (Figure 21.1): (1) an IRT graph expressing construct validity (items are conditionally independent of each other and of exogenous variables), and (2) A Rasch graph adding the score S separating items from Θ. Note that edges between items are added because items are not conditionally independent given the score. The only requirement of construct validity that is not an explicit part of the IRT graph is that the relationship between the latent variable and items must be monotonous. The IRT graph also describes relationships among exogenous variables.

It follows from the Markov properties of the IRT and Rasch graphs that the distribution (21.2) reappears as the conditional distribution of item responses given Θ and X,

$$P(Y_1 = y_1, \ldots, Y_k = y_k | \Theta\theta, X_1 = x_1, \ldots, X_m = x_m) = \qquad (21.4)$$

$$\exp\left(\alpha_0 + \sum_{i=1}^{k} (\theta y_i + \alpha_{iy_i})\right) \qquad (21.5)$$

Marginalizing over Θ in the Rasch graphs results in a *marginal Rasch graph* (not shown) defining a chain-graph model for the manifest variables (Whittaker, 1990, p. 395). The marginal Rasch graph contains edges or arrows between any pair of variables connected to Θ by an arrow originating from Θ.

The IRT and Rasch graphs (Figure 21.1) define the model and provide a visual display of the model structure. The moralized Rasch graph (Figure 21.2) provides information on conditional independencies among the manifest variables of the model. The moral Rasch graph is an undirected graph defined by the marginal Rasch graph where separation implies conditional

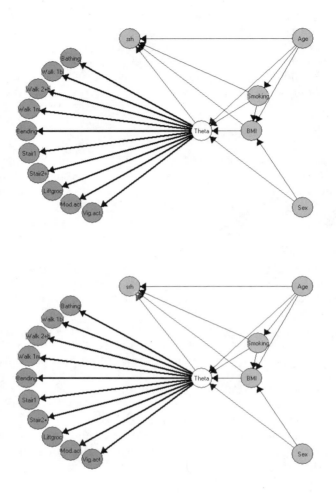

Fig. 21.1. The IRT and Rasch graphs defining the graphical RM for the ten PF items. The IRT describes relationships among exogenous variables: sex and age are marginally independent, smoking and sex are conditionally independent given age, SRH and sex are conditionally independent given Θ, BMI, smoking, and age.

independence due to the global Markov properties of chain-graph models. It follows from this that all pairs of items and exogenous variables are conditionally independent given S. This result lies behind the Mantel–Haenszel test for DIF (Holland & Thayer, 1988) and the global Markov properties of the Rasch graph shows that the result applies to all types of items and exogenous variables in graphical RMs.

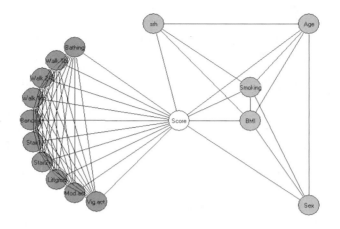

Fig. 21.2. The moral Rasch graph of the graphical model for the ten PF items

DIF is absent in graphical RMs in two ways: items and exogenous variables are conditionally independent given Θ and given S. This property appears to be unique to the RMs. We refer to Kreiner & Christensen (2002, 2004) for further discussions of properties of graphical RMs derived from the global Markov properties of Rasch graphs.

21.5.1 Inference in Graphical Rasch Models

Graphical RMs address two problems: (1) the quality of measurement (regarded as optimal if item responses fit the graphical RM) and (2) latent regression analysis

$$\theta = X_1\beta_1 + \cdots + X_m\beta_m + \epsilon, \qquad \epsilon \sim N(0, \sigma^2)$$

describing the association between the latent variable and covariates $X_1, \ldots,$ X_m. Since the pioneering work of Andersen & Madsen (1977), models of this kind have been studied extensively (Zwinderman, 1991, 1997; Andersen, 1994; Hoijtink, 1995; Kamata, 2001; Maier, 2001 Christensen et al, 2004; De Boeck & Wilson, 2004; Adams & Wu, this volume).

In this chapter, item analysis is separated from latent regression and we are thus able to distinguish between lack of fit of the measurement model and misspecified latent structure (Zwinderman & van den Wollenberg, 1990; Christensen et al., 2004). This means conditional item analysis is used, because marginal inference relies on assumptions about the distribution of the latent variable.

Conditional inference in graphical RMs may be carried out in two ways. The first is a parametric approach fitting the conditional distribution of item responses given the total score, comparing item parameters in different sub-populations and calculating item-fit statistics. The presence of exogenous variables in the graphical RM defines explicit requirements of groups to be compared during the analysis. The second approach is nonparametric, testing the assumptions expressed by the moral Rasch graph. Mantel–Haenszel tests (Holland & Thayer, 1988) can be used for testing conditional independence for pairs of dichotomous items and dichotomous exogenous variables. Partial gamma coefficients (Agresti, 1984, p. 171) may be used when items or exogenous variables are ordinal. The tests of conditional independence will often be tests in large sparse tables and and Monte Carlo tests (Kreiner, 1987; von Davier, 1997) can be used to avoid the problem of inadequate approximation of p-values by conventional asymptotic methods.

The RM applies for any subset of items and therefore LD between an item, Y_i, and the other items can be tested as conditional independence given the rest score, $R_i = S - Y_i$ (Kreiner & Christensen, 2004). This test is one example of a less than conventional approach suggested by the graphical structure of these models.

A starting point for the latent structure analysis can be obtained by nonparametric analysis of manifest variables based on the moral graphs. For the SF-36, analysis of the effect of a covariate on physical disability may be performed as a test of conditional independence in a multi-way table containing these two variables together with the variables separating the two in the moral graph. If conditional independence is rejected the covariate should be included in the latent-regression model.

21.6 Graphical Loglinear Rasch Models

A graphical loglinear RM (GLLRM) adds interaction parameters to the conditional distribution of item responses (21.4): DIF parameters describing interaction between an item and an exogenous variable and LD parameters describe interactions between two items. It is convenient to distinguish between second-order DIF and LD parameters and general higher order interaction parameters. The only restriction imposed on the interaction parameters in GLLRMs is that they must not depend on the latent-trait variable. To simplify the discussion of validity and objectivity in GLLRMs, we first consider models with DIF parameters and present three ways to look at these models. Following this, we then consider models with LD parameters and finally the general family of GLLRM.

21.6.1 Uniform DIF

The model (21.6) adds interaction between items Y_a and X_b

$$P(Y_1 = y_1, \ldots, Y_k = y_k | \Theta = \theta, X_1 = x_1, \ldots, X_m = x_m)$$

$$= \exp \left(\alpha_0 + \sum_{i=1}^{k} \left((\theta y_i + \alpha_{iy_i}) + \delta_{ab}(y_a, x_b) \right) \right) \tag{21.6}$$

For the parameters to be identifiable, we must impose additional restrictions on the δ-parameters in addition to those already imposed on the item main effect parameters. One convenient way to do so is to assume that $\delta_{ab}(0,x) = 0$ and $\delta_{ab}(y,1) = 0$ where we assume that categories of exogenous variables are integer coded from 1 to the number of categories of the variables. We regard the model defined by (21.6) as a model describing uniform DIF, where item parameter of Y_a in the subpopulation given by $X_a = x$ is equal to $\alpha_a(y) + \delta_{ab}(y,x)$. Alternatively, Y_b can be interpreted as a set of "virtual" items given only in a subpopulation (Tennant et al., 2004). Finally, of course, (21.6) is an example of a mixed RM. The mixture is manifest, but apart from that, the model satisfies all assumptions underlying the mixed RM.

21.6.2 Uniform LD

Adding interaction between two items, Y_a and Y_b, to (21.4) leads to a model with LD between the items:

$$P(Y_1 = y_1, \ldots, Y_k = y_k | \Theta = \theta, X_1 = x_1, \ldots, X_m = x_m)$$

$$= \exp \left(\alpha_0 + \sum_{i=1}^{k} \left((\theta y_i + \alpha_{iy_i}) + \lambda_{ab}(y_a, y_b) \right) \right) \tag{21.7}$$

We once again assume that the interaction parameter do not depend on θ and set $\lambda_{ab}(0,y) = \lambda_{ab}(y,0) = 0$. If we remove Y_b from the score and treat it as an exogenous variable it follows from (21.7) that the conditional distribution of the items remaining in the rest score follows a loglinear RMs similar to (21.6) with uniform DIF of Y_a relative to Y_b. We have therefore coined the term uniform LD to cover the kind of local dependence implied by the interaction parameter in (21.7).

21.6.3 Graphical Loglinear Rasch Models

Expanding model (21.6) and (21.7) to models with several cases of uniform DIF and LD as well as higher order interactions terms is straightforward. A general GLLRM is defined by three types of loglinear generators. First, DIF generators, $D = (D_1, \ldots, D_r)$, where $D_i = (A_i, Z_i)$ with $A_i \in \{Y_1, \ldots, Y_k\}$ and $Z_i \in \{X_1, \ldots, X_m\}$. Second, LD generators, $L = (L_1, \ldots, L_s)$ consisting of pairs of items $L_i = (U_i, V_i)$ where $\{U_i, V_i\} \subset \{Y_1, \ldots, Y_k\}$. Finally higher order interactions, $G = (G_1, \ldots, G_s)$, where each $G_i \subset \{Y_1, \ldots, Y_k, X_1, \ldots, X_m\}$ contains at least three variables one of which has to be an item. The GLLRM defined by these generators is given by

$$P(Y_1 = y_1, \ldots, Y_k = y_k | \Theta = \theta, X_1 = x_1, \ldots, X_m = x_m)$$
$$=$$
$$\exp \left(\alpha_0 + \sum_{i=1}^{k} (\theta y_i + \alpha_{iy_i}) + \sum_i \delta_i(a_i, z_i) + \sum_i \lambda_i(u_i, v_i) + \sum_i \mu_i(g_i) \right) \quad (21.8)$$
$$=$$
$$\exp \left(\alpha_0 + s\theta + \sum_{i=1}^{k} \alpha_{iy_i} + \sum_i \delta_i(a_i, z_i) + \sum_i \lambda_i(u_i, v_i) + \sum_i \mu_i(g_i) \right)$$

where s $= \Sigma_i y_i$ and (a_i, z_i), (u_i, v_i) and g_i is the observed outcomes of the variables in the generators. It is usually assumed that the model is hierarchical. We refer to the δ and λ parameters as DIF and LD parameters, respectively, even though the interpretation in these terms is questionable when G is not empty. Note that while the main effects, $\theta y + \alpha_{iy}$, are increasing functions of θ, not all marginal relationships between Θ and items are monotonously increasing when items may be negatively locally dependent. Items fitting a general GLLRM violate all but one of the assumptions of criterion related construct validity and conventional psychometric considerations would reject the scale as invalid. The measurement properties of items fitting a GLLRM models are discussed below based on the example.

21.6.4 Inference in GLLRMs

GLLRM's have moral Rasch graphs that may be used as a starting point for the same kind of tests as for the GRMs. The separation properties are a little more complicated in moral Rasch graphs from GLLRMs but graph theoretical algorithms exist that will take care of these problems.

Item, DIF, LD, and interaction parameters can be estimated by conditional maximum likelihood estimates evaluated by item-fit statistics comparing observed and expected item-characteristic curves and tested by conditional likelihood ratio tests (Kelderman, 1984, 1992, 1995). The Martin-Löf test of unidimenisonality (Martin-Löf, 1970; Glas & Verhelst, 1995; Verhelst, 2001; Christensen et al., 2002) generalize with few problems to GLLRMs (Kreiner & Christensen, 2004).

In a GLLRM the distribution of S given Θ is a power-series distribution similar to (21.3) with score parameters depending on item, DIF, LD, and interaction parameters. Estimation of person parameters and latent regression where estimates of score parameters are inserted can be done in the same way as in conventional models.

21.7 SF-36 Analysis

Data for this example originated in a Danish health survey including 2334 persons responding to the SF-36 items and the five exogenous variables (self-reported health, BMI, smoking status, sex, and age) included in the analysis.

All variables are potential sources of DIF and self-reported health is also used as a criterion variable. The primary purpose of the study is not validation of the measurement instrument, but rather to examine the effect of BMI on physical functioning. This is done using latent regression analysis (Christensen et al., 2004) controlling for the confounding effect of the other variables. Rather than a pure validity study the item analysis is meant to check that the result of the latent regression analysis is not confounded by systematic measurement errors.

The item "vigorous activities" (PF01) discriminates very poorly, $U = -5.94$, $p < 0.001$ (Molenaar, 1983) and is excluded. Presumably this has to do with problems responding when one does not participate in vigorous activities for other reasons than poor health (Fayers & Machin, 2000, p. 19). The complete analysis leading to the model will not be documented here, but evidence against the conventional RM and results supporting the adequacy of the GLLRM for the remaining nine items model is presented.

Conditional likelihood ratio tests (Andersen, 1973c), comparing item parameters in different groups, show evidence against the model (Table 21.1, columns marked RM). The reason for the discrepancy between model and data is not clear from overall test statistics.

Table 21.1. Conditional likelihood ratio tests of homogeneity of item parameters in subpopulations. Results presented for the RM and for the graphical loglinear RM.

	RM			GLLRM		
Variable Defining Subpopulations	CLR	df	P	CLR	df	P
Score groups (1-17, 18-19)	105.1	19	< 0.0005	70.0	67	0.379
SRH—five categories	261.2	76	< 0.0005	212.4	208	0.402
BMI—six categories	125.0	95	0.021	309.3	285	0.154
Smoking—three categories	50.5	38	0.085	168.6	134	0.023
Sex	72.5	19	< 0.0005	70.3	65	0.304
Age—six categories	179.0	95	< 0.0005	311.0	285	0.139

The risk of type I error is inherent in testing for LD of 36 item pairs and for DIF with 45 combinations of items and exogenous variables, and the level of significance is adjusted in order to control the false discovery rate at a 5% level (Benjamini & Hochberg, 1995). Moreover DIF or LD can lead to spurious evidence of DIF and/or LD for other items and/or exogenous variables and subsequent analyses are needed.

Partial gamma coefficients (Agresti, 1984, p. 171) showed strong evidence of LD for the item pairs (PF1, PF2), (PF2, PF3), (PF4, PF5), (PF7, PF8), and (PF8, PF9). Two-sided Monte Carlo estimates of exact conditional p-values were used. Table 21.2 shows evidence of DIF, only evidence from analysis taking several potential DIF sources into account are shown.

Table 21.2. Evidence of DIF disclosed by partial gamma coefficients. p-values are two-sided Monte Carlo estimates of exact conditional p-values. The false discovery rate has been controlled at 5% and only evidence from analysis taking several potential DIF sources into account support the evidence of DIF relative to variables written with bold letters.

Item	Exogenous Variable	Gamma	p
Vigourous activities (PF1)	Sex	0.23	0.012
Moderate activities (PF2)	BMI	0.31	0.000
Lifting groceries (PF3)	Sex	−0.45	0.000
Stairs—2+ flights (PF4)	Smoking	0.23	0.013
Stairs—1 flight (PF5)	Age	−0.24	0.008
Bending (PF6)	BMI	−0.17	0.012

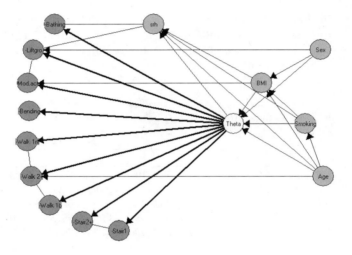

Fig. 21.3. The IRT graph of the final GLLRM for items PF2-PF10

All significant interactions were added to yielding a relatively simple GLLRM for the nine PF items. Figures 21.3 and 21.4 show the IRT graph and moral Rasch graph of this model. Significance levels are shown in Table 21.3. Conditional likelihood ratio tests comparing parameter estimates in subpopulations shows that this model fits the data better (Table 21.1, columns marked GLLRM). Observed and expected item-mean scores in each score group were compared and this also showed a good model fit.

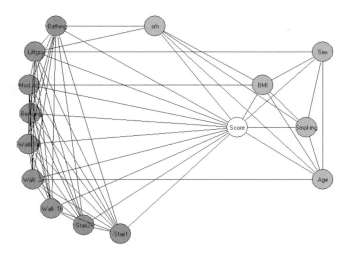

Fig. 21.4. The moral Rasch graph of the final GLLRM for items PF2-PF10

Table 21.3. Tests of vanishing DIF and LD parameters

Type of Interaction	Variables	CLR	df	p
Local dependence	PF2 & PF3	168.2	4	< 0.00005
	PF4 & PF5	116.5	4	< 0.00005
	PF7 & PF8	77.8	4	< 0.00005
	PF8 & PF9	203.5	4	< 0.00005
DIF	PF2 & BMI	34.9	10	0.00001
	PF3 & SRH	22.4	8	0.00430
	PF3 & Sex	20.1	2	< 0.00005
	PF8 & Age	27.6	10	0.00210
	PF10 & SRH	23.7	8	0.00260

21.7.1 Interpretation of Parameters

One item, "Bending and kneeling" (PF6), behaves like an ordinary RM item. Threshold parameters, for a partial-credit interpretation, are -1.83 and 0.11, implying a range of latent-trait values where each response is the most probable.

The items PF4 and PF5 concerning stair walking are locally dependent, but function in the same way relative to all other variables. Locally dependent items can be grouped together as a composite item defined as the sum of item scores. If there is no DIF composite items are distributed as items from an RM. Item parameters for the composite item $PF_{4+5} = PF_4 + PF_5$ can be computed from the item and LD parameters, $\alpha_{4y_4} + \alpha_{5y_5} + \lambda_{45}(y_4, y_5)$. Reparametrization, for a partial interpretation, thresholds show that thresholds are nicely ordered $(-1.75, -0.61, -0.09, 1.39)$.

DIF can be presented as loglinear-item and DIF parameters, but the effect is easier to interpret in terms of virtual items. The item "bathing" (PF10) is biased relative to self-reported health, but no evidence of LD was found. Partial credit thresholds of five "virtual" items in the subpopulations defined by self-reported health are shown in Table 21.4. Apart from some response categories not being used in the healthiest groups these appear to present a consistent picture with decreasing thresholds with failing health.

Table 21.4. Estimated thresholds of five virtual PF10-items in groups defined by self-reported health

SRH	Thresholds 1	2
Very good	0.93	+ inf.
Good	0.92	0.80
Fair	0.82	4.26
Bad	−0.21	1.92
Very bad	−0.27	2.48

For items with both DIF and LD, the situation is complicated and "virtual composite items" do not present an easy interpretation. As an example, consider $PF_{2+3} = PF_2+PF_3$ with DIF of PF2 (relative to BMI) and of PF3 (relative to SRH and sex): thresholds would have to be calculated for 60 virtual items to get a comprehensive description. The items relating to walking are a simpler example: the composite item, PF_{7+8+9}, is biased relative to age because DIF was disclosed for one of the three items. Disordered thresholds are common for "virtual composite items" and while the GLLRM appears to provide adequate description of the relationship between the variables of the model. An easy interpretation is not at hand.

21.7.2 The Effect of DIF on the Score

The score distribution (21.3) applies in GLLRM with the reservation that the score parameters depend on the exogenous variable (the sources of DIF)

$$P(S = s|\Theta = \theta, X = x) = \frac{\exp(\theta s + \varphi_s(x))}{\Phi(x)} \tag{21.9}$$

The score parameters are functions of item, DIF, and LD parameters and can be used to calculate estimates of θ or of the parameters of the distribution of Θ in the same way as for RMs.

Person parameters and their distribution can be compared on the latent-trait scale and this is preferable to the raw scores because the latent-trait scale may be regarded as an interval scale. It can, however, be difficult to decide whether a difference on the latent-trait scale is relevant. DIF equation of true scores between groups can be useful: Let $T_0(\theta) = E(S \mid \Theta = \theta, X = \text{ref})$ be the true score of a person from the reference group and let $\hat{\theta}(s, x)$ be the estimate of θ for a person with S=s in the group defined by X=x. The DIF equated score of this person is equal to $T_0\left(\hat{\theta}(s, x)\right)$.

Figure 21.5 illustrates the effect of DIF w.r.t BMI of the item "Moderate activities" (PF2): persons with high BMI underestimate the degree of physical disability due to health. This is probably of minor consequence for those with BMI $= 22.5 - 25.0$, where the largest adjustment by DIF equation adds about .2 points to low scores, but of some consequence for those with BMI > 30 where DIF equation adds 0.44–0.65 point to scores between 2 and 13.

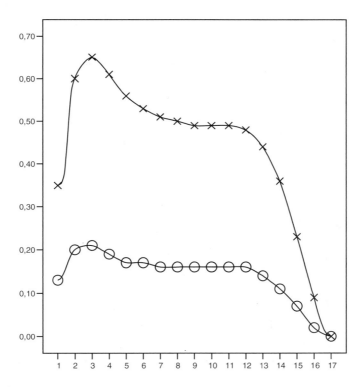

Fig. 21.5. DIF equated adjustment of scores for two groups of 18-to-29-year-old males with very good health (x = BMI $= 22.5$–25.0, o = BMI $= 30+$. The reference group consists of 18-to-29-year-old males with very good health and BMI ≤ 20.

21.7.3 Latent Regression

We now examine the effect of BMI on physical disability. Tests of conditional independence of the score and exogenous variables given the separators of the moral Rasch graph (Figure 21.4) yields a list of covariates that should be included. These show strong effects for all variables except smoking and can be seen as a stronger requirement of criterion validity (insisting that the association does not disappear when covariates related to both variables are taken into account—a requirement that is obviously met here). The estimated score parameters in (21.9) are used for latent regression (Christensen et al., 2004) using SAS (Christensen & Bjorner, 2003): A significant effect of BMI on physical functioning when controlling for sex, age, and self-reported health was found (LRT = 12.5, $df = 5, p = 0.03$).

Table 21.5. Difference between BMI groups controlled for sex, age, and self-reported health

BMI Group	Difference	95% CI
≤ 20	0.02	(−0.25, 0.30)
20.1–22.5	0.06	(−0.17, 0.29)
22.6–25.0	0	-
25.1–27.5	0.21	(−0.02, 0.44)
27.6–30.0	0.14	(−0,15, 0.43)
30.1 +	0.45	(0.18, 0.72)

Table 21.5 shows the estimated differences at the latent-trait scale between the six BMI groups. Physical disability appears to be at a minimum in the reference groups (BMI = 22.5–25.0) with a marked increase in physical disability when BMI is larger than 30. The evidence of increased disability in groups with BMI less than 22.5 is of course not significant.

21.8 Essential Validity and Objectivity

The previous section illustrates how LD and DIF may be dealt with if item responses fit a GLLRM. Latent-trait parameters can be estimated and compared as in the RMs. The question remains, however, whether measurement by these items can be regarded as valid and objective: All assumptions defining criterion-related construct validity except unidimensionality has been violated. We claim that validity and objectivity essentially has been preserved in GLLRMs. We return to the simple models given by (21.6) and (21.7) for the arguments supporting these claims and notice that the arguments carry over without problems to the general class of GLLRM.

The model defined by (21.7) includes one pair of uniformly locally dependent items, Y_a and Y_b. Replacing these two items by the composite item

$Y_{a+b} = Y_a + Y_b$ however results in a set of items satisfying all requirements of ideal scales except, perhaps, monotonicity of the composite item. Given the fact that the total scores are the same it is difficult to argument that Y_a and Y_b violates validity in any important way. The total score is sufficient for θ such that person and item parameters—among which we include the LD interaction parameters—may be separated during the analysis. The fundamental property of RMs supporting claims of objectivity therefore survives intact in (21.7), with one restriction compared to Rasch's definition of specific objectivity: we can not select items in a completely arbitrary way. One has to either include or exclude both items because an item subset including but one of the two dependent items does not fit an RM. This is, in our mind, a small price to pay during construction of a summary scale. Measurement may not be construct valid and objective according to conventional psychometric thinking, but it makes no sense to claim that measurement is invalid and biased or prone to systematic errors due to some arbitrary decision by the person constructing the test.

The model (21.6) with uniform DIF of Y_i relative to X_j, is a little more complicated. One may of course eliminate Y_i to obtain a smaller set of items satisfying requirements of ideal measurement. The set of items therefore is inherently valid and objective. When addressing problems relating to one of the groups defined by X_j, one would prefer to keep Y_i to increase reliability, because measurements are valid and objective in this specific population. From the point of view of the virtual Y_i we may also claim that test equating actually satisfies the requirements of specific objectivity because missing item responses is no hindrance to validity and objectivity. Regarding DIF parameters as item rather than incidental person parameters implies that conditioning with respect to the total score separates item parameters from the latent-trait parameters; the technicalities of objective analysis thus survives. Again a restriction applies: we are no longer free to make completely arbitrary choices during the design of the study. If we decide to include Y_i, we also have to include data on X_j, but apart from this measurements are essentially valid and essentially objective.

All arguments relating to models (21.6) and (21.7) apply without restriction to the general family of GLLRMs. The model may, of course, turn up to be so complicated that we prefer to reject the scale either because it is not practical to work with or because it is so far away from a conventional RM that we may be concerned that the substantive arguments behind the items do not hold water. If the GLLRM appears to fit the data, we should use these arguments and not arguments that measurements are invalid and systematically biased.

21.9 Discussion

This chapter discussed validity assumptions arguing from the point of view of a GLLRM fitting responses to the nine PF items. The SF-36 items violate conventional requirements of validity and objectivity due to unfortunate item-writing. Rather than rejecting the scale, we have taken a second look at requirements of valid and objective scales, partly because the items of SF-36 have a certain degree of face validity, but also because most scales we have worked with in health research suffer from similar problems. Our conclusion is that most requirements can be relaxed and that GLLRMs provide a sensible framework where all but a few properties of valid and objective measurements survive. Of the two types of departures from construct validity permitted by GLLRMs, the presence of uniform local dependency seems to be the least problematic. Regarding two locally dependent items as one composite item is a very small price to pay for the added reliability of the total score compared to the rest score without the items. Uniform DIF is a little more problematic. We may deal with uniform DIF, but it requires that all sources of DIF have to be included among the observations. The results of the analysis presented in this chapter implies that measurements of physical disability by the PF items will to some extent be confounded if sex, age, BMI, and SRH is not observed and taken into account. In addition, interpretation of the DIF of items relating to SRH is difficult. Is self-reported health worse because the person has problems bathing and/or carrying groceries home, or do these two tasks appear particular difficult because health as such is perceived as poor.

Quality of measurement is important and may be the only purpose of analysis. The widespread use of SF-36 is sufficient reason to examine validity, objectivity, and reliability. Often the measurement problem is subordinate to latent-structure analysis, as illustrated by analysis of the effect of BMI on physical disability. In this analysis, the evidence against the Rasch model is inescapable, even though four items fit an RM. The price to pay in terms of reliability is unacceptable because items appear to be face valid. The nine PF items provide essentially valid and objective measurements of physical disability. We base latent regression analysis on these nine items, taking DIF and LD into account and argue that this is better than using four items, even though these provide valid and objective measurements in the strict sense.

Applications of Generalized Rasch Models in the Sport, Exercise, and the Motor Domains

Gershon Tenenbaum[1], Bernd Strauss[2], and Dirk Büsch[3]

[1] Florida State University
[2] University of Münster
[3] University of Bremen

22.1 Introduction

This chapter provides an overview of the applications of Rasch models (RMs) and their generalizations in the sport, exercise, and motor domains. More specifically, it covers the main areas where Rasch analyses advanced the knowledge base on issues such as (1) examining and developing state and trait-type measures such as motivation for physical activity, anxiety and precompetition anxiety, flow, goal orientation, and running discomfort, or other measures like self-concept or fan identification, (2) testing the stability of introspective and actual measures, (3) testing accumulation of perceived exertion during gradual effort increase, and (4) examining motor abilities, detecting motor components, and strategies used in motor control and development. Based on the current use of generalized RMs in the sport, exercise, and motor domains, the chapter outlines the potential areas where applications of the RMs can be used by both scientists and practitioners.

Research in the field of sport psychology has often ignored probabilistic test models (see Strauss, 1999; Tenenbaum, 1999), even though they reveal several advantages over classical test theory (see Lord & Novick, 1968). Though Duda's (1998) edited book on measurement in sport psychology does mention some applications of probabilistic models, its primary focus is on classical approaches. In addition, the few sport psychological studies applying probabilistic models usually refer to the unidimensional RM in its original form.

This chapter provides a short overview of studies that have used RMs in sport, exercise, and motor domains. For illustrative reasons, some studies are described in more detail. However, because the structure of the chapter is domain-oriented, the probabilistic models are not presented in a logically derived order. The sections cover studies on (1) running discomfort, (2) anxiety and precompetition anxiety, (3) flow experience, (4) goal orientation, (5) contrasting actual and retrospective measures of introspection, (6) aspects of the self-concept, (7) perceived exertion, and (8) examining motor abilities, and detecting motor components and strategies.

22.2 Perceived Discomfort in Running

The running discomfort scale (RDS) has been developed by Tenenbaum, Fogarty, Stewart, et al. (1999). The RDS integrates facets of the three-dimensional
construct of pain (i.e., sensory-discriminative, motivational-affective, and
cognitive-affective; Melzack & Wall, 1965) and the perceptions of runners during practice and competitive events. The first version of the RDS consisted
of 36 items and was administered to 142 male and 29 female runners in nine
different races during a competitive road-running season.

The 36 items was then subjected to principal component analysis, resulting in nine factors, which accounted for 66.6% of the total discomfort variance.
Oblique rotation has reduced the number of dimensions to eight, with low to
moderate correlations among them. The eight dimensions were proprioceptive
symptoms, leg symptoms, respiratory difficulties, disorientation, dryness
and heat, task completion thoughts, mental toughness, and head or stomach
symptoms. Of the remaining 32 items, 10 items loaded on the first factor
(proprioceptive symptoms) and accounted for about 50% of the total variance because most of the designated original symptoms were of this nature.
Because the sample size in this study was very small, we present here only
the results for the scale that was established by the first factor. The following analyses will therefore focus on the 10 items that were best represented
by the first factor. A Rasch rating scale analysis was performed for the scale
using the ASCORE program (Andrich et al., 1991). This RDS dimension was
regarded as unidimensional, and item parameters were estimated to examine
the spread of the items on the latent continuum, and item-fit statistics were
computed to indicate how well each item response vector was represented by
the expected responses given that the RM holds. The most easily endorsed
item was "looking forward to finish," a psychological symptom, while the most
difficult to endorse item was "ringing in the ears," a proprioceptive symptom
that was hardly ever experienced by the subjects in the sample. It appears
that physically demanding effort that is believed to elicit more physiological
awareness, by activating the "neural gating circuits" in the dorsal horns of
the spinal cord as suggested by GCT (Melzack & Wall, 1965; Pinel, 1990),
affects most psychological experiences in the form of completion thoughts and
coping strategies. However, all symptoms intensify as physical effort becomes
extremely demanding. Separate item-difficulty estimates for male and female
runners used for the graphical model test suggested by Rasch showed that
the vast majority of the items were located within confidence bounds of the
identity line.

22.3 Evaluation of Trait-State Anxiety Scales

Anxiety is one of the most essential and most researched areas in psychology.
It attracted most of the research attention in the sport psychology domain for

many years (Tenenbaum & Bar-Eli, 1995). However, a very common measurement tool, i.e., the State-Trait Anxiety Inventory (STAI; Spielberger et al., 1970), used in these studies was subjected mainly to classical item-analyses methods. Tenenbaum et al. (1985) were the first to use the rating scale RM (Andrich, 1988; Wright & Masters, 1982) to evaluate whether the items of the STAI can reliably measure anxiety trait and state in athletes. One hundred young students-athletes responded to the trait scales and 55 high-level athletes responded to the state scales within 30 minutes prior to a competition.

Rasch estimates of both person and item parameters for the trait-anxiety scale indicated that the item parameters were clustered and not equally spread across the latent dimension of the trait-anxiety measure. A sufficient number of items exist to differentiate high trait-anxious athletes but not low trait-anxious athlete; 6 of the 20 items showed insufficient item-fit values; several items had almost identical locations on the latent continuum. A similar analysis performed on the state anxiety scale uncovered similar concerns. Item parameters were clustered with insufficient coverages of the low anxiety region of the latent continuum; 15 of the 20 items were located within less than one logit range, thus limiting the discrimination between athletes high and low on state anxiety; six items did not fit the RM. Rasch analysis indicates that the STAI scales need further work in order to be suitable for measuring trait and state anxiety in athletes.

Fig. 22.1. X–Y plot for anxiety items' actual and retrospective estimates

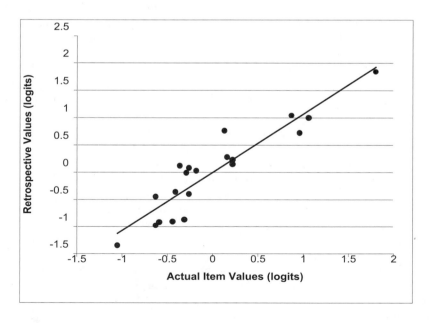

22.4 The Multidimensional Process of the Flow Experience

Flow is an optimal psychological state that has been described by Csik-szentmihalyi (1993) and adapted to sport and physical activity (see Jackson, 1996a,b). Nine areas of flow were operationally defined: challenge-skill balance, action-awareness merging, clear goals, concentration on task at hand, loss of self-consciousness, transformation of time, and autotelic experience. Jackson (1996b) as well as Jackson (1996a) supported these areas using both qualitative and quantitative methods using a 36 items scale; Each of the nine areas is represented by 4 items (i.e., flow-state scale; FSS). Exploratory and confirmatory factor analyses was used to establish the nine-dimensional structure. However, the scale developers reported low communalities of the *transformation of time* and *self-consciousness* factors within the sport domain, and moderate loading of the *autotelic experience* on the second-order first factor.

Rasch analysis was applied to the FSS in order to examine whether such a high-dimensional structure is necessary to describe the response behavior of examinees in the FSS in the sports domain (Tenenbaum, Fogarty, & Jackson, 1999).

A sample of 394 athletes (264 males and 130 females) from 41 sports disciplines was combined with a sample of 398 participants in the World Master games competition. All athletes were administered the FSS, a 36 items scale with 5-Likert type response format. These data was subjected to rating scale Rasch analysis using ASCORE package (Andrich et al., 1991). Person fit statistics resulted in eliminating 62 cases from the final analysis because of response patterns that were very unlikely under a unidimensional model. This may be a first indication that the construct is not unidimensional or homogeneous in this sample, i.e., that the sample consists of more than one population of respondents. The unidimensional analysis revealed that the most easy to endorse item ($\delta = -1.16$ logits) was "I found the experience extremely rewarding," while the most difficult to endorse item was "I was worried about my performance during the event" ($\delta = 1.24$ logits). The other items were spread along the latent continuum between these two items without apparent clusters of items.

Four out of the 5 misfit items resulted from the Rasch analysis were located in the upper end of the latent dimension. The flow experiences they represent were felt only rarely by the sample of athletes in their respective sport experiences. The fifth misfit item was also located within the upper region of the continuum. This misfit results when athletes who differ in their responses to flow experience items at the same time respond in similar ways to items talking about states they have not experienced. Estimates of item difficulties based on separate calibrations of the elite and the nonelite subsamples were used in Rasch's graphical-model test and revealed that item parameters are invariant across the two samples. More importantly, some aspects of flow are more frequently experienced than others or occur at different periods of the entire flow experience. Autotelic experiences, which capture enjoyment, are extensively felt. This would follow by clear goals, competency in meeting demands, total concentration, total control, knowledge of what a person is doing, and focus on the task. Loss of consciousness and transformation of time were less experienced though they are indicators of the "deep" flow experience; one that is almost unfelt, automatic, fluent, and uncontrolled.

22.5 Goal (Task and Ego) Orientation within Motivational Theory

One of the most frequently used questionnaires for measuring goal orientation in sport and exercise is the "task and ego orientation in sport" questionnaire (TEOSQ; Duda & Nicholls, 1992). It consists of 13 items; 7 items comprise a task orientation and 6 comprise an ego orientation. The item response format is a 5-point Likert-type rating scale. Goal orientation is believed to be a strong determinant of motivational orientation, and thus was, and still is, a major concern in the sport and exercise sciences. The TEOSQ was analyzed frequently with respect to its reliability and validity using classical methods. This scale was first subjected to an analysis with the RM by Tenenbaum & Fogarty (1996). The sample used consisted of 1,591 adolescents who participated in sport and fitness activities in Australia, New Zealand, and the United States.

The assumption that the two scales are independent was verified by the moderate correlation between them. A CFA analysis has indicated that the two-factor model fits the data very well; thus, the assumption that the items define their respective dimension was tenable. Also, the item-total correlations were in a magnitude that indicated sufficient homogeneity within the task and ego dimensions. Rating scale Rasch analyses (Andrich, 1988) for the items were performed separately for males and females samples as well as for the entire sample to check for the stability of item parameters estimates across different samples.

The item parameters locations on their respective linear dimension indicate how "easy" and "hard" it was to rate each item highly, but more importantly, the spacing among the items also indicate how narrow or wide is the scale. The spread of item parameters for the ego subscale is comparably narrow (δ range: $-.34 - .69$ logits). The spread of parameters for the task-orientation scale is also very narrow (δ range: $-.44 - .27$ logits). Whereas ego-orientation items did not misfit, the task-orientation scale included three items with unacceptable item misfit, though some were more prominent in one gender than the other one. The raw score distributions further indicated that task scale was negatively skewed, especially for the female-athletes subsample.

22.6 Self-Concept

The self-concept of a person refers to those opinions, attitudes, or beliefs that individuals have about themselves. Shavelson et al. (1976), for example, have proposed that an individual's self-concept may be broken down into an academic part and a nonacademic component. In the nonacademic part of the self-concept, they further distinguish among social, emotional, and physical domains. It is precisely this final aspect that is of particular interest for sport. It refers to how individuals rate themselves in physical terms. Marsh and Redmayne's (1994) hierarchic concept of the physical self-concept distinguishes between a global component, namely, general physical ability, and further specific components such as stamina, power, coordination, and so forth. Marsh et al. (1994) developed a measurement instrument for assessing these components. Their physical self-description questionnaire (PSDQ) is a reliable and valid instrument that is applied frequently. It consists of 11 subscales composed of 70 items, each rated on 6-point scales.

Fletcher & Hattie (2004) (see also Fletcher, 1999) used the graded-response model (Samejima, 1969) to study the item structure and the goodness of fit of the PSDQ items. They administered the PSDQ to 868 examinees aged 13–17 years. Applying this polytomous IRT model enabled them to show which items were more or less representative of the underlying latent variable, and also that the PSDQ discriminated better between (1) persons with a low physical self-concept than between (2) persons with a high self-concept. This meant that fewer items were needed to assess the former compared with the latter.

Another aspect of the self-concept—the self-concept of sport spectators—was studied by Wann & Branscombe (1993) and by Strauss (1994, 1995). Wann & Branscombe (1993) have proposed a 7-item scale to measure sport spectators' identification with their team. This can be viewed as part of a person's social self-concept. Wann & Branscombe (1993) only used classical methods such as factor analysis to demonstrate the unidimensionality of the scale. Strauss (1995) translated Wann and Branscombe's identification scale into German. Each item in the German version was rated on a 5-point scale with the poles *minimum* (1) and *maximum* (5). These were presented to a random sample of 404 citizens of the German city Kiel. Whereas classical analyses confirmed Wann and Branscombe's (1993) results, unidimensionality was also tested with RMs for ordered responses using the mixed RM (MRM) framework (Rost, 1990, 1991). As described in other chapters, if the assumption of unidimensionality holds for the entire sample, the analysis with the MRM should indicate a satisfactory fit for the ordinary RM (one class MRM) and not require a two-class MRM. Using information indices (Akaike, 1973; Schwarz, 1978) as well as bootstrapping procedures for goodness of fit statistics (von Davier, 1997), it was established that a mixture distribution RM did not provide better fit than the ordinary RM for of the German identification scale.

22.7 Motor Abilities and Motor Strategies

22.7.1 Gross-Motor Coordination

Motor abilities in sport, that is, particularly coordination, strength, and endurance, represent a major field of motor research. However, despite the long tradition in this field, coordinative abilities still remain very controversial. The discussion ranges from one extreme assuming that motor abilities in sport are factors determining performance on several motor skills (Fleishman, 1972; Mechling, 1999) to the opposite extreme that rejects the ability construct completely on the basis of insufficient evidence (i.e., the low correlations between the items, the dependence of the number of abilities operationalized on the researchers examining them, and the preference for carrying out exploratory factor analyses (Burton & Miller, 1998; Büsch & Strauss, 2005; Cratty, 1973; Magill, 2003; Schmidt & Lee, 1999; Singer, 1980).

Spray (1987) has argued that IRT models should not be viewed as an alternative in motor research but as a meaningful extension of classical test theory. She pointed out that even though IRT models have been neglected almost completely up to now, they "might hold the future of measurement research in physical education" (p. 208; see, also, Safrit et al., 1989). This led Zhu & Kurz (1994), for example, to use the partial-credit model (Masters, 1982) to develop a test of motor competence in children 3 to 9 years olds. In addition, Hands & Larkin (2001) used Andrich's (1988) rating-scale model to study general motor abilities in children. They gathered data on 24 different motor tasks from 332 children aged 5–6 years. These tasks covered fundamental movement skills such as running, jumping, or balancing. Results produced two separate unidimensional scales for boys and girls. In German-language motor research, Bös & Roth (1978) were the first to explicate the potentials, special features, and advantages of applying probabilistic models. Roth (1982) applied Fischer's (1974) linear-logistic test model (LLTM) to test the unidimensionality of his factors. In this study, 482 children aged 9–14 years also performed different fundamental movement skills. Roth supposed two factors: the *ability to coordinate under time pressure* and the *ability to control movements precisely*. For the dichotomized raw data, he was able to confirm Rasch homogeneity for the ability to control movements precisely (see also Bös & Mechling, 1983). However, he was only able to confirm the unidimensionality of the ability to coordinate under time pressure in the obstacle races used in his study after eliminating the movement task of "dynamic balancing."

Büsch & Strauss (2005) reanalyzed Roth's (1982) coordination model, which postulated the ability to control movements precisely and the ability to coordinate under time pressure. Five-hundred and three participants (249 women and 254 men) with a mean age of 24.5 years ($SD = 4.0$) were asked to perform fundamental movement skills. The raw data were analyzed by means of the mixed RM (MRM; Rost, 1991) and latent-class analysis (LCA) using the WINMIRA 2001 program (von Davier, 2001). The analyses confirmed

Fig. 22.2. Expected values for the two-class solution: (1) latent-class analysis (LCA) and (2) mixed-Rasch analysis (MRM). Class 1 represents the speed strategy (S strategy), and class 2 represents the speed-accuracy strategy (SA strategy)

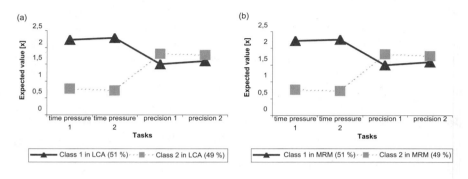

two-class solutions; this did not correspond to Roth's (1982) model (see Figure 22.2). In contrast to the Roth's (1982) ability concept, these results could be interpreted as indicating that persons performing gross-motor tasks may be differentiated according to which coordination strategy or movement tactic they apply. This interpretation corresponds with the assumption that gross-motor tasks should probably be viewed as multidimensional on the ability level (Spray, 1990). From this perspective, precision tasks are mastered with one strategy (see also Bös & Mechling, 1983; Roth, 1982), whereas time-pressure tasks are mastered with two different strategies—either a speed strategy (S) or a speed-accuracy strategy (SA; see Büsch & Strauss, 2005).

22.7.2 Ball Coordination

In a study of 704 Spanish boys aged 7–14 years, Sanchez–Banuelos and Roth (as cited in Bös & Roth, 1978) applied Fischer's (1974) linear-logistic test model to the dichotomized data from 18 different ball tasks assessing movement skills such as throwing, catching, bouncing, or rolling. They found that the latent variable "ball coordination" could be scaled most successfully through the movement tasks containing successive or simultaneous combinations of the movement skills throwing and catching. A further study on ball coordination tested whether movement tasks with and without a ball are determined by different skill levels (Büsch et al., 2001) or by different coordination strategies (Büsch & Strauss, 2005). Should the former be true, one would expect a unidimensional RM; for the latter, two latent classes in which Rasch homogeneity holds could be anticipated. A total of 305 participants (155 ball-game athletes and 150 non-ball-game athletes) with a mean age of 24.6 years ($SD = 3.9$) performed three time-pressure tasks with no ball and three time-pressure tasks with a ball. The tasks with a ball involved the movement skill of dribbling. The raw scores were analyzed with the mixed RM (Rost, 1990) and the latent-class analysis (Lazarsfeld & Henry, 1968) using the WINMIRA 2001 program (von Davier, 2001). Acceptable model fit was obtained for both the latent-class and the mixed-Rasch analyses. From a formal perspective, however, it was not possible to decide unequivocally between a Rasch-homogeneous one-class solution and a latent two-class solution. From a theoretical perspective, the two-class solution would seem preferable, because the classes are not associated with the skill level but rather with two different coordination strategies (Büsch, 2004).

22.7.3 Motor Development

Zhu & Cole (1996) examined the advantages and potential applications of the many-facet RM by analyzing performance on the much-evaluated and repeatedly applied Test of Gross Motor Development (TGMD; Ulrich, 1985). They administered the TGMD to 909 children (451 boys) aged 3–10 years. This test battery contains two motor categories: "locomotion" and "object control." The former contains seven subtests assessed through four performance criteria, and the latter five subtests assessed through three performance criteria. To calibrate the TGMD over the many-facet RM (Linacre, 1994a,b), eight facets were defined; that is, five examinee-related facets (disability status, ethnicity group, age, gender, examinee) and three item-related facets (subtest, item, category). Results showed a clear age ($\delta = -2.77$ logits for 3-year-olds to $\delta = 2.28$ logits for 10-year-olds) and gender effect ($\delta = 0.81$ logits for males and $\delta = 0.65$ logits for females). Furthermore, the fundamental movement skills in the object-control category were more difficult ($\delta = -0.04$ logits) than those in the locomotion category ($\delta = 0.04$ logits). The authors used these analyses to formulate a recalibrated new scoring form for the TGMD that provides the experimenter with information on which is the easiest and the most difficult item for a certain child, and how this skill-oriented information should be judged in relation to (gross-motor) coordination ability in motor development.

22.7.4 Motor Tests

Further applications of the RM, particularly for test construction and test validation, can be found, e.g., in research on adapted physical education (Cole et al., 1991) and rehabilitation (Dickson & Köhler, 1996; Fisher, Jr., 1993; Fisher, 1993). Another example is a study reported by Safrit et al. (1992). They used the Rasch Poisson counts model to examine how difficulty varied in 18 different sit-ups tests for training abdominal muscles. A total of 426 college students performed the 18 tests within an 8-week period. The number of attempts within 1 min was recorded, and data were analyzed with the FACETS program (Linacre, 1994a,b). The simplest item was performance with hands on thighs and feet anchored ($\delta = -4.02$ logits), whereas the most difficult item was performance with hands clasped behind the neck and feet not anchored, and elbows pointed forward ($\delta = -3.57$ logits). An example of a useful application of sit-ups tests of varying difficulty is adaptive testing in the clinical domain.

22.8 Final Remark

Probabilistic measurement models in sport psychology were devoted mainly for testing properties of questionnaires and on several research questions in the motor domain. However, the use of these models is rare but very fruitful from both a methodological and a content-related perspective in sport sciences. The studies presented in this chapter underline this very clearly. Recently, von Davier & Strauss (2003) provided an overview on new developments in testing probabilistic models that will further enhance the measurement of constructs in sport psychology and in movement science. Despite the advantages that the RMs offer to scientists and practitioners, their use is not widely spread. It remains to be seen to what extent scholars in the field will apply the valuable concept and methodology in the future.

References

Ackerman, P. L., Beier, M. E., & Boyle, M. O. (2005). Working memory and intelligence: The same or different constructs? *Psychological Bulletin, 131,* 30–60.

Ackerman, T. A. (1994). Using multidimensional item response theory to understand what items and tests are measuring. *Applied Measurement in Education, 7,* 255–278.

Adams, R. J., & Wilson, M. R. (1996). Formulating the Rasch model as a mixed coefficients multinomial model. In G. Engelhard Jr. & M. R. Wilson (Eds.), *Objective measurement: Theory into practice* (Vol. 3, pp. 143–166). Norwood, New Jersey: Ablex.

Adams, R. J., Wilson, M. R., & Wang, W. (1997). The multidimensional random coefficients multinomial logit model. *Applied Psychological Measurement, 21,* 1–23.

Adams, R. J., Wilson, M. R., & Wu, M. L. (1997). Multilevel item response modelling: An approach to errors in variables regression. *Journal of Educational and Behavioral Statistics, 22,* 47–76.

Adams, R. J., & Wu, M. L. (Eds.). (2002). *Pisa 2000 technical report.* Paris: Organisation for Economic Co-Operation and Development (OECD) Publications.

Adams, R. J., & Wu, M. L. (2004). *The construction and implementation of user-defined fit tests for use with marginal maximum likelihood estimation and generalised item response models.* Paper presented at the International Meeting of the Psychometric Society, Pacific Grove, California.

Agresti, A. (1984). *Analysis of ordinal categorical data.* New York: Wiley.

Agresti, A. (1990). *Categorical data analyses.* Wiley: New York.

Aitchison, J., & Silvey, S. D. (1958). Maximum likelihood estimation of parameter subject to restraints. *Annals of Mathematical Statistics, 29,* 813–828.

Akaike, H. (1973). Information theory and an extension of the maximum likelihood principle. In B. N. Petroy & F. Csaki (Eds.), *The second international symposium on information theory.* Budapest, Romania: Akadmiai Kiado.

Akaike, H. (1981). Likelihood of a model and information criteria. *Journal of Econometrics, 16*, 3–14.

Akaike, H. (1983). Statistical inference and measurement of entropy. In H. Akaike & C.-F. Wu (Eds.), *Scientific inference, data analysis, and robustness* (pp. 165–189). New York: Academic Press.

Albert, J. H. (1992). Bayesian estimation of normal ogive item response functions using Gibbs sampling. *Journal of Educational Statistics, 17*, 251–269.

Andersen, E. B. (1970). Asymptotic properties of conditional maximum likelihood estimators. *Journal of the Royal Statistical Society, 32*, 283–301.

Andersen, E. B. (1971). *Conditional inference for multiple choice questionaires (report no. 8.)*. Copenhagen, Denmark: Copenhagen School for Economics and Business Administration.

Andersen, E. B. (1972). The numerical solution of a set of conditional estimation equations. *Journal of the Royal Statistical Society, 34*, 42–54.

Andersen, E. B. (1973a). *Conditional inference and models for measuring*. Copenhagen, Denmark: Mentalhygiejnisk Forlag.

Andersen, E. B. (1973b). Conditional inference and multiple choice questionnaires. *British Journal of Mathematical and Statistical Psychology, 26*, 31–44.

Andersen, E. B. (1973c). A goodness of fit test for the Rasch model. *Psychometrika, 38*, 123–140.

Andersen, E. B. (1977). Sufficient statistics and latent trait models. *Psychometrika, 42*, 69–81.

Andersen, E. B. (1980). *Discrete statistical models with social science applications*. Amsterdam: North Holland.

Andersen, E. B. (1985). Estimating latent correlations between repeated testings. *Psychometrika, 50*, 3–16.

Andersen, E. B. (1991). Longitudinal studies for discrete data based on latent structure models. In D. Magnusson, L. R. Bergman, G. Rudinger, & B. Törestad (Eds.), *Problems and methods in longitudinal research: Stability and change* (pp. 308–322). Cambridge, England: Cambridge University Press.

Andersen, E. B., & Madsen, M. (1977). Estimating the parameters of the latent population distribution. *Psychometrika, 42*, 357–374.

Anderson, C. J., & Vermunt, J. K. (2000). Log-multiplicative association models as latent variable models for nominal and/or ordinal data. *Sociological Methodology, 30*, 81–121.

Andrich, D. (1978). A rating formulation for ordered response categories. *Psychometrika, 43*, 561–573.

Andrich, D. (1982). An extension of the Rasch model for ratings providing both location and dispersion parameters. *Psychometrika, 47*, 105–113.

Andrich, D. (1985). A latent trait model for items with response dependencies: Implications for test construction and analysis. In S. E. Embretson (Ed.), *Test design—Developments in psychology and psychometrics*. New York: Academic Press, Inc.

Andrich, D. (1988). *Rasch models for measurement.* Thousand Oaks, CA: Sage Publications.

Andrich, D. (1995a). Further remarks on nondichotomization of graded responses. *Psychometrika, 60,* 37–46.

Andrich, D. (1995b). Models for measurement, precision, and the nondichotomization of graded responses. *Psychometrika, 60,* 7–26.

Andrich, D., De Jong, J. H., & Sheridan, B. (1997). Diagnostic opportunities with the Rasch model for ordered response categories. In J. Rost & R. Langeheine (Eds.), *Applications of latent trait and latent class models in the social sciences* (pp. 59–70). Münster, Germany: Waxmann.

Andrich, D., Sheridan, B., & Lyne, A. (1991). *ASCORE: Manual of procedures.* Perth, Australia: University of Western Australia.

Armon, C. (1984). *Ideals of the good life: Evaluative reasoning in children and adults.* Unpublished doctoral dissertation, Harvard, Boston.

Arnold, S. F. (1988). Sufficient statistics. In S. Kotz & N. L. Johnson (Eds.), *Encyclopedia of statistical sciences. vol 9.* (pp. 72–80). New York: John Wiley & Sons.

Bachman, L. F. (1990). *Fundamental considerations in language testing.* Oxford: Oxford University Press.

Barratt, E. S. (1953). An analysis of verbal reports of solving spatial problems as aid in defining spatial factors. *The Journal of Psychology, 36,* 17–25.

Beaton, A. E. (1987). *Implementing the new design: The NAEP 1983-84 technical report* (Tech. Rep. No. 15-TR-20). Princeton, NJ: Educational Testing Service.

Béguin, A. A., & Glas, C. A. W. (2001). Mcmc estimation and some fit analysis of multidimensional IRT models. *Psychometrika, 66,* 541–562.

Bejar, I. (2002). Generative testing: From conception to implementation. In S. H. Irvine & P. C. Kyllonen (Eds.), *Item generation for test development* (pp. 199–217). Hillsdale, NJ: Erlbaum.

Béland, A., & Mislevy, R. J. (1996). Probability-based inference in a domain of proportional reasoning tasks. *Journal of Educational Assessment, 33,* 3–27.

Benjamini, Y., & Hochberg, Y. (1995). Controlling the false discovery rate: A practical and powerful approach to multiple testing. *Journal of the Royal Statistical Society, Series B, 57,* 289–300.

Bickel, P., & Doksum, K. (1977). *Mathematical statistics.* Englewood Cliffs, NJ: Prentice Hall.

Birnbaum, A. (1968). Some latent trait models and their use in inferring an examinee's ability. In F. M. Lord & M. R. Novick (Eds.), *Statistical theories of mental test scores* (pp. 397–479). Reading, MA: MIT Press.

Blackwood, L. G., & Bradley, E. L. (1989). The equivalence of two methods of parameter estimation for the Rasch model. *Psychometrika, 54,* 751–754.

Bock, R. D. (1972). Estimating item parameters and latent ability when responses are scored in two or more nominal categories. *Psychometrika, 37,* 29–51.

Bock, R. D., & Aitkin, M. (1981). Marginal maximum likelihood estimation of item parameters: An application of the EM algorithm. *Psychometrika*, *46*, 443-4-59.

Bock, R. D., Gibbons, R. D., & Muraki, E. (1988). Full-information factor analysis. *Applied Psychological Measurement*, *12*, 261–280.

Bock, R. D., & Lieberman, M. (1981). Fitting a response model for *n* dichotomously scored items. *Psychometrika*, *35*, 179–187.

Bock, R. D., & Mislevy, R. J. (1989). *Duplex design: Giving students a stake in educational assessment*. Chicago: NORC, Methodology Research Center.

Bock, R. D., Muraki, E., & Pfeiffenberger, W. (1988). Item pool maintenance in the presence of item parameter drift. *Journal of Educational Measurement*, *25*, 275–285.

Bock, R. D., & Schilling, S. G. (1997). High dimensional full-information item factor analysis. In M. Berkane (Ed.), *Latent variable modeling and applications of causality*. New York: Springer Verlag.

Bock, R. D., & Zimowski, M. F. (1997). Multiple group IRT. In W. van der Linden & R. Hambleton (Eds.), *Handbook of modern item response theory* (pp. 433–448). New York: Springer Verlag.

Bolt, D. M., Cohen, A. S., & Wollack, J. A. (2001). A mixture item response model for multiple choice data. *Journal of Educational and Behavioral Statistics*, *26*, 381–409.

Bolt, D. M., Cohen, A. S., & Wollack, J. A. (2002). Item parameter estimation under conditions of test speededness: Application of a mixture Rasch model with ordinal constraints. *Journal of Educational Measurement*, *39*(4), 331–348.

Bond, T. G. (1995a). Piaget and measurement II: Empirical validation of the Piagetian model. *Archives de Psychologie*, *63*, 155–185.

Bond, T. G. (1995b). Piaget and measurement I: The twain really do meet. *Archives de Psychologie*, *63*, 71–87.

Bond, T. G., & Bunting, E. M. (1995). Piaget and measurement III: Reassessing the methode critique. *Archives de Psychologie*, *63*, 231–255.

Bös, K., & Mechling, H. (1983). *Dimensionen sportmotorischer Leistungen [Dimensions of motor performances]*. Schorndorf, Germany: Hofmann.

Bös, K., & Roth, K. D. (1978). Möglichkeiten der anwendung probabilistischer modelle im bereich sportmotorischer und sportpsychologischer forschung. [Applications of probabilistic models in motor research and sport psychology]. *Sportwissenschaft*, *8*, 407–421.

Boughton, K. A., Larkin, K. A., & Yamamoto, K. Y. (2004). *Modeling differential speededness using a hybrid psychometric approach*. Paper presented at the annual meeting of the American Educational Research Association, San Diego, CA, USA.

Boughton, K. A., & Yamamoto, K. Y. (2004). *Recovery of item parameters and switching distributions in the hybrid model for test speededness: A comparison of marginal maximum likelihood estimation and markov chain monte carlo estimation.* Paper presented at the annual meeting of the National Council on Measurement in Education, San Diego, CA, USA.

Box, G., & Tiao, G. (1973). *Bayesian inference in statistical analysis.* Reading, MA: Addison-Wesley Publishing Company.

Bradley, R. A., & Terry, M. E. (1952). The rank analysis of incomplete block designs I: The method of paired comparisons. *Biometrika, 39,* 324.

Bradlow, E. T., Wainer, H., & Wang, X. (1999). A Bayesian random effects model for testlets. *Psychometrika, 64,* 153–168.

Breslow, N. (2003). *"Whither PQL?"* (Tech. Rep. No. Working Paper 192). UW: Biostatistics.

Brown, J. S., & van Lehn, K. (1980). Repair theory: A generative theory of bugs in procedural skills. *Cognitive Science, 2,* 379-426.

Burnham, K. P., & Anderson, D. R. (2002). *Model selection and multimodel inference.* New York: Springer Verlag.

Burton, A. W., & Miller, D. E. (1998). *Movement skill assessment.* Champaign, IL: Human Kinetics.

Büsch, D. (2004). Unterschiede im fertigkeitsniveau—Ein qualitativer oder "nur" ein quantitativer unterschied? Eine re-analyse. [Differences in the skill level—A qualitative or only a quantitative difference? A re-analysis]. *Zeitschrift für Sportpsychologie, 11,* 137–146.

Büsch, D., Hagemann, N., & Thielke, S. (2001). Gibt es eine ballfähigkeit? [Does ball ability exist?]. *Psychologie und Sport, 8,* 57–66.

Büsch, D., & Strauss, B. (2005). Qualitative differences in performing coordination tracks. *Measurement in Physical Education and Exercise Science, 9*(3), 161–180.

Campbell, N. R. (1920). *Physics: The elements.* Cambridge, England: Cambridge University Press.

Carpenter, P. A., Just, M. A., & Shell, P. (1990). What one intelligence test measures: A theoretical account of processing in the Ravens's progressive marices test. *Psychological Review, 97,* 404–531.

Carroll, J. B. (1976). Psychometric tests as cognitive tasks: A new structure of intellect. In L. B. Resnick (Ed.), *The nature of intelligence* (pp. 27–57). Hillsdale, NJ: Erlbaum.

Carstensen, C. H. (2000). *Ein mehrdimensionales testmodell mit anwendungen in der pädagogisch-psychologischen diagnostik [A multidimensional test model with applications in psychological diagnostics].* Dissertation, Christian Albrechts Universität zu Kiel, Germany.

Carstensen, C. H., & Rost, J. (2001). *MULTIRA—A program system for multidimensional Rasch models* [Computer software]. Kiel, Germany: IPN—Leibniz Institute for Science Education.

Case, R. (1985). *Intellectual development: Birth to adulthood.* Orlando, FL: Academic Press.

Cheong, Y. F. (2006). Analysis of school context effects on differential item functioning using hierarchical generalized linear models. *International Journal of Testing, 6,* 57–79.

Cheong, Y. F., & Raudenbush, S. W. (2000). Measurement and structural models for children's problem behaviors. *Psychological Methods*, *5*, 477–495.

Christensen, K. B., & Bjorner, J. B. (2003). *SAS macros for Rasch based latent variable modelling* (Research Rep. No. 03/13). Copenhagen, Denmark: University of Copenhagen, Department of Biostatistics.

Christensen, K. B., Bjorner, J. B., Kreiner, S., & Petersen, J. H. (2002). Testing unidimensionality in polytomous Rasch models. *Psychometrika*, *67*, 563–574.

Christensen, K. B., Bjorner, J. B., Kreiner, S., & Petersen, J. H. (2004). Latent regression in loglinear Rasch models. *Communications in Statistics. Theory and Methods*, *33*, 1295–1313.

Chu, K., & Kamata, A. (2005). Test equating in the presence of DIF items. *Journal of Applied Measurement*, *6*, 342–354.

Clogg, C. C., & Goodman, L. A. (1984). Latent structure analyses of a set of multidimensional contingency tables. *Journal of the American Statistical Association*, *79*, 762–771.

Cole, E. L., Wood, T. M., & Dunn, J. M. (1991). Item response theory: A useful test theory for adapted physical education. *Adapted Physical Activity Quarterly*, *8*, 317–332.

Commons, M. L., Trudeau, E. J., Stein, S. A., Richards, F. A., & Krause, S. R. (1998). Hierarchical complexity of tasks shows the existence of developmental stages. *Developmental Review*, *18*, 237–278.

Cooper, L. A., & Shepard, R. N. (1973). Chronometric studies of the rotation of mental images. In W. G. Chase (Ed.), *Visual information processing* (pp. 75–176). London: Academic Press.

Cornfield, J., Kannel, W., & Truett, J. (1967). A multivariate analysis of the risk of coronary heart disease in Framingham. *Journal of Chronic Disease*, *20*, 511–524.

Costa, P., & McRae, R. (1992). *Revised NEO personality inventory (NEO-PI-R) and NEO five factor inventory (NEO-FFI): Professional manual*. Odessa, FL.

Cratty, B. J. (1973). *Teaching motor skills*. Englewood Cliffs, NJ:: Prentice-Hall.

Cressie, N., & Holland, P. W. (1983). Characterizing the manifest probabilities of latent trait models. *Psychometrika*, *48*, 129–141.

Cronbach, L. (1957). The two disciplines of scientific psychology. *American Psychologist*, *12*, 671–684.

Croon, M. (1990). Latent class analysis with ordered latent classes. *British Journal of Mathematical and Statistical Psychology*, *43*, 171–192.

Csikszentmihalyi, M. (1993). *The evolving self*. Harper and Row, New York.

Dagohoy, A. (2005). *Explanatory item response models: A generalized linear and nonlinear approach*. Unpublished doctoral dissertation, University of Twente, The Netherlands.

Dawson, T. (2002). New tools, new insights. Kohlberg's moral reasoning stages revisited. *International Journal of Behavior Development, 26*, 154–166.

Dawson, T., Goodheart, E., Draney, K., Wilson, M. R., & Commons, M. L. (1997). *Assessment of stage transitions in performance on Commons' balance beam instrument.* Paper presented at the International Objective Measurement Workshop, Chicago.

Dawson-Tunik, T. L. (2002). A good education is... The development of evaluative thought across the life-span. *Genetic, Social, and General Psychology Monographs, 130*, 4–112.

Dayton, C. M., & Macready, G. B. (1976). A probabilistic model for validation of behavioral hierarchies. *Psychometrika, 41*, 189–204.

De Boeck, P., & Wilson, M. R. (2004). *Explanatory item response models: A generalized linear and nonlinear approach.* New York: Springer Verlag.

Demetriou, A., & Efklides, A. (1989). The person's conception of the structures of developing intellect: Early adolescence to middle age. *Genetic, Social, and General Psychology Monographs, 115*, 371–423.

Demetriou, A., & Efklides, A. (1994). Structure, development, and dynamics of mind: A meta-Piagetian theory. In A. Demetriou & A. Efklides (Eds.), *Intelligence, mind, and reasoning: Structure and development. Advances in psychology.* Amsterdam: North-Holland/Elsevier Science.

Demetriou, A., Efklides, A., Papadaki, M., Papantoniou, G., & Economou, A. (1993). Structure and development of causal-experimental thought: From early adolescence to youth. *Developmental Psychology, 29*, 480–497.

Deming, W. E., & Stephan, R. R. (1940). On a least squares adjustment of a sampled frequency table when the expected marginal totals are known. *Annals of Mathematical Statistics, 11*, 427–444.

Dempster, A. P., Laird, N. M., & Rubin, D. B. (1977). Maximum likelihood from incomplete data via the EM algorithm. *Journal Royal Statistical Society Series B, 39*, 1–38.

Dickson, H. G., & Köhler, F. (1996). The multi-dimensionality of the fim motor items preludes an interval scaling using Rasch analysis. *Scandinavian Journal of Rehabilitation Medicine, 26*, 159–162.

Digman, J. M. (1990). Personality structure: Emergence of the five-factor model. *Annual Review of Psychology, 41*, 417–440.

Donovan, J. J., Dwight, S. A., & Hurtz, G. M. (2003). An assessment of the prevalence, severity, and verifiability of entry-level applicant faking using the randomized response technique. *Human Performance, 16*, 81–106.

Draney, K. (1996). *The polytomous saltus model: A mixture model approach to the diagnosis of developmental differences.* Unpublished doctoral dissertation, University of California, Berkeley.

Duda, J. L. (1998). *Advances in sport and exercise psychology measurement.* Morgantown, WV: FIT.

Duda, J. L., & Nicholls, J. G. (1992). Dimensions of achievement motivation in schoolwork and sport. *Journal of Educational Psychology, 84*, 290–299.

Duncan, O. D. (1984). Rasch measurement: Further examples and discussion. In C. F. Turner & E. Martin (Eds.), *Surveying subjective phenomena* (Vol. 2, pp. 367–403). New York: Russell Sage Foundation.

Duncan, O. D., & Stenbeck, M. (1987). Are Likert scales unidimensional? *Social Science Research, 16* (245-259).

Edwards, A. L. (1957). *The social desirability variable in personality assessment and research.* New York: Dryden.

Efron, B. (1979). Bootstrap methods: Another look at the jackknife. *The Annals of Statistics, 7,* 1–26.

Efron, B. (1982). *The jackknife, the bootstrap and other resampling plans.* Philadelphia: SIAM—Society for Industrial and Applied Mathematics.

Eid, M., & Rauber, M. (2000). Detecting measurement invariance in organizational surveys. *European Journal of Psychological Assessment, 16,* 20–30.

Elliot, C. D. (1990). *Differential ability scales (DAS).* New York: Psychological Corporation.

Elliot, C. D., Smith, P., & McCulloch, K. (1996). *British ability scales II (BAS II).* Windsor, England: NFER-Nelson.

Embretson, S. E. (1983). Construct validity: Construct representation versus nomothetic span. *Psychological Bulletin, 93,* 179–197.

Embretson, S. E. (1985a). A general latent trait model for response processes. *Psychometrika, 49,* 175–186.

Embretson, S. E. (1985b). Multicomponent latent trait models for test design. In S. E. Embretson (Ed.), *Test design: Developments in psychology and psychometrics* (pp. 195–218). Orlando, FL: Academic Press.

Embretson, S. E. (1991). A multidimensional latent trait model for measuring learning and change. *Psychometrika, 56,* 495–515.

Embretson, S. E. (1994). Applications of cognitive design systems to test development. In C. Reynolds (Ed.), *Advances in cognitive assessment: An interdisciplinary perspective* (pp. 107–135). New York: Plenum Publishing Company.

Embretson, S. E. (1995a). A measurement model for linking individual learning to processes and knowledge: Applications to mathematical reasoning. *Psychometrika, 32,* 277–294.

Embretson, S. E. (1995b). Working memory capacity versus general central processes in intelligence. *Intelligence, 20,* 169–189.

Embretson, S. E. (1997). Multicomponent latent trait models. In W. van der Linden & R. Hambleton (Eds.), *Handbook of modern item response theory* (p. 305-322). New York: Springer Verlag.

Embretson, S. E. (1998). A cognitive design system approach to generating valid tests: Application to abstract reasoning. *Psychological Methods, 3,* 380–396.

Embretson, S. E. (2000). Multidimensional measurement from dynamic tests: Abstract reasoning under stress. *Multivariate Behavioral Research, 35,* 505–542.

Embretson, S. E. (2002). Generating abstract reasoning items with cognitive theory. In S. Irvine & P. C. Kyllonen (Eds.), *Generating items for cognitive tests: Theory and practice* (pp. 305–322). Mahwah, NJ: Erlbaum.

Embretson, S. E. (2004). Application of two IRT models for construct validation issues about spatial ability. *Metodologia de las Ciencias del Comportamiento*, *5*, 159–180.

Embretson, S. E., Schneider, L. M., & Roth, D. L. (1986). Multiple processing strategies and the construct validity of verbal reasoning tests. *Journal of Educational Measurement*, *23*, 13–32.

Everitt, B., & Hand, D. (1981). *Finite mixture distributions*. New York: Chapman & Hall.

Fahrenberg, J., Hampel, R., & Selg, H. (1984). *Das Freiburger Persönlichkeitsinventar FPI [Freiburg personality inventory FPI]* (5th ed.). Göttingen, Germany: Hogrefe.

Fayers, P., & Machin, D. (2000). *Quality of life. assessment, analysis and interpretation*. Chichester, England: John Wiley & Sons, Ltd.

Fienberg, S. E. (1980). *The analyses of cross-classified categorical data*. Boston: MIT Press.

Fieuws, S., Spiessens, B., & Draney, K. (2004). Mixture models. In P. De Boeck & M. R. Wilson (Eds.), *Explanatory item response models: A generalized linear and nonlinear approach*. New York: Springer Verlag.

Fischer, G. H. (1968). *Psychologische Testtheorie*. Bern, Germany: Huber.

Fischer, G. H. (1973). The linear logistic model as an instrument in educational research. *Acta Psychologica*, *37*, 359-374.

Fischer, G. H. (1974). *Einführung in die theorie psychologischer tests. [Introduction to the theory of psychological tests]*. Bern, Germany: Huber.

Fischer, G. H. (1976). Some probabilistic models for measuring change. In D. N. M. de Gruijter & L. J. T. van der Kamp (Eds.), *Advances in psychological and educational measurement* (pp. 97–110). New York: Wiley.

Fischer, G. H. (1983). Logistic latent trait models with linear constraints. *Psychometrika*, *48*, 3–26.

Fischer, G. H. (1989). An IRT-based model for dichotomous longitudinal data. *Psychometrika*, *54*, 599–624.

Fischer, G. H. (1995a). Derivations of the Rasch model. In G. H. Fischer & I. W. Molenaar (Eds.), *Rasch models—Foundations, recent developments and applications* (pp. 15–38). New York: Springer Verlag.

Fischer, G. H. (1995b). Linear logistic models for change. In G. H. Fischer & I. W. Molenaar (Eds.), *Rasch Models: Foundations, Recent Developments, and Applications* (pp. 157–180). New York: Springer Verlag.

Fischer, G. H. (1995c). Linear logistic models for change. In G. H. Fischer & I. W. Molenaar (Eds.), *Rasch models—Foundations, recent developments, and applications* (p. 157-180). New York: Springer Verlag.

Fischer, G. H. (1995d). The linear logistic test model. In G. H. Fischer & I. W. Molenaar (Eds.), *Rasch Models: Foundations, Recent Developments, and Applications* (pp. 131–155). New York: Springer Verlag.

Fischer, G. H. (2003). The precision of gain scores under an item response theory perspective: A comparison of asymptotic and exact conditional inference about change. *Applied Psychological Measurement*, *27*, 3–26.

Fischer, G. H., & Allerup, P. (1968). Rechentechnische Fragen zu Raschs eindimensionalem Modell. In G. H. Fischer (Ed.), *Psychologische Testtheorie*. Bern, Germany: Verlag Hans Huber.

Fischer, G. H., & Formann, A. K. (1982). Some applications of logistic latent trait models with linear constraints on the parameters. *Applied Psychological Measurement*, *4*, 397–416.

Fischer, G. H., & Molenaar, I. W. (1995). *Rasch models—Foundations, recent developments, and applications*. New York: Springer Verlag.

Fischer, G. H., & Parzer, P. (1991). An extension of the rating scale model with an application to the measurement of change. *Psychometrika*, *56*, 637–651.

Fischer, G. H., & Ponocny, I. (1994). An extension of the partial credit model with an application to the measurement of change. *Psychometrika*, *59*, 177–192.

Fischer, G. H., & Ponocny, I. (1995). Extended rating scale and partial credit models for assessing change. In G. Fischer & I. Molenaar (Eds.), *Rasch models: Foundations, recent developments and applications* (pp. 353–370). New York: Springer Verlag.

Fischer, G. H., & Ponocny-Seliger, E. (1998). *Structural Rasch modeling. Handbook of the usage of LPCM-WIN 1.0*. Groningen, The Netherlands: ProGAMMA.

Fischer, G. H., & Scheiblechner, H. (1970). Algorithmen und programme für das probabilistische testmodell von Rasch [Algorithms and computer programs for testing the Rasch model]. *Psychologische Beiträge*, *12*, 23–51.

Fischer, K. W., Hand, H. H., & Russel, S. (1984). Mixture models. In M. L. Commons, F. A. Richards, & C. Armon (Eds.), *Beyond formal operations: Late adolescent and adult cognitive development* (pp. 43–73). New York: Praeger.

Fischer, K. W., Pipp, S. L., & Bullock, D. (1984). Detecting discontinuities in development: Methods and measurement. In *Continuities and discontinuities in development*. Norwood, NJ: Ablex.

Fisher, A. G. (1993). The assessment of IADL motor skills: An application of many-faceted Rasch analysis. *The American Journal of Occupational Therapy*, *47*, 319–329.

Fisher, Jr., W. P. (1993). Measurement-related problems in functional assessment. *The American Journal of Occupational Therapy*, *47*, 331–338.

Fleishman, A. (1972). Structure and measurement of psychomotor abilities. In R. N. Singer (Ed.), *The psychomotor domain movement behavior* (pp. 78–106). Philadelphia: Lea & Febiger.

Fletcher, R. B. (1999). Incorporating recent advances in measurement in sport and exercise psychology. *Journal of Sport and Exercise Psychology*, *21*, 24–38.

Fletcher, R. B., & Hattie, J. A. (2004). An examination of the psychometric properties of the physical self-description questionnaire using a polytomous item response model. *Psychology of Sport and Exercise, 5*, 423–446.

Follmann, D. (1988). Consistent estimation in the Rasch model based on nonparametric margins. *Psychometrika, 53*, 553-562.

Folstein, M. F., Folstein, S. E., & McHugh, P. R. (1975). "mini-mental state." A practical method for grading the cognitive state of patients for the clinician. *Journal of Psychiatric Research, 12*, 189–198.

Formann, A. K. (1982). Linear logistic latent class analysis. *Biometrical Journal, 24*, 171–190.

Formann, A. K. (1985). Constrained latent class models: Theory and applications. *British Journal of Mathematical and Statistical Psychology, 38*, 87–111.

Formann, A. K. (1989). Constrained latent class models: Some further applications. *British Journal of Mathematical and Statistical Psychology, 42*, 37–54.

Formann, A. K. (1992). Linear logistic latent class analysis for polytomous data. *Journal of the American Statistical Association, 87*, 476–486.

Formann, A. K. (2003). Latent class model diagnosis from a frequentist point of view. *Biometrics, 59*, 189–196.

Formann, A. K., & Kohlmann, T. (1998). Structural latent class models. *Sociological Methods and Research, 26*, 530–565.

Fox, J. P., & Glas, C. A. W. (2001). Bayesian estimation of a multilevel IRT model using Gibbs sampling. *Psychometrika, 66*, 271–288.

Franke, G. H. (2002). Faking bad in personality inventories: Consequences for the clinical context. *Psychologische Beiträge, 44*, 50–61.

Fuller, W. A. (1987). *Measurement error models.* New York: Wiley.

Gelfand, A. E., & Smith, A. F. M. (1990). Sampling based approaches to calculating marginal densities. *Journal of American Statical Association, 85*, 398–409.

Gelman, A., Carlin, J. B., Stern, H. S., & Rubin, D. B. (1995). *Bayesian data analysis.* London: Chapman & Hall.

Gibby, R. E. (2004). *Identifying fakers on personality tests and the properties that make personality items fakable.* Unpublished doctoral dissertation, Bowling Green State University, Ohio.

Gilks, W. R., Richardson, S., & Spiegelhalter, D. J. (1996). *Markov chain Monte Carlo in practice.* London: Chapman and Hall.

Gillis, J. R., Rogers, R., & Dickens, S. E. (1990). The detection of faking bad response styles on the MMPI. *Canadian Journal of Behavioural Science, 22*, 408–416.

Gilula, Z., & Haberman, S. J. (1994). Models for analyzing categorical panel data. *Journal of the American Statistical Association, 89*, 645–656.

Gilula, Z., & Haberman, S. J. (1995). Prediction functions for categorical panel data. *The Annals of Statistics, 23*, 1130–1142.

Gilula, Z., & Haberman, S. J. (2000). Density approximation by summary statistics: An information-theoretic approach. *Scandinavian Journal of Statistics*, *27*, 521–534.

Gitomer, D. H., & Yamamoto, K. Y. (1991). Performance modeling that integrates latent trait and class theory. *Journal of Educational Measurement*, *28*, 173–189.

Gittler, G. (1990). *Dreidimensionaler Würfeltest: Ein Rasch-Skalierter Test zur Messung des räumlichen Vorstellungsvermögens [Three-dimensional cube test: A rasch calibrated test for the measurement of spatial abilities]*. Göttingen, Germany: Beltz Test.

Gittler, G., & Glück, J. (1998). Differential transfer of learning: Effects of instruction in descriptive geometry on spatial test performance. *Journal for Geometry and Graphics*, *2*, 71–84.

Glas, C. A. W. (1988). The derivation of some tests for the Rasch model from the multinomial distribution. *Psychometrika*, *53*, 525–546.

Glas, C. A. W. (1992). A Rasch model with a multivariate distribution of ability. In M. R. Wilson (Ed.), *Objective measurement: Theory into practice* (Vol. 1, p. 236-258). Norwood, New Jersey: Ablex Publishing Corporation.

Glas, C. A. W. (1997). Testing the generalized partial credit model. In M. R. Wilson, G. Engelhard Jr., & K. Draney (Eds.), *Objective measurement: Theory into practice* (Vol. 4, p. 237-260). Norwood, New Jersey: Ablex Publishing Corporation.

Glas, C. A. W. (1999). Modification indices for the 2-pl and the nominal response model. *Psychometrika*, *64*, 273–294.

Glas, C. A. W., & Meijer, R. R. (2003). A Bayesian approach to person fit analysis in item response theory models. *Applied Psychological Measurement*, *27*(3), 217–233.

Glas, C. A. W., & Suarez-Falcon, J. C. (2003). A comparison of item-fit statistics for the three-parameter logistic model. *Applied Psychological Measurement*, *27*, 87–106.

Glas, C. A. W., & Verhelst, N. D. (1989). Extensions of the partial credit model. *Psychometrika*, *54*, 635–659.

Glas, C. A. W., & Verhelst, N. D. (1995). Testing the Rasch model. In G. H. Fischer & I. W. Molenaar (Eds.), *Rasch Models: Foundations, Recent Developments, and Applications* (pp. 69–95). New York: Springer Verlag.

Glück, J., & Indurkhya, A. (2001). Assessing changes in the longitudinal salience of items in constructs. *Journal of Adolescent Research*, *16*, 169–187.

Glück, J., Machat, R., Jirasko, M., & Rollett, B. (2002). Training-related changes in solution strategy in a spatial test: An application of item response models. *Learning and Individual Differences*, *13*, 1–22.

Glück, J., & Spiel, C. (1997). Item response models for repeated measures designs: Application and limitations of four different approaches. *MPR-Online*, *2*(1), 1–20.

Glück, J., & Spiel, C. (in press). Using item response models to analyze change: Advantages and limitations. In A. O. &. M. van Dulmen (Ed.), *Handbook of positive psychology*. Oxford: Oxford University Press.

Goldstein, H., Bonnet, G., & Rocher, T. (2005). A study of procedures for the analysis of PISA 2000 reading data. *Submitted for publication*.

Gollwitzer, M., Eid, M., & Jürgensen, R. (2005). Response styles in the assessment of anger expression. *Psychological Assessment*, 56–69.

Goodman, L. A. (1974). Exploratory latent structure analysis using both identifiable and unidentifiable models. *Biometrika, 61*, 215–231.

Goodman, L. A. (1979). Simple models for the analysis of association in cross-classifications having ordered categories. *Journal of the American Statistical Association, 74*, 537–552.

Goodman, L. A. (1991). Measures, models, and graphical displays in the analysis of cross-classified data. *Journal of the American Statistical Association, 86*, 1085–1111.

Graham, J. R. (2000). *MMPI-2: Assessing personality and psychopathology*. New York: Oxford University Press.

Guilford, J. P. (1967). *The nature of human intelligence*. New York: McGraw-Hill.

Gustafsson, J. (1980). A solution of the conditional estimation problem for long tests in the Rasch model for dichotomous items. *Educational and Psychological Measurement, 40*, 337–385.

Haberman, S. J. (1973). Log-linear models for frequency data: Sufficient statistics and likelihood equations. *The Annals of Statistics, 1*, 617–632.

Haberman, S. J. (1974). *The analysis of frequency data (statistical research monographs)*. University of Chicago Press.

Haberman, S. J. (1977a). Log-linear models and frequency tables with small expected cell counts. *Annals of Statistics, 5*, 1148–1169.

Haberman, S. J. (1977b). Maximum likelihood estimates in exponential response models. *The Annals of Statistics, 5*, 815–841.

Haberman, S. J. (1978a). *Analyses of qualitative data* (Vol. 1). New York: Academic Press.

Haberman, S. J. (1978b). *Analysis of qualitative data: Introductory topics*. Academic Pr.

Haberman, S. J. (1979). *Analyses of qualitative data* (Vol. 2). New York: Academic Press.

Haberman, S. J. (2004). *Joint and conditional maximum likelihood estimation for the Rasch model for binary responses* (ETS Research Rep. No. RR-04-20). Princeton, NJ: Educational Testing Service.

Hands, B., & Larkin, D. (2001). Using the Rasch measurement model to investigate the construct of motor ability in young children. *Journal of Applied Measurement, 2*, 101–120.

Harker, R., & Tymms, P. (2003). The effects of student composition on school outcomes. *School Effectiveness and School Improvement, 15*, 177–199.

Hedeker, D., & Gibbons, R. D. (1993). *MIXOR: A computer program for mixed-effects ordinal probit and logistic regression analysis.* (Unpublished manuscript, University of Illinois at Chicago.)

Heinen, T. (1993). *Discrete latent variable models.* Tilburg: University Press.

Heinen, T. (1996). *Latent class and discrete latent trait models, similarities and differences.* Thousand Oaks, CA: Sage Publications.

Hestenes, D., Wells, M., & Swackhamer, G. (1992). Force concept inventory. *The Physics Teacher, 30*(3), 141–151.

Hiele, P. M. van. (1986). *Structure and insight: A theory of mathematics education.* Orlando, FL: Academic Press.

Hochberg, J., & Gellman, L. (1977). The effort of landmark features on mental rotation times. *Memory and Cognition, 5*, 23–26.

Hoijtink, H. (2001). Testing the Rasch model. In A. Boomsma, M. A. J. van Duijn, & T. A. B. Snijders (Eds.), *Essays on item response theory* (pp. 109–130). New York: Springer Verlag.

Hoijtink, H., & Boomsma, A. (1996). Statistical inference based on latent ability estimates. *Psychometrika, 61*, 37–52.

Hoijtink, H., & Molenaar, I. W. (1997). A multidimensional item response model: Constrained latent class analysis using the gibbs sampler and posterior predictive checks. *Psychometrika, 62*, 171–189.

Holland, P. W. (1990a). The dutch identity: a new tool for the study of item response models. *Psychometrika, 55*, 5–18.

Holland, P. W. (1990b). On the sampling theory foundations of item response theory models. *Psychometrika, 55*(4), 577–601.

Holland, P. W., & Thayer, D. T. (1988). *Differential item performance and the mantel-haenszel procedure.* Lawrence Erlbaum Associates.

Holland, P. W., & Thayer, D. T. (2000). Univariate and bivariate loglinear models for discrete test score distributions. *Journal of Educational and Behavioral Statistics, 25*, 133–183.

Holland, P. W., & Wainer, H. (1993). *Differential item functioning.* Hillsdale, NJ: Lawrence Erlbaum Associates.

Horn, J., & Cattell, R. (1966). Refinement and test of the theory of fluid and crystalized intelligence. *Journal of Educational Psychology, 57*, 253–270.

Hoskins, M., & De Boeck, P. (1995). Componential IRT models for polytomous items. *Journal of Educational Measurement, 32*, 364–384.

Hout, M., Duncan, O. D., & Sobel, M. E. (1987). Association and heterogeneity: structural models of similarities and differences. *Sociological Methodology, 17*, 145–184.

Huang, C.-W. (2003). *Psychometric analyses based on evidence-centered design and cognitive science of learning to explore students' problem-solving in physics.* (Unpublished manuscript, University of Maryland, College Park.)

Huang, G.-H., & Bandeen-Roche, K. (2004). Building an identifiable latent class model with covariate effects on underlying and measured variables. *Psychometrika, 69*, 5–32.

Inhelder, B., & Piaget, J.(1958). *The growth of logical thinking from childhood to adolescence.* New York: Basic.

Ippel, M. J., & Beem, A. L. (1987). A theory of antagonistic strategies. In E. De Corte, R. Lodewijks, Parmentier, & P. Span (Eds.), *Learning and instruction: European research in an international context* (Vol. 1, pp. 111–121). Oxford UK: Pergamon Press.

Jackson, S. A. (1996a). Development and validation of a scale to measure optimal experience: The flow state scale. *Journal of Sport and Exercise Psychology, 18,* 17–35.

Jackson, S. A.(1996b). Toward a conceptual understanding of the flow state in elite athletes. *Research Quarterly for Exercise and Sport, 67,* 76–90.

Jäger, A. O., Süß, H. M., & Beauducel, A.(1997). *Berliner Intelligenzstruktur-Test, Form 4.* Göttingen: Hogrefe.

Jannarone, R. J.(1986). Conjunctive item response theory kernels. *Psychometrika, 51,* 357–373.

Jansen, M. G. H., & Glas, C. A. W. (2001). Conditional independence and differential item functioning in the two-parameter logistic model. In A. Boomsma, M. A. J. van Duijn, & T. A. B. Snijders (Eds.), *Essays on item response theory* (pp. 109–130). New York: Springer Verlag.

Jansen, P. G. W., & Roskam, E. E. (1986). Latent trait models and dichotomization of graded responses. *Psychometrika, 51,* 69–91.

Janssen, R., & De Boeck, P.(1997). Psychometric modeling of componentially designed synonym tasks. *Applied Psychological Measurement, 21,* 37–50.

Janssen, R., Tuerlinckx, F., Meulders, M., & De Boeck, P.(2000). A hierarchical IRT model for criterion-referenced measurement. *Journal od Educational and Behavioral Statistics, 25,* 285–306.

Judd, C. M., & McClelland, G. H.(1989). *Data analysis: A model-comparison approach.* Orlando, FL: Harcourt, Brace and Jovanovich.

Judkins, D. R. (1990). Fay's method for Variance Estimation. *Journal of Official Statistics, 6,* 223–229.

Junker, B. W.(1999). *Some statistical models and computational methods that may be useful for cognitively-relevant assessment.* (Paper prepared for the Committee on the Foundations of Assessment, National Research Council)

Junker, B. W., & Sijtsma, K.(2001). Cognitive assessment models with few assumptions, and connections with non-parametric item response theory. *Applied Psychological Measurement, 25,* 258–272.

Just, M. A., & Carpenter, P. A. (1985). Cognitive coordinate systems: Accounts of mental rotation and individual differences in spatial ability. *Psychological Review, 92,* 137–172.

Kamata, A.(2001). Item analysis by the hierarchical generalized linear model. *Journal of Educational Measurement, 38,* 79–93.

Kaufman, A. S., & Kaufman, N. L.(1983). *Kaufman asssessment battery for children (k- abc).* Circle Pines, Minn.: American Guidance Service.

Keats, J. A.(1971). *An introduction to quantitative psychology.* Sydney: John Wiley Publisher.

Kelderman, H. (1984). Loglinear Rasch model tests. *Psychometrika*, *49*, 223–245.

Kelderman, H. (1988). *An IRT model for item responses that are subject to omission and/or intrusion errors* (Research Rep. No. 88-16). Enschede, The Netherlands: University of Twente.

Kelderman, H. (1989). Item bias detection using loglinear IRT. *Psychometrika*, *54*, 681–697.

Kelderman, H. (1992). Computing maximum likelihood estimates of loglinear models from marginal sums with special attention to loglinear item response theory. *Psychometrika*, *57*, 437–450.

Kelderman, H. (1995). The polytomous Rasch model within the class of generalized linear symmetry models. In G. H. Fischer & I. W. Molenaar (Eds.), *Rasch Models: Foundations, Recent Developments, and Applications* (pp. 307–324). New York: Springer Verlag.

Kelderman, H. (1996). Multidimensional Rasch models for partial credit scoring. *Applied Psychological Measurement*, *20*, 155–168.

Kelderman, H., & Macready, G. B. (1990). The use of loglinear models for assessing differential item functioning across manifest and latent examinee groups. *Journal of Educational Measurement*, *27*, 307–327.

Kelderman, H., & Rijkes, C. M. P. (1994). Loglinear multidimensional IRT models for polytomously scored items. *Psychometrika*, *59*, 149–176.

Kelderman, H., & Steen, R. (1993). *Logimo: Loglinear (IRT) modelling.*

Kempf, W. (1983). Some theoretical concerns about applying latent trait models in educational testing. In S. B. Anderson & J. S. Helmick (Eds.), *On educational testing*. San Francisco: Josey-Bass.

Kiefer, J., & Wolfowitz, J. (1956). Consistency of the maximum likelihood estimator in the presence of infinitely many incidental parameters. *The Annals of Statistics*, *69*, 887–906.

Klahr, D. (1978). Information-processing models of cognitive development. In J. M. Scandura & C. J. Brainerd (Eds.), *Structural/process models of complex human behavior*. Alphen aan den Rijn: Sijthoff and Noordhoff.

Klauer, K. (1989). An exact and optimal standardized person test for assessing consistency with the Rasch model. *Psychometrika*, *56*, 213–228.

Klein, M. F., Birenbaum, M., Standiford, S. N., & Tatsuoka, K. K. (1981). *Logical error analysis and construction of tests to diagnose student "bugs" in addition and subtraction of fractions* (Research Report No. 81-6). Urbana, IL: University of Illinois, Computer-Based Education Research Laboratory.

Kohlberg, L., & Candee, D. (1984). The six stages of justice development. In L. Kohlberg (Ed.), *The psychology of moral development: The nature and validity of moral stages* (Vol. 2, pp. 621–683). San Francisco: Jossey-Bass.

Kolmogoroff, A. (1942). Definitions of center of dispersion and measure of accuracy from a finite number of observations. *Izv. Akad. Nauk. SSSR Ser. Mat.*, *6*, 3–32.

Kreiner, S. (1987). Analysis of multidimensional contingency tables by exact conditional tests: Techniques and strategies. *Scand. Journ. Stat.*, *14*, 97–112.

Kreiner, S., & Christensen, K. B. (2002). Graphical Rasch models. In M. Mesbah, F. C. Cole, & M. T. Lee (Eds.), *Statistical methods for quality of life studies* (pp. 187–203). Dordrecht: Kluwer Academic Publishers.

Kreiner, S., & Christensen, K. B. (2004). Analysis of local dependence and multidimensionality in graphical loglinar Rasch models. *Communications in Statistics. Theory and Methods*, *33*, 1239–1276.

Kreiner, S., Hansen, M., & Hansen, C. R. (2006). On local homogeneity and stochastically ordered mixed Rasch models. *Applied Psychological Measurement*, *30*(6), 271–297.

Kreiner, S., Simonsen, E., & Mogensen, J. (1990). Validation of a personality inventory scale: The mcmi p scale (paranoia). *Journal of Personality Disorders*, *4*, 303–311.

Kubinger, K. D. (1989). Aktueller Stand und kritische Würdigung der probabilistischen Testtheorie [Critical evaluation of latent trait theory. In K. D. Kubinger (Ed.), *Moderne Testtheorie—Ein Abriss samt neuesten Beiträgen. [Modern psychometrics—A brief survey with recent contributions]* (pp. 19–83). München: Psychologie Verlags Union.

Kubinger, K. D., & Wurst, E. (2000). *Adaptives intelligenz diagnosticum—Version 2.1 (AID 2).[Adaptive intelligence diagnosticum—Version 2.1.]*. Göttingen, Germany: Beltz.

Kyllonen, P. C., & Christal, R. (1990). Reasoning ability is (little) more than working-memory capacity?! *Intelligence*, *14*, 389–433.

Kyllonen, P. C., Lohman, D. F., & Snow, R. E. (1984). Effects of aptitudes, strategy training, and test facets on spatial task performance. *Journal of Educational Psychology*, *76*, 130–145.

Kyllonen, P. C., Lohman, D. F., & Woltz, D. J. (1984). Componential modeling of alternative strategies for performing spatial tasks. *Journal of Educational Psychology*, *76*, 1325–1345.

Langeheine, R., Pannekoek, J., & van de Pol, F. (1996). Bootstrapping goodness-of-fit measures in categorical data analysis. *Sociological Methods and Research*, *24*(4), 492–516.

Langeheine, R., & van de Pol, F. (1994). Discrete-time mixed Markov latent class models. In A. D. . R. B. Davies (Ed.), *Analyzing social and political change. A casebook of methods* (pp. 170–197). London: Sage Publications.

Lauritzen, S. L. (1996). *Graphical models.* London: Clarendon Press.

Lazarsfeld, P. F. (1950a). The interpretation and computation of some latent structures. In S. A. Stouffer (Ed.), *Measurement and prediction in World War II.* Princeton, NJ: Princeton University Press.

Lazarsfeld, P. F. (1950b). Logical and mathematical foundations of latent structure analysis. In S. A. Stouffer (Ed.), *Studies in social psychology in World War II, IV.* Princeton, NJ: Princetion University Press.

Lazarsfeld, P. F., & Henry, N. W. (1968). *Latent structure analysis*. Boston: Houghton Mifflin.

Leeuw, J. de, & Verhelst, N. D. (1986). Maximum likelihood estimation in generalized Rasch models. *Journal of Educational Statistics, 11* (183-196).

Lehman, E. L. (1986). *Testing educational hypotheses* (2nd ed.). New York: Springer Verlag.

Leunbach, G. (1976). *A probabilistic measurement model for assessing whether two tests measure the same personal factor* (Tech. Rep. No. 1976.19). Copenhagen, Denmark: The Danish Institute of Educational Research.

Lim, J., & Butcher, J. N. (1996). Detection of faking on the MMPI-2: Differentiation among faking-bad, denial, and claiming extreme virtue. *Journal of Personality Assessment, 67*, 1–25.

Linacre, J. M. (1989). *Many-faceted Rasch measurement*. Chicago: MESA Press.

Linacre, J. M. (1994a). *FACETS: A computer program for many-faceted Rasch measurement (Version 2.7) [computer software and software manual]*. Chicago, IL: MESA Press.

Linacre, J. M. (1994b). *FACETS: A user's guide*. Chicago, IL: Mesa Press.

Linden, W., Paulhus, D. L., & Dobson, K. (1986). Effects of response styles on the report of psychological and somatic distress. *Journal of Consulting and Clinical Psychology, 54*, 309–313.

Lindsay, B., Clogg, C. C., & Grego, J. (1991). Semiparametric estimation in the Rasch model and related exponential response models, including a simple latent class model for item analysis. *Journal of the American Statistical Association, 86*, 96–107.

Linn, R. L. (1989). *Educational measurement*. New York: American Council on Education/Macmillan.

Liou, M. (1994). More on the computation of higher-order derivatives of the elementary symmetric functions in the Rasch model. *Applied Psychological Measurement, 18*, 53–62.

Lord, F. M. (1980). *Applications of item response theory to practical testing problems*. Hillsdale, NJ: Erlbaum.

Lord, F. M., & Novick, M. R. (1968). *Statistical theories of mental test scores*. Reading, MA: Addison-Wesley.

Lourenço, O., & Machado, A. (1996). In defense of Piaget's theory: A reply to 10 common criticisms. *Psychological Review, 103*, 143–164.

Luce, R. D., & Tukey, J. W. (1964). Simultaneous conjoint measurement: A new type of fundamental measurement. *Journal of Mathematical Psychology, 1*, 1–27.

Macaskill, G., Adams, R. J., & Wu, M. L. (1998). Scaling methodology and procedures for the mathematics and science literacy, advanced mathematics and physics scales. In M. Martin & D. L. Kelly (Eds.), *Third international mathematics and science study, technical report volume 3: Implementation and analysis*. Chestnut Hill, MA: Center for the Study of Testing, Evaluation and Educational Policy, Boston College.

Magill, R. A. (2003). *Motor learning and control: Concepts and applications* (7th ed.). Boston: McGraw-Hill.

Maris, E. (1999). Estimating multiple classification latent class models. *Psychometrika, 64* (2), 187–212.

Marsh, H. W., & Redmayne, R. S. (1994). A multidimensional physical self-concept and its relations to multiple components of physical fitness. *Journal of Sport and Exercise Psychology, 16*, 43–55.

Marsh, H. W., Richards, G. E., Johnson, S., Roche, L., & Tremayne, P. (1994). Psychometric properties and a multitrait-multimethod analysis of relations with existing instruments. *Journal of Sport and Exercise Psychology, 15*, 270–305.

Martin, J. D., & van Lehn, K. (1995). A Bayesian approach to cognitive assessment. In P. Nichols, S. Chipman, & R. Brennan (Eds.), *Cognitively diagnostic assessment* (pp. 141–165). Hillsdale, NJ: Erlbaum.

Martin-Löf, P. (1970). *Statistiska modeller. Anteckninger från seminarier läsåret 1969-70 [Statistical models. Notes from the academic year 1969-70]*. Stockholm: Institut för försäkringsmatematik och matematisk statistik.

Marvelde, J. M. te, Glas, C. A. W., Landeghem, V., & van Damme, J. (2006). Applications of multidimensional IRT models to longitudinal data. *Educational and Psychological Mesasurement, 66*, 5–34.

Masters, G. N. (1982). A Rasch model for partial credit scoring. *Psychometrika, 47*, 149–174.

McFarland, L. A., & Ryan, A. M. (2000). Variance in faking across noncognitive measures. *Journal of Applied Psychology, 85*, 812–821.

McGee, M. C. (1979). Human spatial abilities: Environmental, genetic, hormonal, and neurological influences. *Psychological Bulletin, 86*, 889–918.

McLachlan, G., & Basford, K. (1988). *Mixture models: Inference and applications to clustering*. New York: Marcel Dekker.

McLachlan, G., & Peel, D. (2000). *Finite mixture models*. New York: Wiley.

Mechling, H. (1999). Co-ordinative abilities. In Y. V. Auweele, F. Bakker, S. Biddle, M. Durand, & R. Seiler (Eds.), *Psychology for physical educators* (pp. 159–186). Champaign, IL: Human Kinetics.

Meijer, R. R. (2003). Diagnosing item score patterns on a test using IRT based person-fit statistics. *Psychological Methods, 85*, 72–88.

Meijer, R. R., & Sijtsma, K. (2001). Methodology review: evaluating person fit. *Applied Psychology Measurement, 25*, 107–135.

Meiser, T. (1996). Loglinear Rasch models for the analysis of stability and change. *Psychometrika, 61*, 629–645.

Meiser, T. (2005). Log-linear Rasch models for stability and change. In B. S. Everitt & D. C. Howell (Eds.), *Encyclopedia of statistics in behavioral science, vol. 2* (pp. 1093–1097). Chichester, England: Wiley.

Meiser, T., Hein-Eggers, M., Rompe, P., & Rudinger, G. (1995). Analyzing homogeneity and heterogeneity of change using Rasch and latent class models: A comparative and integrative approach. *Applied Psychological Measurement, 19*, 377–391.

Meiser, T., & Rudinger, G. (1997). Modeling stability and regularity of change: Latent structure analysis of longitudinal discrete data. In J. Rost & R. Langeheine (Eds.), *Applications of latent trait and latent class models in the social sciences* (pp. 170–197). Münster, Germany: Waxmann.

Meiser, T., Stern, E., & Langeheine, R.(1998). Latent change in discrete data: Unidimensional, multidimensional, and mixture distribution Rasch models for the analysis of repeated observations. *MPR-Online, 3*, 75–93.

Mellenbergh, G. J.(1989). Item bias and item response theory. *International Journal of Educational Research, 13*, 127–143.

Mellenbergh, G. J.(1994). A unidimensional latent trait model for continuous item responses. *Multivariate Behavioral Research, 29*, 223–236.

Mellenbergh, G. J.(2001). Outline of a faceted theory of item response data. In A. Boomsma, M. A. J. van Duijn, & T. A. B. Snijders (Eds.), *Essays on item response theory.* New York: Springer Verlag.

Mellenbergh, G. J., & Vijn, P.(1981). The Rasch model as a loglinear model. *Applied Psychological Measurement, 5*, 369–376.

Melzack, K., & Wall, P. D.(1965). Pain mechanisms: A new theory. *Science, 105*, 971–979.

Messick, S.(1994). The interplay of evidence and consequence in the validation of performance assessments. *Educational Researcher, 23*(2), 13–23.

Messick, S., & Jackson, D. N.(1961). Acquiescence and the factorial interpretation of the MMPI. *Psychological Bulletin, 58*, 299–304.

Michell, J.(1997). Quantitative science and the definition of measurement in psychology. *British Journal of Psychology, 88*, 355–383.

Michell, J.(1999). *Measurement in psychology: A critical history of a methodological concept.* New York: Cambridge University Press.

Michell, J. (2000). Normal science, pathological science and psychometrics. *Theory & Psychology, 10*, 639–667.

Millsap, R. E.(1997). Invariance in measurement and prediction: Their relationship in the single-factor case. *Psychological Methods, 2*, 248–260.

Mislevy, R. J. (1983). Item response models for grouped data. *Journal of Educational Statistics, 8*, 271–288.

Mislevy, R. J. (1984). Estimating latent distributions. *Psychometrika, 49*, 359–381.

Mislevy, R. J. (1985). Estimation of latent group effects. *Journal of the American Statistical Association, 80*(392), 993–997.

Mislevy, R. J.(1986). Bayes modal estimation in item response models. *Psychometrika, 51*, 177–195.

Mislevy, R. J. (1987). Exploiting auxiliary information about examinees in the estimation of item parameters. *Applied Psychological Measurement, 11*, 81–91.

Mislevy, R. J. (1991). Randomization-based inference about latent variables from complex samples. *Psychometrika, 56*(2), 177–196.

Mislevy, R. J.(1994). Evidence and inference in educational assessment. *Psychometrika, 59*, 439–483.

Mislevy, R. J. (2003). Substance and structure in assessment arguments. *Law, Probability, and Risk, 2*, 237–258.

Mislevy, R. J., Beaton, A. E., Kaplan, B., & Sheehan, K. M. (1992). Estimating population characteristics from sparse matrix samples of item responses. *Journal of Educational Measurement, 29*, 133–161.

Mislevy, R. J., & Bock, R. D. (1989). A hierarchical item-response model for educational testing. In R. Bock (Ed.), *Multilevel analysis of educational data* (pp. 57–74). San Diego, CA: Academic Press.

Mislevy, R. J., & Gitomer, D. H. (1996). The role of probability-based inference in an intelligent tutoring system. *User-Modeling and User-Adapted Interaction, 5*, 253–282.

Mislevy, R. J., & Sheehan, K. M. (1989). Information matrices in latent-variable models. *Journal of Educational Statistics, 14*(4), 335–350.

Mislevy, R. J., Steinberg, L. S., & Almond, R. G. (2002). Design and analysis in task-based language assessment. *Language Assessment, 19*, 477–496.

Mislevy, R. J., Steinberg, L. S., Breyer, F. J., Almond, R. G., & Johnson, L. (2002). Making sense of data from complex assessments. *Applied Measurement in Education, 15*.

Mislevy, R. J., & Verhelst, N. D. (1990). Modeling item responses when different subjects employ different solution strategies. *Psychometrika, 55*(2), 195–215.

Mislevy, R. J., & Wilson, M. R. (1996). Marginal maximum likelihood estimation for a psychometric model of discontinuous development. *Psychometrika, 61*, 41–71.

Mislevy, R. J., Wingersky, M. S., Irvine, S. H., & Dann, P. L. (1991). Resolving mixtures of strategies in spatial visualization tasks. *British Journal of Mathematical and Statistical Psychology, 44*, 265–288.

Mislevy, R. J., Yamamoto, K. Y., & Anacker, S. (1992). Toward a test theory for assessing student understanding. In R. A. Lesh & S. Lamon (Eds.), *Assessments of authentic performance in school mathematics* (pp. 293–318). Washington, DC: American Association for the Advancement of Science.

Molenaar, I. W. (1983). Some improved diagnostics for failure in the Rasch model. *Psychometrika, 48*, 49–72.

Molenaar, I. W. (1997). Lenient or strict application of IRT with an eye on practical consequences. In J. Rost & R. Langeheine (Eds.), *Applications of latent trait and latent class models in the social sciences* (pp. 38–49). Münster, Germany: Waxmann.

Monseur, C., & Adams, R. J. (2002). *Plausible values—How to deal with their limitations.* Paper presented at the International Objective Measurement Workshop, New Orleans, LA.

Moreno, K. E., Wetzel, C. D., McBride, J. R., & Weiss, D. J. (1984). Relationships between corresponding armed services vocational aptitude battery and computerized adaptive testing (cat). *Applied Psychological Measurement, 8*, 155–163.

Mosenthal, P. B., & Kirsch, I. S. (1991). Resolving mixtures of strategies in spatial visualization tasks. *Toward an explanatory model of document process, 14*, 147–180.

Moses, T., von Davier, A. A., & Casabianca, J. (2004). *Loglinear smoothing: An alternative numerical approach using [SAS]* (ETS Research Rep. No. RR-04-27). Princeton, NJ: Educational Testing Service.

Müller, H. (1995). Threshold discriminations, nondichotomization, and precision in a Rasch model for continuous responses: A comment on a debate between Roskam and Andrich. In *Arbeiten aus dem Institut für Psychologie.* Frankfurt, Germany: J.W. Goethe University, Institute for Psychology.

Muraki, E. (1992). A generalized partial credit model: Application of an EM algorithm. *Applied Psychological Measurement, 16*(2), 159–177.

Newell, A., & Simon, H. A. (1972). *Human problem solving.* Englewood Cliffs, NJ: Prentice-Hall.

Neyman, J., & Scott, E. (1948). Consistent estimates based on partially consistent observations. *Econometrica, 16*, 1–32.

Nichols, P. D., Chipman, S. F., & Brennan, R. L. (1995). *Human problem solving.* Hillsdale, NJ: Erlbaum.

Noelting, G. (1980a). The development of proportional reasoning and the ratio concept—Part I: Differentiation of stages. *Educational Studies in Mathematics, 11*, 217–253.

Noelting, G. (1980b). The development of proportional reasoning and the ratio concept—Part II: Problem-structure at successive stages;problem-solving strategies and the mechanism of adaptive restructuring. *Educational Studies in Mathematics, 11*, 331–363.

Noelting, G., Coudé, G., & Rousseau, J. P. (1995). *Rasch analysis applied to multiple-domain tasks.* Paper presented at the twenty-fifth annual symposium of the Jean Piaget Society, Berkeley, CA.

OECD. (2001). *Knowledge and skills for life: First results from pisa 2000.* Paris: Organisation for Economic Co-Operation and Development (OECD) Publications.

OECD. (2004). *Learning for tomorrow's world: First results from pisa 2003.* Paris: Organisation for Economic Co-Operation and Development (OECD) Publications.

OECD. (2005). *Pisa 2003 technical report.* Paris: Organisation for Economic Co-Operation and Development (OECD) Publications.

Orlando, M., & Thissen, D. (2000). Likelihood-based item-fit indices for dichotomous item response theory models. *Applied Psychological Measurement, 24*, 50–64.

Oshima, T. C. (1994). The effect of speededness on parameter estimation in item response theory. *Journal of Educational Measurement, 31*, 200–219.

Pastor, D. A., & Beretvas, S. N. (2006). Longitudinal Rasch modeling in the context of psychotherapy outcomes assessment. *Applied Psychological Measurement, 30*, 100–120.

Patz, R., & Junker, B. W. (1999a). Applications and extensions of mcmc in IRT: Multiple item types, missing data, and rated responses. *Journal of Educational and Behavioral Statistics*, *24*, 342–366.

Patz, R., & Junker, B. W. (1999b). A straightforward approach to Markov chain Monte Carlo methods for item response models. *Journal of Educational and Behavioral Statistics*, *24*, 146–178.

Paulhus, D. L. (1983). Sphere specific measures of perceived control. *Journal of Personality and Social Psychology*, *44*, 1253–1265.

Paulhus, D. L. (1984). Two-component models of socially desirable responding. *Journal of Personality and Social Psychology*, *46*, 598–609.

Paulson, J. A. (1986). *Latent class representation of systematic patterns in test responses* (Tech. Rep. No. ONR-1). Portland, OR: Portland State University.

Perline, R., Wright, B. D., & Wainer, H. (1979). The Rasch model as additive conjoint measurement. *Applied Psychological Measurement*, *3*, 237–255.

Piaget, J. (1950). *The psychology of intelligence.* London: Lowe & Brydone.

Pinel, J. P. J. (1990). *Biopsychology.* Boston, MA: Allyn and Bacon.

Pirolli, P., & Wilson, M. R. (1998). A theory of the measurement of knowledge content, access, and learning. *Psychological Review*, *105*, 58–82.

PISA. (2003). *Australian data.* Available from the PISA Web site, http://www.pisa.oecd.org.

Ponocny, I. (2000). Exact person fit indexes for the Rasch model for arbitrary alternatives. *Psychometrika*, *65*, 29–42.

Ponocny, I. (2001). Nonparametric goodness-of-fit tests for the Rasch model. *Psychometrika*, *66*, 437–459.

Ponocny, I., & Ponocny-Seliger, E. (1999). *T-Rasch 1.0.* Groningen, The Netherlands: ProGAMMA.

Portney, S. (1988). Asymptotic behavior of likelihood methods for exponential families when the number of parameters tends to infinity. *The Annals of Statistics*, *16*, 356–366.

Prenzel, M., Baumert, J., Blum, W., Lehmann, R., Leutner, D., Neubrand, M., et al. (2004). *PISA 2003. Der Bildungsstand der Jugendlichen in Deutschland—Ergebnisse des zweiten internationalen Vergleichs.* Münster, Germany: Waxmann.

Prenzel, M., Carstensen, C. H., Rost, J., & Senkbeil, M. (2002). Naturwissenschaftliche Grundbildung im Ländervergleich. In M. Weiß (Ed.), *PISA 2000—Die Länder der Bundesrepublik Deutschland im Vergleich* (pp. 129–158). Opladen: Leske + Budrich.

Puchhammer, M. (1989). Die Berücksichtigung von Rateparametern im Modell von Rasch. [A Rasch model with guessing parameter.]. In K. D. Kubinger (Ed.), *Moderne Testtheorie- Ein Abriss samt neuesten Beiträgen. [Modern psychometrics – A brief survey with recent contributions.]* (pp. 271–280). München: Psychologie Verlags Union.

Raju, N. S., van der Linden, W. J., & Fleer, P. F. (1995). IRT-based internal measures of differential functioning of items and tests. *Applied Psychological Measurement, 19*, 353–368.

Rasch, G. (1960). *Probabilistic models for some intelligence and attainment tests.* Copenhagen, Denmark: Nielsen and Lydiche.

Rasch, G. (1968). An individualistic approach to item analysis. In P. F. Lazarsfeld & N. W. Henry (Eds.), *Readings in mathematical social science* (pp. 89–107). Cambridge: MIT Press.

Rasch, G. (1980). *Probabilistic models for some intelligence and attainment tests.* Chicago: University of Chicago Press (original work published 1960).

Raudenbush, S. W., & Bryk, A. S. (2002). *Hierarchical linear models: Applications and data analysis methods.* Thousand Oaks, CA: Sage Publications, Inc.

Raudenbush, S. W., & Sampson, R. (1999). Assessing direct and indirect effects in multilevel designs with latent variables. *Sociological Methods and Research, 28*(2), 123–153.

Raudenbush, S. W., Yang, M., & Yosef, M. (2000). Maximum likelihood for generalized linear models with nested random effects via high-order, multivariate laplace approximation. *Journal of Computational and Graphical Statistics, 9*, 141–157.

Raven, J. C. (1938). *Guide to progressive matrices.* London: London: H.K. Lewis.

Rigdon, S. E., & Tsutakawa, R. K. (1983). Parameter estimation in latent trait models. *Psychometrika, 48*, 567–574.

Rijmen, F., & De Boeck, P. (2002). The random weights linear logistic test model. *Applied Psychological Measurement, 26*, 271–285.

Rijmen, F., & De Boeck, P. (2003). A latent class model for individual differences in the interpretation of conditionals. *Applied Psychological Measurement, 14*, 271–282.

Rijmen, F., Tuerlinckx, F., De Boeck, P., & Kuppens, P. (2003). A nonlinear mixed model framework for item response theory. *Psychological Methods, 8*, 185–205.

Rindskopf, D. (1990). Nonstandard log-linear models. *Psychological Bulletin, 108*, 150–162.

Robinson, P. (1984). Task complexity, cognitive resources, and syllabus design. In P. Robinson (Ed.), *Cognition and second language acquisition* (pp. 287–318). Cambridge, England: Cambridge University Press.

Rosenbaum, P. (1989). Criterion-related construct validity. *Psychometrika, 54*, 625–633.

Roskam, E. E. (1995). Graded responses and joining categories: A rejoinder to Andrich's "Models for measurement, precision and nondichotomization of graded responses". *Psychometrika, 60*, 27–35.

Roskam, E. E., & Jansen, P. G. W. (1984). A new derivation of the Rasch model. In E. Degreef & J. van Bruggenhaut (Eds.), *Trends in mathematical psychology* (pp. 293–307). Amsterdam: North-Holland.

Roskam, E. E., & Jansen, P. G. W. (1989). Conditions for rasch- dichotomizability of the unidimensional polytomous Rasch model. *Psychometrika, 54,* 317–332.

Rost, J. (1988). Test theory with qualitative and quantitative latent variables. In R. Langeheine & J. Rost (Eds.), *Latent trait and latent class models.* New York: Plenum Press.

Rost, J. (1989). Rasch models and latent class models for measuring change with ordinal variables. In R. C. &. S. Bolasco (Ed.), *Multiway data analysis* (pp. 473–483). Amsterdam: Elsevier.

Rost, J. (1990). Rasch models in latent classes: an integration of two approaches to item analysis. *Applied Psychological Measurement, 14,* 271–282.

Rost, J. (1991). A logistic mixture distribution model for polychotomous item responses. *British Journal of Mathematical and Statistical Psychology, 44,* 75–92.

Rost, J. (1996). *Lehrbuch Testtheorie Testkonstruktion.* Bern, Germany: Huber.

Rost, J. (2004). *Lehrbuch Testtheorie—Testkonstruktion* (2 ed.). Bern, Germany: Huber.

Rost, J., & Carstensen, C. H. (2002). Multidimensional Rasch measurement via item component models and faceted designs. *Applied Psychological Measurement, 26*(1), 42–56.

Rost, J., Carstensen, C. H., & von Davier, M. (1997). Applying the mixed Rasch model to personality questionnaires. In J. Rost & R. Langeheine (Eds.), *Applications of latent trait and latent class models in the social sciences* (pp. 324–332). New York: Waxmann.

Rost, J., & Spada, H. (1983). Die Quantifizierung von Lerneffekten anhand von Testdaten. *Zeitschrift für Differentielle und Diagnostische Psychologie, 4,* 29–49.

Rost, J., & von Davier, M. (1993). Measuring different traits in different populations with the same items. In K. F. W. R. Steyer & K. Widaman (Eds.), *Psychometric methodology. Proceedings of the 7th European meeting of the Psychometric Society in Trier* (pp. 446–450). Gustav Fischer Verlag.

Rost, J., & von Davier, M. (1994). A conditional item fit index for Rasch models. *Applied Psychological Measurement, 18,* 171–182.

Rost, J., & von Davier, M. (1995). Mixture distribution Rasch models. In I. W. Molenaar (Ed.), *Rasch models—Foundations, recent developments and applications* (pp. 257–268). New York: Springer Verlag.

Rost, J., & Walter, O. (2005). Multimethod item response theory. In M. Eid & E. Diener (Eds.), *Handbook of psychological measurement: A mulitmethod perspective.* American Psychological Association.

Rost, J., Walter, O., Carstensen, C. H., Senkbeil, M., & Prenzel, M. (2004). Naturwissenschaftliche Kompetenz. In U. Schiefele (Ed.), *PISA 2003. Der Bildungsstand der Jugendlichen in Deutschland—Ergebnisse des zweiten internationalen Vergleichs* (pp. 111–146). Münster, Germany: Waxmann.

Roth, K. D. (1982). *Strukturanalyse koordinativer fähigkeiten (analysis of coordination abilities)*. Bad Homburg, Germany: Limpert.

Royall, R. (1997). *Statistical evidence. A likelihood paradigm*. London: Chapman & Hall.

Rubin, D. B. (1987). *Multiple imputations for non-response in surveys*. New York: John Wiley & Sons.

Safrit, M. J., Cohen, A. S., & Costa, M. G. (1989). Item response theory and the measurement of motor behavior. *Research Quarterly for Exercise and Sport, 60*, 325–335.

Safrit, M. J., Zhu, W., Costa, M. G., & Zhang, L. (1992). The difficulty of sit ups tests: an empirical investigation. *Research Quarterly for Exercise and Sport, 63*, 227–283.

Samejima, F. (1969). Estimation of latent ability using a pattern of graded scores. *Psychometric Monograph, 17*.

Samejima, F. (1983). *A latent trait model for differential strategies in cognitive processes* (Tech. Rep. No. ONR/RR-83-1). Knoxville, TN: University of Tennessee.

Sanathanan, L., & Blumenthal, S. (1978). The logistic model and estimation of latent structure. *Journal of the American Statistical Association, 73*, 794–799.

Scheiblechner, H. (1972). Das Lernen und Lösen komplexer Denkaufgaben [learning and solving complex cognitive problems]. *Zeitschrift fuer Experimentelle und Angewandte Psychologie, 19*, 476–506.

Schmidt, R. A., & Lee, T. D. (1999). *Motor control and learning*. Champaign, IL: Human Kinetics.

Schmitt, M. J., & Ryan, A. M. (1993). The big five in personnel selection: Factor structure in applicant and nonapplicant populations. *Journal of Applied Psychology, 78*, 966–974.

Schnipke, D. L., & Scrams, D. J. (1997). Modeling item response times with a two-state mixture model: A new method of measuring speededness. *Journal of Educational Measurement, 34*, 213–232.

Schultz-Larsen, K., Kreiner, S., & Lomholt, R. K. (2005a). Comparison of two scoring systems of the mmse as a screening test for dementia. a community-based population study of elderly. *Journal of Clinical Epidemiology, in press*.

Schultz-Larsen, K., Kreiner, S., & Lomholt, R. K. (2005b). Scaling the mini-mental state examination using item response theory (IRT): an exploration of cognitive dimensions and diagnostic cut-points. *Journal of Clinical Epidemiology, in press*.

Schum, D. (1994). *The evidential foundations of probabilistic reasoning*. New York: Wiley.

Schwarz, G. (1978). Estimating the dimensions of a model. *Annals of Statistics, 6*, 461–464.

Shafer, G. (1976). *A mathematical theory of evidence*. Princeton, NJ: Princeton University Press.

Shannon, C. E. (1948). A mathematical theory of communication. *Bell System Technical Journal, 27*, 379–423, 623–656.

Shavelson, R. J., Hubner, J. J., & Stanton, G. C. (1976). Self-concept validation of construct interpretations. *Review of Educational Research, 46*, 407–441.

Sheehan, K. M., & Mislevy, R. J. (1990). Integrating cognitive and psychometric models in a measure of document literacy. *Journal of Educational Measurement, 27*, 255–272.

Shepard, R. N., & Meltzer, J. (1971). Mental rotation of three-dimensional objects. *Science, 171*, 701–703.

Siegler, R. S. (1981). Developmental sequences within and between concepts. *Monograph of the Society for Research in Child Development, Serial No. 189, 46*.

Siegler, R. S. (1987). Strategy choices in substraction. In J. Sloboda & D. Rogers (Eds.), *Cognitive process in mathematics* (pp. 81–106). Oxford: Oxford University Press.

Siegler, R. S. (1991). Strategy choice and strategy discovery. *Learning and Instruction, 1*, 89–102.

Siegler, R. S., & Campbell, J. (1989). Diagnosing individual differences in strategy choice procedures. In N. Frederiksen, R. Glaser, A. Lesgold, & M. G. Shafto (Eds.), *Diagnostic monitoring of skill and knowledge acquisition* (pp. 113–139). Hillsdale, NJ: Erlbaum.

Siegler, R. S., & McGilly, K. (1989). Strategy choices in children's time-telling. In I. Levin & D. Zakay (Eds.), *Psychological time: A life span perspective*. Elsevier: The Netherlands.

Sijtsma, K., & Molenaar, I. W. (2002). *Introduction to nonparametric item response theory, vol. 5*. SAGE Publications.

Simon, H. A. (1975). The functional equivalence of problem solving skills. *Cognitive Psychology, 7*, 268–288.

Singer, R. N. (1980). *Motor learning and human performance*. New York: Macmillan.

Sinharay, S. (2003). *Practical applications of posterior predictive model checking for assessing fit of common item response theory models*. (ETS Research Rep. No. RR-03-33). Princeton, NJ: Educational Testing Service.

Sinharay, S., & Johnson, M. S. (2003). *Simulation studies applying posterior predictive model checking for assessing fit of the common item response theory models* (ETS Research Rep. No. RR-03-28). Princeton, NJ: Educational Testing Service.

Skrondal, A., & Rabe-Hesketh, S. (2004). *Generalized latent variable modeling*. London: Chapman & Hall.

Smit, A., Kelderman, H., & van der Flier, H. (1999). Collateral information and mixed Rasch models. *MPR-Online, 4*, 1–12.

Smit, A., Kelderman, H., & van der Flier, H. (2000). The mixed Birnbaum model: Estimation using collateral information. *MPR-Online, 5*, 31–43.

Smit, A., Kelderman, H., & van der Flier, H. (2003). Latent trait latent class analysis of an Eysenck personality questionnaire. *MPR-Online*, *8*, 23–50.

Smith, R. M. (1985). A comparison of Rasch person analysis and robust estimators. *Educational and psychological measurement*, *45*, 433–444.

Smith, R. M. (1986). Person fit in the Rasch model. *Educational and Psychological Measurement*, *46*, 359–372.

Snijders, T. (2001). Exact person fit indexes for the Rasch model for arbitrary alternatives. *Psychometrika*, *66*, 331–342.

Snow, R. E., & Lohman, D. F. (1989). Implications of cognitive psychology for educational measurement. In R. L. Linn (Ed.), *Educational measurement* (3rd ed. ed., pp. 263–331). New York: American Council on Education/Macmillan.

Spada, H., & Kluwe, R. H. (1980). Two models of intellectual development and their reference to the theory of Piaget. In R. H. Kluwe & H. Spada (Eds.), *Developmental models of thinking*. New York: Academic Press.

Spada, H., & McGaw, B. (1985). The assessment of learning effects with linear logistic test models. In S. E. Embretson (Ed.), *Test design: Developments in psychology and psychometrics* (pp. 169–194). Orlando, FL: Academic Press.

Spearman, C. (1923). *The nature of intelligence and the principles*. London: Macmillan.

Spearman, C. (1927). *The abilities of man*. New York: Macmillan.

Spiegelhalter, D. J., Thomas, A., Best, N. G., & Gilks, W. R. (1996). *BUGS 0.5 examples (vol. 1)*. Cambridge, England: University of Cambridge, Institute of Public Health, Medical Research Council Biostatistics Unit.

Spiegelhalter, D. J., Thomas, A., Best, N. G., & Lunn, D. (2003). *WinBUGS Version 1.4 users manual* (Tech. Rep.). Cambridge, MA: MRC Biostatistics Unit.

Spiel, C. (1994). Latent trait models for measuring change. In A. van Eye & C. C. Clogg (Eds.), *Latent variables analysis: Applications for developmental research* (pp. 274–293). Thousand Oaks, CA: Sage Publications.

Spiel, C., Gittler, G., Sirsch, U., & Glück, J. (1997). Application of the Rasch model for testing Piaget's theory of cognitive development. In J. Rost & R. Langeheine (Eds.), *Applications of latent trait and latent class models in the social sciences* (pp. 111–117). Münster, Germany: Waxmann.

Spiel, C., Glück, J., & Gössler, H. (2001). Stability and change of unidimensionality—The sample case of deductive reasoning. *Journal of Adolescent Research*, *16*, 150–168.

Spiel, C., Glück, J., & Gössler, H. (2004). Messung von Leistungsprofil und Leistungshöhe im Schlussfolgerndem Denken im SDV—Die Integration von Piagets Entwicklungskonzept und Item-response Modellen. [Measurement of performance profile and level in deductive reasoning by use of the SDV—An integration of Piaget's developmental theory and item response models.]. *Diagnostica*, *50*, 145–152.

Spielberger, C., Gorsuch, R., & Lushene, R. (1970). *STAI manual for the state-trait anxiety inventory.* Palo Alto, CA: Consulting Psychologist Press.

Spray, J. A. (1987). Recent developments in measurement and possible applications to the measurement of psychomotor behavior. *Research Quarterly for Exercise and Sport, 58,* 203–209.

Spray, J. A. (1990). One-parameter item response theory models for psychomotor tests involving repeated, independent attempts. *Research Quarterly for Exercise and Sport, 61,* 162–168.

SPSS. (2003). *SPSS for Windows, Release 12.0.1.* Chicago: SPSS.

Sternberg, R. J. (1977). *Intelligence, information-processing, and analogical reasoning: The componential analysis of human abilities.* New York: Erlbaum.

Sternberg, R. J. (1985). *Beyond iq: A triarchic theory of human intelligence.* New York: Cambridge University Press.

Stocking, M. L., & Lord, F. M. (1983). Developing a common metric in item response theory. *Applied Psychological Measurement, 7,* 201–210.

Strauss, B. (1994). Orientierungen von Sportzuschauern [Orientations of sports spectators]. *Psychologie und Sport, 1,* 19–25.

Strauss, B. (1995). Die Messung der Identifikation mit einer Sportmannschaft: Eine deutsche Adaptation der "Team Identification Scale" von Wann und Branscombe [Measuring identification with a sports team: A German adaptation of Wann und Branscombe's Team Identification Scale]. *Psychologie und Sport, 2,* 132–145.

Strauss, B. (1999). IRT models in sport psychology. *International Journal of Sport Psychology, 30,* 17–40.

Streiner, D. (2003). Diagnosing tests: Using and misusing diagnostic and screening tests. *Journal of Personality Assessment, 81,* 209–219.

Stroud, A. H., & Sechrest, D. (1966). *Gaussian quadrature formulas.* Englewood Cliffs, NJ: Prentice Hall.

Swanson, D. B., Clauser, B. E., Case, S. M., Nungester, R. J., & Featherman, C. (2002). Analysis of differential item functioning (dif) using hierarchical logistic regression models. *Journal of Educational and Behavioral Statistics, 27,* 53–75.

Takane, Y., & Leeuw, J. de. (1987). On the relationship between item response theory and factor analysis of discretized variables. *Psychometrika, 52,* 393–408.

Tatsuoka, K. K. (1983). Rule space: An approach for dealing with misconceptions based on item response theory. *Journal of Educational Measurement, 20,* 345–354.

Tatsuoka, K. K., Linn, R. L., Tatsuoka, M. M., & Yamamoto, K. Y. (1988). Differential item functioning resulting from the use of different solution strategies. *Journal of Educational Measurement, 25,* 301–319.

Tenenbaum, G. (1999). The implementation of Thurstone's and Guttman's measurement ideas in Rasch analysis. *International Journal of Sport Psychology, 30,* 3–16.

Tenenbaum, G., & Bar-Eli, M. (1995). Contemporary issues and future directions in exercise and sport psychology. In S. J. H. Biddle (Ed.), *Exercise and sport psychology: A European perspective* (pp. 292–323). Champaign, IL: Human Kinetics.

Tenenbaum, G., & Fogarty, G. J. (1996). Application of the Rasch analysis to sport and exercise psychology measurement. In J. Duda (Ed.), *Advances in sport and exercise psychology measurement* (pp. 410–421). Morgantown, WV: Fitness Information Technology.

Tenenbaum, G., Fogarty, G. J., & Jackson, S. A. (1999). Stages of the flow experience: A Rasch analysis of jackson's flow state scale. *Journal of Outcome Measurement, 3*, 278–294.

Tenenbaum, G., Fogarty, G. J., Stewart, E., Calcagnini, N., Kirker, B., Thorne, G., et al. (1999). Perceived discomfort in aerobic-type tasks: Scale development and theoretical considerations. *Journal of Sport Sciences, 17*, 183–196.

Tenenbaum, G., Furst, D., & Weingarten, G. (1985). A statistical re-evaluation of the stai anxiety questionnaire. *Journal of Clinical Psychology, 41*, 239–244.

Tennant, A., Penta, M., Tesio, L., Grimby, L., Thonnard, J.-L., Slade, A., et al. (2004). Assessing and adjusting for cross-cultural validity of impairment and activity limitation scales through differential item functioning within the framework of the Rasch model. *Medical Care, 42*, 37–48.

The SAS Institute. (2002). *SAS [Version 9]*. Cary, NC: The SAS Institute.

Thissen, D. (1982). Marginal maximum likelihood estimation for the one-parameter logistic model. *Psychometrika, 47*, 175–186.

Thissen, D., Steinberg, L. S., & Wainer, H. (1993). Detection of differential item functioning using the parameters of item response models. In P. W. Holland & H. Wainer (Eds.), *Differential item functioning* (pp. 67–113). Hillsdale, NJ: Lawrence Erlbaum Associates.

Thomas, N. (2000). Assessing model sensitivity of the imputation methods used in the National Assessment of Educational Progress. *Journal of Educational and Behavioral Statistics, 25*, 351–371.

Thurstone, L. L., & Thurstone, T. G. (1941). *Factorial studies of intelligence*. Chicago: The University of Chicago Press.

Titterington, D. M., Smith, A. F. M., & Makov, U. E. (1985). *Statistical analysis of finite mixture distributions*. New York: Wiley.

Tjur, T. (1982). A connection between rasch's item analysis model and a multiplicative poisson model. *Scandinavian Journal of Statistics,, 9*, 23–30.

Toulmin, S. (1958). *The uses of argument*. New York: Cambridge University Press.

Ulrich, D. A. (1985). *Test of gross motor development*. Austin, TX: ProEd.

van de Pol, F., & Langeheine, R. (1990). Mixed Markov latent class models. In C. C. Clogg (Ed.), *Sociological methodology 1990, vol. 20* (pp. 213–247). Oxford: Blackwell.

van den Wollenberg, A. L. (1982). Two new tests for the Rasch model. *Psychometrika*, *47*, 123–140.

van der Linden, W. J., & Hambleton, R. K. (1997). Item response theory: Brief history, common models, and extensions. In W. J. van der Linden & R. K. Hambleton (Eds.), *Handbook of item response theory* (pp. 1–28). New York: Springer Verlag.

van Kuyk, J. J. (1988). Verwerven van grootte-begrippen [Acquiring size concepts.]. *Pedagogische Studiën*, *65*, 1–10.

van Maanen, L., Been, P., & Sijtsma, K. (1989). The linear logistic test model and heterogeneity of cognitive strategies. In E. E. Roskam (Ed.), *Mathematical psychology in progress*. Berlin, Germany: Springer Verlag.

Verguts, T., & De Boeck, P. (2001). Some mantel-haenszel tests of Rasch model assumptions. *British Journal of Mathematical and Statistical Psychology*, *54*, 21–37.

Verhelst, N. D. (1992). *Het sere model geschat met een pseudolikelihood methode [The sere model estimated with a pseudo likelihood method]* (Internal report). Enschede, The Netherlands: University of Twente.

Verhelst, N. D. (2001). Testing the unidimensionality assumption of the Rasch model. *MPR-Online*, *6(3)*, 231–271.

Verhelst, N. D., & Glas, C. A. W. (1995). The one parameter logistic model. In G. H. Fischer & I. W. Molenaar (Eds.), *Rasch models—Foundations, recent developments, and applications*. New York: Springer Verlag.

Vermunt, J. K. (1997a). *ℓEM: A general program for the analysis of categorial data [Computer program]*. Tilburg, The Netherlands: Tilburg University. (Internet: www.uvt.nl/faculteiten/fsw/organisatie/departementen/mto/software2.html)

Vermunt, J. K. (1997b). *Log-linear models for event histories*. Thousand Oaks, CA, USA: Sage Publications, Inc.

Volodin, N., & Adams, R. J. (1995). *Identifying and estimating a D-dimensional Rasch model*. Unpublished manuscript, Australian Council for Educational Research, Camberwell, Victoria, Australia.

von Davier, M. (1994). *WINMIRA—A Windows-program for analyses with the Rasch model, with the latent class analysis and with the mixed Rasch model* (Tech. Rep.). Kiel, Germany: IPN Software, Institute for Science Education.

von Davier, M. (1996). Mixtures of polytomous Rasch models and latent class models for ordinal variables. In F. Faulbaum & W. Bandilla (Eds.), *Softstat 95—advances in statistical software 5*. Stuttgart, Germany: Lucius and Lucius.

von Davier, M. (1997). *Methoden zur Prüfung probabilistischer Testmodelle* (Vol. 157). Olshausenstrasse 62, 24098 Kiel, Germany: IPN.

von Davier, M. (2001). *WINMIRA 2001—A Windows-program for analyses with the Rasch model, with the latent class analysis and with the mixed Rasch model [computer software]* (Tech. Rep.). Groningen, The

Netherlands: ASC—Assessment Systems Corporation USA and Science Plus Group.

von Davier, M. (2005). *A general diagnostic model applied to language testing data* (ETS Research Report No. RR-05-16). Princeton, NJ: Educational Testing Service.

von Davier, M. (2006). Book review: Introduction to Rasch Measurement, edited by E. V. Smith and R. M. Smith. *Applied Psychological Measurement, 30*(5), 443–446.

von Davier, M., DiBello, L., & Yamamoto, K. Y. (2006). *Reporting test outcomes with models for cognitive diagnosis* (ETS Research Report No. RR-06-28). Princeton, NJ: Educational Testing Service.

von Davier, M., & Molenaar, I. W. (2003). A person-fit index for polytomous Rasch models, latent class models, and their mixture generalizations. *Psychometrika, 68*, 213–228.

von Davier, M., & Rost, J. (1995). Polytomous mixed Rasch models. In G. H. Fischer & I. W. Molenaar (Eds.), *Rasch Models: Foundations, Recent Developments, and Applications* (pp. 371–379). New York: Springer Verlag.

von Davier, M., & Strauss, B. (2003). New developments in testing probabilistic models. *International Journal of Sport and Exercise Psychology, 1*, 61–82.

von Davier, M., & Yamamoto, K. Y. (2004a). *A class of models for cognitive diagnosis.* Presented at the 4th Spearman Conference, Philadelphia, PA.

von Davier, M., & Yamamoto, K. Y. (2004b). Partially Observed Mixtures of IRT Models: An Extension of the Generalized Partial Credit Model. *Applied Psychological Measurement, 28*(6), 389–406.

Waldherr, K. (2001). *Differential Item Functioning-Analysen mittels der Familie der Rasch-Modelle. (Differential item functioning analyses within the family of Rasch models).* Unpublished doctoral dissertation, Universitt Wien, Vienna, Austria.

Walter, O. (2005). *Kompetenzmessung in den PISA-Studien.* Lengerich, Germany: Pabst.

Wang, W. (1999). Direct estimation of correlations among latent traits within IRT framework. *MPR-Online, 4*(2), 47–68.

Wann, D. L., & Branscombe, N. R. (1993). Sports fans: Measuring degree of identification with their team. *International Journal of Sport Psychology, 24*, 1-17.

Ware Jr., J. E., Snow, K. K., Kosinski, M., & Gandek, B. (1993). *Sf-36 health survey. manual and interpretation guide.* Boston: The Health Institute, New England Medical Center.

Warm, T. A. (1985). *Weighted maximum likelihood estimation of ability in item response theory with tests of finite length* (Tech. Rep. No. CGI-TR-85-08). Oklahoma City: U.S. Coast Guard Institute.

Warm, T. A. (1989). Weighted likelihood estimation of ability in item response theory. *Psychometrika, 54*, 427–445.

Weber, G., Glück, J., Schäfer, L., Wehinger, K., Heiss, C., & Sassenrath, . (2005). *Esaw – europäische studie zum wohlbefinden im alter: Hauptergebnisse unter besonderer berücksichtigung der situation in Österreich. esaw – european study of adult well-being: Main results with a special focus on the austrian situation.* Vienna: WUV.

Weinert, F. E., & Helmke, A. (1997). *Entwicklung im grundschulalter [Development in primary school.* Weinheim: FRG: Psychologie Verlags Union.

Westers, P., & Kelderman, H. (1991). Examining differential item functioning due to item difficulty and alternative attractiveness. *Psychometrika, 57*, 107-118.

White, L. A., Nord, R. D., Mael, F. A., & Young, M. C. (1993). The assessment of background and life experiences (able). In T. H. Trent Laurence (Ed.), *Adaptability screening for the armed forces* (pp. 101–162). Washington, DC: Office of the Assistant Secretary of Defense.

Whitely, S. E. (1976). Solving verbal analogies: Some cognitive components of intelligence test items. *Journal of Educational Psychology, 68*, 234-242.

Wilkening, F., & Anderson, N. H. (1982). Comparison of two rule-assessment methodologies for studying cognitive development and cognitive structure. *Psychological Bulletin, 92*, 215–237.

Wilkinson, G. N., & Rogers, C. E. (1973). Symbolic descriptions of factorial models in analysis of variance. *Applied Statistics, 22*, 392–399.

Wilson, M. R. (1989). Saltus: a psychometric model of discontinuity in cognitive development. *Psychological Bulletin, 105*, 276–289.

Wilson, M. R. (2005). *Constructing measures: An item response modeling approach.* Mahwah, NJ: Lawrence Erlbaum Associates.

Wood, R. (1978). Fitting the Rasch model–a heady tale. *British Journal of Mathematical and Statistical Psychology, 31*, 27–32.

Wright, B. D., & Masters, G. N. (1982). *Rating scale analysis.* Chicago: MESA Press.

Wright, B. D., & Stone, M. H. (1979). *Best test design.* Chicago: MESA Press.

Wu, M. L. (1997). *The development and application of a fit test for use with marginal maximum likelihood estimation and generalised item response models.* Melbourne: Unpublished Masters thesis, University of Melbourne.

Wu, M. L., & Adams, R. J. (2002). *Plausible values–Why are they important.* Paper presented at the International Objective Measurement Workshop, New Orleans, LA.

Wu, M. L., Adams, R. J., & Wilson, M. R. (1997). *ConQuest: Multi-Aspect Test Software.* Camberwell, Australian: Australian Council for Educational Research.

Xie, Y. (1992). The log-multiplicative layer effect model for comparing mobility tables. *American Sociological Review, 57*, 380–395.

Xu, X., & von Davier, M. (2006). *Appying the general diagnostic model to data from large scale educational surveys* (ETS Research Report No. RR-06-08). Princeton, NJ: Educational Testing Service.

Yamamoto, K. Y. (1987). *A model that combines IRT and latent class models*. Unpublished doctoral dissertation, University of Illinois Urbana-Champaign.

Yamamoto, K. Y. (1989). *HYBRID model of IRT and latent class models* (ETS Research Report No. RR-89-41). Princeton, NJ: Educational Testing Service.

Yamamoto, K. Y. (1990). *HYBILm: A computer program to estimate HYBRID model parameters*. Princeton, NJ: Educational Testing Service.

Yamamoto, K. Y. (1995). *Estimating the effects of test length and test time on parameter estimation using the HYBRID model* (TOEFL Technical Report No. TOEFL-TR-10). Princeton, NJ: Educational Testing Service.

Yamamoto, K. Y., & Everson, H. T. (1995). *Modeling the mixture of IRT and pattern responses by a modified HYBRID model* (ETS Research Rep. No. RR-95-16). Princeton, NJ: Educational Testing Service.

Yamamoto, K. Y., & Everson, H. T. (1997). Modeling the effects of test length and test time on parameter estimation using the HYBRID model. In J. Rost & R. Langeheine (Eds.), *Applications of latent trait and latent class models in the social sciences* (pp. 89–98). Münster, Germany: Waxmann.

Yen, W. (1985). Increasing item complexity: A possible cause of scale shrinkage for unidimensional item response theory. *Psychometrika, 50,* 399–410.

Zhu, W., & Cole, E. L. (1996). Many-faceted Rasch calibration of a gross motor instrument. *Research Quarterly for Exercise and Sport, 67,* 24–34.

Zhu, W., & Kurz, K. A. (1994). Rasch partial credit analysis of gross motor competence. *Perceptual and Motor Skills, 79,* 947–961.

Zickar, M. J. (2001). Conquering the next frontier: Modeling personality data with item response theory. In B. R. &. R. Hogan (Ed.), *Applied personality psychology: The intersection of personality and i/o psychology.* Washington, DC: American Psychological Association.

Zickar, M. J., Gibby, R. E., & Robie, C. (2004). Uncovering faking samples in applicant, incumbent, and experimental data sets: An application of mixed model item response theory. *Organizational Research Methods, 7,* 168–190.

Zickar, M. J., & Robie, C. (1999). Modeling faking good on personality items: An item-level analysis. *Journal of Applied Psychology, 84,* 551–563.

Zimowski, M. F., Muraki, E., Mislevy, R. J., & Bock, R. D. (2003). *Bilog mg 3rd manual.* Lincolnwood: Scientific Software International.

Zwinderman, A. H. (1991). A generalized Rasch model for manifest predictors. *Psychometrika, 56,* 589–600.

Zwinderman, A. H., & van den Wollenberg, A. L. (1990). Robustness of marginal maximum likelihood estimation in the Rasch model. *Applied Psychological Measurement, 14,* 73–81.

Author Index

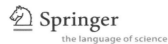

Springer springeronline.com

the language of science

The Kernel Method of Test Equating

A.A. von Davier, P.W. Holland, and D.T. Thayer

Kernel Equating is based on a flexible family of equipercentile-like equating functions and contains the linear equating function as a special case. This book will be an important reference for (a) Statisticians and others interested in the theory behind equating methods and the use of model-based statistical methods for data smoothing in applied work; (b) Practitioners who need to equate tests—including those with these responsibilities in testing companies, state testing agencies and school districts; and (c) Instructors in psychometric and measurement programs.

2004. 229 p. (Statistics for Social Science and Public Policy) Hardcover
ISBN 0-387-01985-5

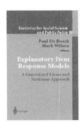

Explanatory Item Response Models

P. De Boeck and M. Wilson

This volume gives a new and integrated introduction to item response models from the viewpoint of the statistical theory of generalized linear and nonlinear mixed models. This new framework allows the domain of item response models to be co-ordinated and broadened to emphasize their *explanatory* uses beyond their standard *descriptive* uses.

2004. 382 p. (Statistics for Social Science and Public Policy) Hardcover
ISBN 0-387-40275-6

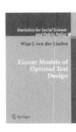

Linear Models for Optimal Test Design

W.J. van der Linden

This book begins with a reflection on the history of test design--the core activity of all educational and psychological testing. It then presents a standard language for modeling test design problems as instances of multi-objective constrained optimization. The main portion of the book discusses test design models for a large variety of problems from the daily practice of testing, and illustrates their use with the help of numerous empirical examples.

2005. 429 p. (Statistics for Social Science and Public Policy) Hardcover
ISBN 0-387-20272-2

Easy Ways to Order▶ Call: Toll-Free 1-800-SPRINGER • E-mail: orders-ny@springer.sbm.com • Write: Springer, Dept. S8113, PO Box 2485, Secaucus, NJ 07096-2485 • Visit: Your local scientific bookstore or urge your librarian to order.

Printed in the United States of America